ıgton Manual®
ıary Medicine
Subspecialty Consult

The Washington Manual® Pulmonary Medicine Subspecialty Consult

Editor
Adrian Shifren, M.D.
Postdoctoral Research Scholar/Instructor
Department of Internal Medicine
Division of Pulmonary and Critical Care Medicine
Washington University School of Medicine
Barnes-Jewish Hospital
St. Louis, Missouri

Series Editor
Tammy L. Lin, M.D.
Adjunct Assistant Professor of Medicine
Division of Medical Education
Washington University School of Medicine
St. Louis, Missouri

Series Advisor
Daniel M. Goodenberger, M.D.
Professor of Medicine
Chief, Division of Medical Education
Washington University School of Medicine
St. Louis, Missouri
Director, Internal Medicine Residency Program
Barnes-Jewish Hospital
St. Louis, Missouri

Lippincott Williams & Wilkins
a Wolters Kluwer business
Philadelphia • Baltimore • New York • London
Buenos Aires • Hong Kong • Sydney • Tokyo

Acquisitions Editors: Danette Somers/Sonya Seigafuse
Developmental Editors: Tanya Lazar/Lauren Aquino
Project Manager: Nicole Walz
Senior Manufacturing Manager: Ben Rivera
Production Editor: Kate Sallwasser, Silverchair Science + Communications, Inc.
Design Coordinator: Holly Reid McLaughlin
Cover Designer: Marie Clifton
Compositor: Silverchair Science + Communications, Inc.
Printer: RR Donnelley–Crawfordsville

Printed in the USA

Library of Congress Cataloging-in-Publication Data

The Washington manual pulmonary medicine subspecialty consult /
editor, Adrian Shifren.
p. ; cm. -- (The Washington manual subspecialty consult series)
Includes bibliographical references and index.
ISBN 0-7817-4376-1
1. Respiratory organs--Diseases--Handbooks, manuals, etc.
I. Shifren, Adrian. II. Title: Pulmonary medicine subspecialty consult.
III. Series.
[DNLM: 1. Lung Diseases--Handbooks. 2. Pulmonary Disease (Specialty)--methods--Handbooks. 3. Respiratory Function Tests --Handbooks. WF 39 W319 2006]
RC732.W366 2006
616.2--dc21
2003054598

Care has been taken to confirm the accuracy of the information presented and to describe generally accepted practices. However, the authors, editors, and publisher are not responsible for errors or omissions or for any consequences from application of the information in this book and make no warranty, expressed or implied, with respect to the currency, completeness, or accuracy of the contents of the publication. Application of this information in a particular situation remains the professional responsibility of the practitioner.

The authors, editors, and publisher have exerted every effort to ensure that drug selection and dosage set forth in this text are in accordance with current recommendations and practice at the time of publication. However, in view of ongoing research, changes in government regulations, and the constant flow of information relating to drug therapy and drug reactions, the reader is urged to check the package insert for each drug for any change in indications and dosage and for added warnings and precautions. This is particularly important when the recommended agent is a new or infrequently employed drug.

Some drugs and medical devices presented in this publication have Food and Drug Administration (FDA) clearance for limited use in restricted research settings. It is the responsibility of health care providers to ascertain the FDA status of each drug or device planned for use in their clinical practice.

10 9 8 7 6 5 4 3 2 1

Contents

Contributing Authors

Nitin J. Anand, M.D.
Fellow
Division of Pulmonary and Critical Care
Boston University School of Medicine
Boston, Massachusetts

Audreesh Banerjee, M.D.
Resident Physician
Department of Internal Medicine
Washington University School of Medicine
Barnes-Jewish Hospital
St. Louis, Missouri

Mario Castro, M.D., M.P.H.
Associate Professor of Medicine and Pediatrics
Department of Internal Medicine
Washington University School of Medicine
Barnes-Jewish Hospital
St. Louis, Missouri

Murali Chakinala, M.D.
Assistant Professor of Medicine
Department of Internal Medicine
Division of Pulmonary and Critical Care Medicine
Washington University School of Medicine
Barnes-Jewish Hospital
St. Louis, Missouri

Alexander C. Chen, M.D.
Fellow
Department of Internal Medicine
Division of Pulmonary and Critical Care Medicine
Washington University School of Medicine
Barnes-Jewish Hospital
St. Louis, Missouri

Ting-hsu Chen, M.D.
Fellow
Division of Pulmonary and Critical Care
Boston University School of Medicine
Boston, Massachusetts

Shan Cheng, M.D.
Fellow
Division of Gastroenterology
University of California, San Francisco, School of Medicine
San Francisco, California

Lance Cohen, M.D.
Attending Physician
Department of Internal Medicine
Christian Northeast Hospital
St. Louis, Missouri

Daniel H. Cooper, M.D.
Resident Physician
Department of Internal Medicine
Washington University School of Medicine
Barnes-Jewish Hospital
St. Louis, Missouri

Shiraz A. Daud, M.D.
Fellow
Division of Pulmonary and Critical Care Medicine
Washington University School of Medicine
Barnes-Jewish Hospital
St. Louis, Missouri

Daniel M. Goodenberger, M.D.
Professor of Medicine
Chief, Division of Medical Education
Washington University School of Medicine
St. Louis, Missouri
Director, Internal Medicine Residency Program
Barnes-Jewish Hospital
St. Louis, Missouri

Ramsey R. Hachem, M.D.
Assistant Professor
Department of Medicine
Division of Pulmonary and Critical Care Medicine
Washington University School of Medicine
Barnes-Jewish Hospital
St. Louis, Missouri

Sujith Kalathiveetil, M.D.
Fellow
Cardiovascular Division
Washington University School of Medicine
Barnes-Jewish Hospital
St. Louis, Missouri

Marin H. Kollef, M.D.
Professor of Medicine
Department of Internal Medicine
Division of Pulmonary and Critical Care Medicine
Washington University School of Medicine
Barnes-Jewish Hospital/Washington University Medical Center
St. Louis, Missouri

Robin Kundra, M.D., Ph.D.
Attending Physician
Department of Internal Medicine
Grant Medical Center
St. Louis, Missouri

Steven L. Leh, M.D.
Fellow
Department of Internal Medicine
Division of Pulmonary and Critical Care Medicine
Washington University School of Medicine
Barnes-Jewish Hospital
St. Louis, Missouri

Faye Lialios, M.D.
Fellow
Cardiovascular Division
Washington University School of Medicine
Barnes-Jewish Hospital
St. Louis, Missouri

Barbara A. Lutey, M.D.
Fellow
Department of Internal Medicine
Division of Pulmonary and Critical Care Medicine
Washington University School of Medicine
St. Louis, Missouri

Santhosh J. Mathews, M.D., M.S.
Postdoctoral Research Scholar
Cardiovascular Division
Washington University School of Medicine
Barnes-Jewish Hospital
St. Louis, Missouri

Martin L. Mayse, M.D.
Assistant Professor of Medicine
Department of Internal Medicine
Division of Pulmonary and Critical Care Medicine
Washington University School of Medicine
Barnes-Jewish Hospital
St. Louis, Missouri

Lee E. Morrow, M.D., M.Sc.
Assistant Professor of Medicine
Department of Medicine
Division of Pulmonary and Critical Care
Creighton University School of Medicine
Creighton University Medical Center
Omaha, Nebraska

Anne K. Nagler, M.D.
Instructor of Medicine
Department of Internal Medicine
Division of Hospital Medicine
Washington University School of Medicine
Barnes-Jewish Hospital
St. Louis, Missouri

Stephen B. Osmon, M.D.
Attending Physician
Department of Medicine
St. Luke's Hospital
St. Louis, Missouri

Jeanie Park, M.D.
Fellow
Division of Gastroenterology
Keck School of Medicine of the University of Southern California
Los Angeles, California

Tonya D. Russell, M.D.
Assistant Professor of Medicine
Department of Internal Medicine
Division of Pulmonary and Critical Care Medicine
Washington University School of Medicine
Barnes-Jewish Hospital
St. Louis, Missouri

Stephen Ryan, M.D.
Fellow
Department of Internal Medicine
Division of Pulmonary and Critical Care Medicine
Washington University School of Medicine
Barnes-Jewish Hospital
St. Louis, Missouri

Randy Sasich, M.D.
Postdoctoral Fellow
Department of Internal Medicine
Division of Pulmonary and Critical Care Medicine
Washington University School of Medicine
Barnes-Jewish Hospital
St. Louis, Missouri

Dan Schuller, M.D.
Associate Professor of Medicine
Division of Pulmonary and Critical Care
Creighton University School of Medicine
Creighton University Medical Center
Omaha, Nebraska

Sanjay Sharma, M.D.
Fellow
Division of Hematology/Oncology
Mount Sinai School of Medicine of New York University
New York, New York

Adrian Shifren, M.D.
Postdoctoral Research Scholar/Instructor
Department of Internal Medicine
Division of Pulmonary and Critical Care Medicine
Washington University School of Medicine
Barnes-Jewish Hospital
St. Louis, Missouri

Latha Sivaprasad, M.D.
Internist
Department of Internal Medicine
Washington University School of Medicine
Barnes-Jewish Hospital
St. Louis, Missouri

K. Cajal Sumino, M.D., Ph.D.
Instructor
Department of Internal Medicine
Division of Pulmonary and Critical Care Medicine
Washington University School of Medicine
Barnes-Jewish Hospital
St. Louis, Missouri

Raghu Tadikamalla, M.D.
Fellow
Division of Cardiology
University of Pittsburgh School of Medicine
Pittsburgh, Pennsylvania

Sabu Thomas, M.D.
Fellow
Division of Cardiology
University of Minnesota Medical School
Minneapolis, Minnesota

Elbert P. Trulock III, M.D.
Rosemary and I. Jerome Flance Professor of Medicine
Department of Internal Medicine
Division of Pulmonary and Critical Care Medicine
Washington University School of Medicine
Barnes-Jewish Hospital
St. Louis, Missouri

Peter G. Tuteur, M.D.
Associate Professor of Medicine
Department of Internal Medicine
Division of Pulmonary and Critical Care Medicine
Washington University School of Medicine
Barnes-Jewish Hospital
St. Louis, Missouri

Sarah Waheed, M.D.
Resident Physician
Department of Internal Medicine
Washington University School of Medicine
Barnes-Jewish Hospital
St. Louis, Missouri

Christine Yeh, M.D.
Fellow
Department of Internal Medicine
Gastroenterology Section
Baylor College of Medicine
Texas Medical Center
Houston, Texas

Roger D. Yusen, M.D., M.P.H.
Assistant Professor of Medicine
Department of Internal Medicine
Division of Pulmonary and Critical Care Medicine
Washington University School of Medicine
Barnes-Jewish Hospital
St. Louis, Missouri

Chairman's Note

Medical knowledge is increasing at an exponential rate, and physicians are being bombarded with new facts at a pace that many find overwhelming. The Washington Manual® Subspecialty Consult Series was developed in this context for interns, residents, medical students, and other practitioners in need of readily accessible practical clinical information. They therefore meet an important unmet need in an era of information overload.

I would like to acknowledge the authors who have contributed to these books. In particular, Tammy L. Lin, M.D., Series Editor, provided energetic and inspired leadership, and Daniel M. Goodenberger, M.D., Series Advisor, Chief of the Division of Medical Education in the Department of Medicine at Washington University, is a continual source of sage advice. The efforts and outstanding skill of the lead authors are evident in the quality of the final product. I am confident that this series will meet its desired goal of providing practical knowledge that can be directly applied to improving patient care.

Kenneth S. Polonsky, M.D.
Adolphus Busch Professor
Chairman, Department of Medicine
Washington University School of Medicine
St. Louis, Missouri

Series Preface

The Washington Manual® Subspecialty Consult Series is designed to provide quick access to the essential information needed to evaluate a patient on a subspecialty consult service. Each manual includes the most updated and useful information on commonly encountered symptoms or diseases and highlights the practical information you need to gather before formulating a plan. Special efforts have been made to organize the information so that these guides will be valuable and trusted companions for medical students, residents, and fellows. They cover everything from questions to ask during the initial consult to issues in subsequent management.

One of the strengths of this series is that it is written by residents and fellows who know how busy a consult service can be, who know what information will be most helpful, and can detail a practical approach to patient care. Each volume is written to provide enough information for you to evaluate a patient until more in-depth reading can be done on a particular topic. Throughout the series, key references are noted, difficult management situations are addressed, and appropriate practice guidelines are included. Another strength of this series is that it was written in concert. All of the guides were designed to work together.

The most important strength of this series is the collection of authors, faculty advisors, and especially lead authors assembled to write this series. In addition, we received incredible commitment and support from our chairman, Kenneth S. Polonsky, M.D. As a result, the extraordinary depth of talent and genuine interest in teaching others at Washington University is showcased in this series. Although there has always been house staff involvement in editing The Washington Manual® series, it came to our attention that many of them also wanted to be involved in writing and making decisions about what to convey to fellow colleagues. Remarkably, many of the lead authors became junior subspecialty fellows while writing their guides. Their desire to pass on what they were learning, while trying to balance multiple responsibilities, is a testament to their dedication and skills as clinicians, teachers, and leaders.

We hope this series fulfills the need for essential and practical knowledge for those learning the art of consultation in a particular subspecialty and for those just passing through it.

Tammy L. Lin, M.D., Series Editor
Daniel M. Goodenberger, M.D., Series Advisor

Preface

This is the first printing of *The Washington Manual® Pulmonary Medicine Subspecialty Consult*. The goal of this book is to provide the medical student, resident, and pulmonary fellow on a pulmonary medicine service with a handbook that will be helpful in the evaluation of patients with pulmonary disease. It is also hoped that it will serve as a quick reference for internists and nonpulmonary physicians in practice. As such, it is not intended as a complete reference of pulmonary medicine, but rather as a focused source of information that will assist in the process of history taking, physical examination, and testing as it pertains to the patient concerned.

Our knowledge of pulmonary medicine has grown exponentially over the last 40 years and is continually expanding. Reflecting this are the increasing complexity and bulk of the current general pulmonary texts. To simplify matters and effectively address our target audience, each chapter has been written with the input of either a medical resident or a pulmonary fellow. The chapters have been further evaluated by attending physicians with expertise in the relevant field to ensure accurate information. At the end of each chapter is a list of references that were chosen for their relevant content. These references will serve as an excellent starting point for further reading.

The chapters have been organized in a simple fashion and, where possible, deal with a single pulmonary entity of the type often faced by the consulting pulmonary team (e.g., solitary pulmonary nodule). When the topic is more complex (e.g., interstitial lung disease), the approach is more generalized.

A book like this is always a collective effort, with many of the contributors working in the background. With that in mind, I would like to thank Kate Sallwasser for all her help, and Lauren Aquino, without whom this book would not have reached completion. Finally, it is my hope that this book enriches both the reader's medical knowledge in general and appreciation of pulmonary medicine in particular. Ideally, the small contribution made to each physician or physician-in-training by this book will result in the improved care of patients.

A.S.

Key to Abbreviations

ABG	arterial blood gas
ACE	angiotensin-converting enzyme
AFB	acid-fast bacilli
AFP	α-fetoprotein
Ag	antigen
AIDS	acquired immune deficiency syndrome
ALT	alanine aminotransferase
ANA	antinuclear antibody
ANCA	antineutrophil cytoplasmic antibody
AP	anteroposterior
aPTT	activated partial thromboplastin time
ARDS	acute respiratory distress syndrome
ASA	aspirin
AST	aspartate aminotransferase
BMI	body mass index
BP	blood pressure
BPM	beats per minute
BUN	blood urea nitrogen
CBC	complete blood count
CDC	Centers for Disease Control and Prevention
CMV	cytomegalovirus
CNS	central nervous system
COPD	chronic obstructive pulmonary disease
CPR	cardiopulmonary resuscitation
CREST	syndrome of calcinosis cutis, Raynaud's phenomenon, esophageal motility disorder, sclerodactyly, telangiectasia
CRP	C-reactive protein
CSF	cerebrospinal fluid
CT	computed tomograph, -graphy
DBP	diastolic blood pressure
DIC	disseminated intravascular coagulation
DLCO	diffusing capacity of lung for CO
DNA	deoxyribonucleic acid
ECG	electrocardiogram, -graphic, -graphy
ENT	ear, nose, and throat
ER	emergency room
ESR	erythrocyte sedimentation rate
ETT	endotracheal tube
FEV_1	forced expiratory volume in 1 second
GABA	γ-aminobutyric acid
GI	gastrointestinal
hCG	human chorionic gonadotropin
Hct	hematocrit
Hgb	hemoglobin
HIV	human immune deficiency syndrome

HLA	human leukocyte antigen
HTN	hypertension
ICP	intracranial pressure
ICU	intensive care unit
Ig	immunoglobulin
INR	international normalized ratio
IV	intravenous, -ly
MAOI	monoamine oxidase inhibitor
MDI	metered-dose inhaler
MRI	magnetic resonance imaging
NG	nasogastric
NIH	National Institutes of Health
NSAIDs	nonsteroidal antiinflammatory drugs, agents
PCR	polymerase chain reaction
PET	positron emission tomography
PO	oral, -ly
PPD	purified protein derivative
PT	prothrombin time
PTH	parathyroid hormone
PTT	partial thromboplastin time
RBC	red blood cell
RNA	ribonucleic acid
RV	right ventricle
SBP	systolic blood pressure
SC	subcutaneous
SIADH	syndrome of inappropriate antidiuretic hormone secretion
SLE	systemic lupus erythematosus
TB	tuberculosis
TMP-SMX	trimethoprim-sulfamethoxazole
UA	urinalysis
U/S	ultrasound
V/Q	ventilation/perfusion
VZV	varicella zoster virus
WBC	white blood cell

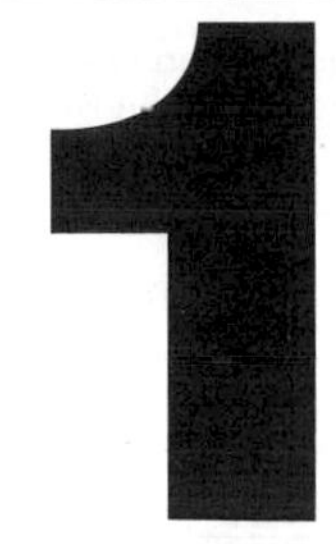

The Chest X-Ray

Sarah Waheed and
Adrian Shifren

INTRODUCTION

This chapter is an introduction to chest radiography that covers basic principles on chest x-rays (CXRs), including how they are obtained and how to interpret them. The only way to become truly proficient at chest film interpretation is through repeated personal review of all chest films ordered. Close interaction with radiology staff is invaluable. We present a systematic approach to the interpretation of CXRs: By repeating the same process for each CXR, one will develop a comprehensive and competent method of reading films.

Ideally, CXRs should be interpreted without an extensive knowledge of the clinical context to allow an unbiased and objective evaluation of the film. However, similar to any medical test, evaluating the CXR in the context of the clinical scenario is very important and allows a focus on specific areas of the film and a detailed search for associated pathologic findings.

The importance of **prior CXRs** for comparison cannot be stressed enough. Comparison allows for the evaluation of the lesion over time and may also allow for the detection of more subtle findings missed on the current or the prior CXRs.

IDENTIFYING DATA

The first step in reviewing a CXR is to make sure that one has the correct study. Therefore, the identifying data should be sought. This information is usually found in one of the corners of the CXR and should include (a) patient name, (b) date of birth, and (c) date of the study. Also, look at the actual study to confirm that it is the one that was ordered. Once this information has been obtained, interpretation can proceed.

FILM QUALITY

Once the film has been identified, it should be evaluated for quality. This evaluation includes assessing the film for the presence of rotation, checking the degree of inspiration, making sure there are no motion artifacts, and assessing the exposure of the film. As a rule, the optimally exposed CXR allows visualization of the vertebral bodies and disk spaces through the mediastinal structures and also allows visualization of the pulmonary vessels through the heart and diaphragmatic shadows. Chest films that are inadequately exposed can lead to faulty interpretation.

STUDY VIEWS

There are a number of different studies that may be obtained to evaluate chest pathology. These include the anteroposterior (AP) view, the lateral (LAT) view, the posteroanterior (PA) view, and the lateral decubitus (LD) view. Some centers also make use of special end-expiratory (EE) views.

The **PA** view is taken with the patient in a standing position during full inspiration. The patient faces the radiograph cassette, which is in contact with his or her chest. The x-ray beam is directed toward the cassette from a distance of 6 ft, which results in minimal magnification and maximum sharpness for evaluation.

The **LAT** film is also taken with the patient standing during full inspiration at a distance of 6 ft. By convention, the patient's left side is placed in contact with the radiograph cassette, and the beam is directed from right to left. LAT views are useful for evaluating lesions behind the heart, diaphragm, or mediastinum that may be hidden on PA views.

AP views are usually taken with portable x-ray machines and are most often used to image the chest in sick patients who cannot have formal PA and LAT views taken in the radiology department. These studies are conducted with the x-ray cassette behind the patient, in contact with his or her back. The x-rays are directed from front to back, often at a distance of <6 ft (more space is usually unavailable in a patient room). The patient is often in a sitting position and therefore unable to perform a full inspiration (which requires erect posture). AP views therefore result in increased lung markings (owing to lack of complete inspiration), magnification of mediastinal and cardiac structures (owing to increased distance between these structures and the cassette), and decreased image sharpness (owing to a shorter distance between the x-ray source and the cassette).

LD views are taken with the patient lying on one side. They are most useful for evaluating three conditions: (a) pleural effusions, (b) pneumothorax, and (c) cavitary lesions. Because free intrapleural fluid gravitates to the most dependent portion of the pleural space, LD films can be used to confirm whether a pleural fluid collection is freely flowing or walled off (loculated). In this situation, the patient is placed on the affected side (a left effusion is evaluated in the left LD position), allowing the fluid to collect in the lowermost portion of the thorax. The mobility of the fluid may have implications for the management of the effusion. Also, the size of the effusion on LD views may influence the clinician's decision to intervene.

The opposite situation occurs with **free air in the pleural space:** It rises to the least dependent portion of the pleural space. Thus, a small pneumothorax that is difficult to see on PA and LAT views may become more obvious in an LD view. In this situation, the patient is placed on the unaffected side (a left pneumothorax is evaluated in the right LD position), allowing the air to collect in the uppermost portion of the thorax. A lung cavity may be evaluated for fluid or a fungal ball in a manner similar to that used to evaluate pneumothorax. In the lateral position, the fluid (lung abscess) or fungal ball shifts to the most dependent part of the cavity. These studies are performed with the patient placed on the affected side (left LD position for a left-sided cavity).

EE views are occasionally used to evaluate for focal air trapping. As air appears black on CXRs, expiratory views of the lungs appear whiter and have smaller volumes than their inspiratory counterparts. Thus, focal air trapping of any cause appears as a darker and occasionally more voluminous area (depending on the extent) on an EE view when compared to the normal portions of the lung. EE views also help accentuate a small pneumothorax because expiration causes the lung on the affected side to pull away from the chest wall, creating a larger dark area of free intrapleural air.

SCHEMA FOR READING THE POSTEROANTERIOR FILM

It is very important to develop a systematic approach to looking at CXRs to avoid missing subtle pathology. Subtle pathologies can be missed for two reasons: (a) Only the process that is suspected is noted, and (b) an obvious but previously unexpected finding commands the viewer's attention. These situations lead one to neglect the rest of the film and miss other pathologies.

There are as many systems for evaluating CXRs as there are physicians. The schema used here is arranged so that often-neglected areas are addressed first, and more common areas that may divert attention are addressed last. The PA CXR is addressed in detail, but any view can be read in a similar or slightly modified fashion.

The first structures surveyed are the **bony structures** of the thorax including the ribs (anterior and posterior aspects), the sternum (including signs of previous sternal splitting surgeries), the shoulder girdle (including the clavicles and scapulae), and the spine (both the vertebrae and the disk spaces). The order followed is the spine, then the ribs from posterior to anterior, the sternum, the clavicles and shoulder girdle, and finally, both humeri if present on the film. Lesions to note include fractures (including compression fractures in the spine), lytic lesions, and deformities (such as scoliosis or kyphosis). While looking at the bony structures, the soft tissue shadows that surround them should also be noted.

Next, the **upper abdomen** is inspected. This is usually done from right to left. Three abdominal structures are usually noted, especially on a PA view. From right to left, these are the liver shadow (a homogeneous density under the right diaphragm), the gastric bubble (a gas collection with an air–fluid interface under the left diaphragm), and the left colic flexure (a gas collection laterally under the left diaphragm). A PA film is also the study of choice for evaluating the presence of free air in the abdomen. Free air is seen as thin dark shadows under the diaphragmatic surfaces. Because upper abdominal disease and lower thoracic disease often imitate each other clinically, close inspection of a CXR may assist the clinician in evaluation of both chest and abdominal complaints.

The **diaphragms** themselves are looked at next. They are smooth hemispherical structures, with the right diaphragm being 2–3 cm higher than the left owing to the presence of the liver below. Again, inspection takes place from the right to the left. The diaphragms should be evaluated for shape (flattened in hyperinflation), sharpness (obscured with pleural effusions), and general symmetry (eventration or paralysis of a single diaphragm leads to asymmetry).

The **mediastinal** structures should now be evaluated. This evaluation is one of the most complex parts of the CXR evaluation because it includes a significant number of thoracic structures. The best method for evaluating the mediastinum is by individually assessing each structure from bottom to top. The mediastinal shadow can initially be examined to look for any gross abnormalities. It is important to distinguish focal mediastinal disease (tumor or abscess) from diffuse disease (hemorrhage or inflammation).

The **cardiac** portion of the mediastinum is assessed first. Its boundaries are formed on the right (from bottom to top) by the right atrium, the ascending aorta, and superior vena cava, and on the left (from bottom to top) by the left ventricle, left auricle, and main pulmonary artery. Both global and chamber enlargement should be noted. Global cardiac enlargement can be determined by calculating the cardio-thoracic ratio—the width of the cardiac shadow should be less than half the internal width of the bony thorax at its widest point. Any ratio >50% signifies cardiac enlargement. Although chamber enlargement is often the cause of an enlarged cardiac shadow, a pericardial effusion gives a similar appearance and should always be considered, especially in the appropriate clinical setting. Other important lesions to note are calcifications of the coronary arteries (indicative of atherosclerotic coronary disease), the cardiac valves, and the pericardium (indicative of constrictive pericarditis).

The **aorta** is examined next. All of its portions (ascending, arch, and descending) should be evaluated for enlargement (possible aneurysm), calcification (atherosclerotic disease), and tortuosity (hypertensive disease). The hila are then evaluated. Their shape, size, and density are important and may indicate the presence of disease. Gross enlargement of one or both hila is generally due to either pathologic lymph node enlargement (malignancy and infection being the most common offenders) or pulmonary vascular disease (typically pulmonary hypertension). Hilar calcification is also very common in certain geographic areas and may be due to old calcified granulomas. The main conducting airways (trachea and mainstem bronchi) are also assessed. Splaying of the main carina indicates a subcarinal lesion (often due to enlarged lymph nodes). The trachea itself may be widened (tracheomalacia), narrowed (strictures), or displaced to either side (large effusion or lung collapse).

The **pleural** (between the parietal and visceral pleurae) and **extrapleural spaces** (between the parietal pleura and chest wall) are then evaluated. First, the pleurae at the base of one lung are inspected from the cardiophrenic angle (formed by the diaphragm meeting the heart border) to the costophrenic angle (formed by the diaphragm meeting the chest wall) in a medial to lateral direction. Then the costophrenic angle is inspected. Next, the pleura lining the lateral margin of the lung is followed upward to the apex, and then over and down the mediastinal contour to the cardiophrenic angle where the inspection began. By following the pleural markings, the fissures of the lungs (including fluid collecting or tracking into them) and even accessory fissures can be evaluated. Careful examination of these spaces allows for the detection of small pleural effusions, pneumothoraces, pleural thickening or calcification, and masses. LAT films are more sensitive than are PA films for the detection of small pleural effusions. Whereas approximately 175 mL of fluid is needed to produce blunting of the costophrenic angles on PA views, as little as 75 mL can be detected in the costophrenic angle on a LAT view.

Extrapulmonary masses (pleural and extrapleural) can be difficult to distinguish from pulmonary masses on PA films. A number of features may assist in differentiating between the two types of masses. First, a second view can be obtained (a mass overlying the lungs on a PA view may be noted to be extrapulmonary on a LAT view). Second, the interface between the lesion and the lung is sharp with an extrapulmonary mass because they are superimposed structures. And third, the angle between the chest wall and an extrapulmonary lesion is obtuse (>90 degrees).

An often-neglected part of CXR evaluation is the meticulous identification and **monitoring of medical appliances.** In current practice, iatrogenic contribution to the CXR abnormalities cannot be overlooked. These appliances have usually been identified by this stage of the exam. They include central venous catheters (including dialysis catheters), various peritoneal shunts, coronary artery stents, pacing and defibrillating devices, chest tubes, and surgical staple lines or wires.

The final structures undergoing evaluation are the **lungs** themselves. Again, a focused, repetitive approach is best. Working from bottom to top, the lungs are compared to each other in a side-to-side ascending sweep. With the exception of the slightly elevated right hemidiaphragm and the asymmetric cardiac shadow, the lungs should be similar in appearance at each level of inspection. Any differences in the density of the film or the vascular markings are an indication of possible pulmonary pathology. Thereafter, each lung is inspected individually in a similar ascending fashion to look for more subtle changes that may have been initially overlooked. Any abnormalities detected on the initial bilateral scan should be paid special attention.

Again, it must be emphasized that once the evaluation is complete, it is essential to **evaluate old films and compare them with the current study.** This comparison allows for a more detailed understanding of the pathology being evaluated and may affect management in a significant fashion (e.g., a rapidly growing mass will be managed differently than a mass that has been stable for a number of years). As a final measure, the film should be **viewed together with a radiologist** to get his or her expert opinion as well as some teaching from a specialist.

KEY POINTS TO REMEMBER

- The importance of prior CXRs for comparison cannot be stressed enough.
- The optimally exposed CXR allows visualization of the vertebral bodies and disk spaces through the mediastinal structures and also allows visualization of the pulmonary vessels through the heart and diaphragmatic shadows.
- Develop a systematic approach to looking at CXRs so as not to miss any subtle pathologies that may be present.

REFERENCES AND SUGGESTED READINGS

Armstrong P, Wilson AG, Dee P, Hamsell DM. *Imaging of diseases of the chest,* 2nd ed. St. Louis: Mosby–Year Book, 1995.

Brant WE, Helms CA. *Fundamentals of diagnostic radiology.* Philadelphia: Lippincott Williams & Wilkins, 1998.

Fishman AP, Elias JA, Fishman JA, et al. *Fishman's pulmonary diseases and disorders,* 3rd ed. New York: McGraw-Hill, 1998.

Fraser RG, Paré JAP, Paré PD, et al. *Diagnosis of diseases of the chest.* Vol. 1, 3rd ed. Philadelphia: WB Saunders, 1998.

Freundlich IM, Bragg DG. *A radiographic approach to diseases of the chest,* 2nd ed. Baltimore: Williams & Wilkins, 1997.

Goodman LR. *Felson's principles of chest roentgenology: a programmed text,* 2nd ed. Philadelphia: WB Saunders, 1999.

Lange S, Stark P. *Teaching atlas of thoracic radiology*. New York: Georg Thieme Verlag, 1993.

Lange S, Walsh G. *Radiology of chest diseases,* 2nd ed. New York: Thieme Medical Publishers, 1998.

Slone RM, Gutierrez FR, Fisher AJ. *Thoracic imaging: a practical approach*. New York: McGraw-Hill, 1999.

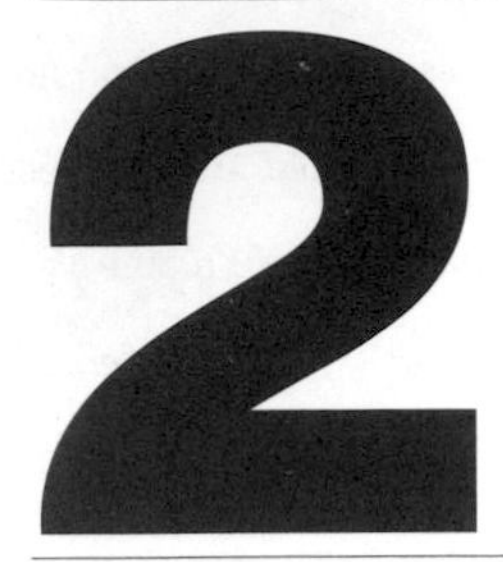

Pulmonary Function Testing

Adrian Shifren

INTRODUCTION

Pulmonary function tests (PFTs) are an integral part of a pulmonary evaluation. They have evolved from tools of physiologic study to clinical tools with a wide variety of applications, including case management, occupational health screening, sports medicine testing, and quantifying impairment, among others. Although a contemporary pulmonary function lab uses a host of sophisticated equipment, the availability of user-friendly testing devices has produced widespread use of PFTs by community physicians and an increased need for formal training in their interpretation.

It is important to remember that PFTs do not make pathologic diagnoses such as emphysema or pulmonary fibrosis. They provide physiologic measurements **identifying obstructive or restrictive ventilatory defects** (among others) and, in doing so, provide support for the existence of the relevant disease process. This text is not intended as an extensive reference on PFTs. It is a guide for the evaluation of basic spirometry and lung volumes that will allow the reader to identify common ventilatory defects using the data provided. In-depth analysis of PFTs and detailed descriptions of the physiologic principles underlying them may be found elsewhere in a number of excellent texts.

DEFINITION OF NORMAL VALUES

The results of PFTs are interpreted by comparing them to predicted values representing "normal" subjects. These predicted or normal values take into account many variables, including age, height, and gender; however, they neglect other influencing variables that have significant effects on predicted values, including race, air pollution, socioeconomic status, and others.

Traditionally, but without scientific basis, pulmonary function labs have arbitrarily set upper and lower limits of normal by comparing measured values with the predicted normal values as a percent (a measured value is interpreted as a percentage of the so-called normal value) and are expressed as "percent of predicted." This method is used in this text because it permits easy instruction and is still commonly used today. Alternative methods of defining normal range include statistical methods for determining 95th percentiles for given population groups or 95% confidence intervals for given population groups.

STANDARDIZATION OF PULMONARY FUNCTION TESTS

To obtain useful information from PFTs, both the adequacy of the equipment and the reproducibility of the results need to be scrutinized. The American Thoracic Society (ATS) publishes guidelines for the standardization of spirometry, including recommendations on equipment calibration, validation of results, measurement of parameters, and acceptability and reproducibility of data obtained. Because most PFTs are obtained from dedicated PFT labs, this text concentrates on the standardized criteria for interpretation of PFT data and not on equipment setup and testing.

ACCEPTABILITY AND REPRODUCIBILITY

Each PFT should initially be assessed for acceptability. Test acceptability is best determined by studying the flow–volume loops. Acceptability criteria for PFTs include the following:

- Freedom from artifacts (coughing, glottic closure, early termination, leak, variable effort)
- Good starts (i.e., the initial portion of the curve that is most dependent on patient effort is free from artifact)
- Satisfactory expiratory time (at least 6 secs of expiration on the volume–time curve, or at least a 1-sec plateau in the volume–time curve)

Once the minimum of three acceptable flow–volume loops have been obtained, the reproducibility of the PFTs should be assessed. **Reproducibility criteria for PFTs** include the following:

- The two largest forced vital capacity (FVC) measurements should be within 0.2 L or 5% of each other.
- The two largest FEV_1 measurements should be within 0.2 L or 5% of each other.

(See next section for explanation of FEV_1 and FVC.)

Only when all the above criteria are met can the PFTs be interpreted with confidence. If these criteria are not met, further testing needs to be performed to obtain accurate results. Up to eight efforts may be performed; after this, patient fatigue affects the data obtained. The best results are always used for interpretation.

NORMAL PULMONARY FUNCTION TESTS

PFTs are best interpreted in relation to an individual's clinical presentation and not in isolation. All parts of the PFTs should be used, including the spirometry (flow–volume loop) and the lung volumes. Normal spirometry is defined by a normal-shaped flow–volume loop (the plot of the FVC maneuver followed by a deep inspiration). A normal flow–volume loop has a rapid peak and a gradual decline in flow back to zero on the expiratory limb. The inspiratory limb should be a rounded shape (Fig. 2-1).

Normal spirometry is also defined by the measured values for the FVC and the FEV_1. **FVC** is defined as the maximum volume of air that is forcefully exhaled after a maximum inspiration. **FEV_1** is defined as the volume of air exhaled during the first second of the FVC maneuver. The measured values for FEV_1 and FVC are compared to the predicted values for FEV_1 and FVC as a percent. Values >80% are considered normal:

FEV_1 >80% of predicted (normal), or
FVC >80% of predicted (normal)

In contrast, lung volumes are defined by comparing the measured values for the volume concerned to the predicted values for that volume as a percent. Values between 80% and 120% are considered normal:

Lung volume = 80–120% of predicted (normal)

The important **lung volumes** in this discussion include residual volume (RV), total lung capacity (TLC), and the slow vital capacity (SVC). **TLC** is defined as the volume of air in the lung after complete maximal inspiration. **RV** is defined as the volume of air left in the lungs after complete maximal expiration. **SVC** is defined as the maximum volume of air that can be exhaled with normal effort after a maximum inspiration. (It is similar to the FVC except performed *without* full force.)

OBSTRUCTIVE VENTILATORY DEFECTS

An obstructive ventilatory defect (OVD) is defined as a disproportionate decrease in the FEV_1 compared to the FVC. An **FEV_1:FVC ratio of <70%** defines an OVD.

FEV_1: FVC <70% (OVD)

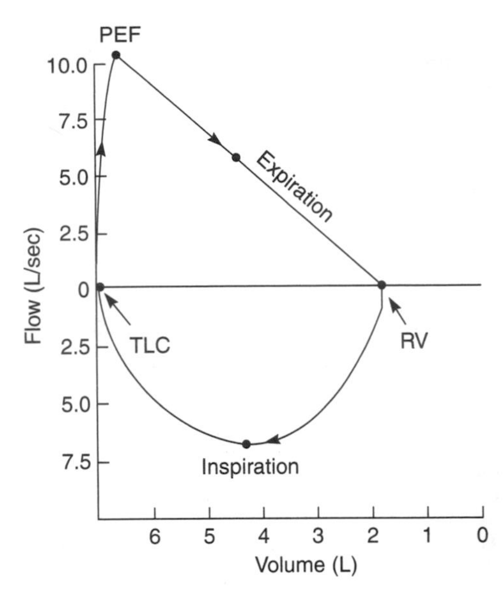

FIG. 2-1. Normal spirometry. PEF, peak expiratory flow; RV, residual volume; TLC, total lung capacity. Modified from Beers MH, Berkow R, eds. *The Merck manual of diagnosis and therapy,* 17th ed. Whitehouse Station, NJ: Merck, 1999:526–527.

The FVC may be reduced in an OVD, but the FEV_1 is always reduced by an even greater amount. The ATS cautions against diagnosing an OVD in individuals who have a decreased FEV_1:FVC ratio but normal FEV_1 and FVC because this pattern can be seen in healthy subjects. OVDs are an indication of airflow limitation and imply airway narrowing during expiration. An OVD is not specific for any pathologic cause of airway narrowing. For example, in emphysema, the narrowing is believed to be the result of decreased elastic support of smaller airways owing to alveolar septal destruction, whereas in chronic bronchitis, mucosal inflammation and excess mucus production are the culprit lesions.

Once the diagnosis of an OVD has been made, the defect needs to be fully characterized by the following:

- Quantifying the severity of the OVD
- Assessing the reversibility of the obstruction
- Determining whether there is hyperinflation
- Determining whether there is air trapping

Quantifying the **severity of the OVD** is done by comparing the measured FEV_1 to the predicted FEV_1 as a percent:

Normal: FEV_1 >80% of predicted
Mild: FEV_1 = 65–80% of predicted
Moderate: FEV_1 = 50–64% of predicted
Severe: FEV_1 <50% of predicted

Assessing the **reversibility** of the obstruction requires spirometry performed both before and after bronchodilator administration. A 12% increase (calculated from prebronchodilator values) *and* a 200-mL increase in either FEV_1 *or* FVC defines a positive bronchodilator response and indicates reversibility of an obstruction. Thus, reversibility is said to be present when, compared with the prebronchodilator values

Postbronchodilator FEV_1 improves by *both* 12% and 200 mL, or
Postbronchodilator FVC improves by *both* 12% and 200 mL

Hyperinflation denotes that, at maximum inspiration and expiration, the lungs are at a larger volume than is expected for an individual. In physiologic terms, the individual's TLC *or* RV is increased. The presence of **hyperinflation** is determined by comparing the measured TLC or RV to the predicted TLC or RV as a percent:

TLC >120% of predicted, or
RV >120% of predicted

Air trapping denotes that during forced (rapid) expiration, there is dynamic collapse of airways with resultant incomplete expiration of air compared with nonforced (slow) expiration. In physiologic terms, the individual's FVC is smaller than the SVC. Air trapping occurs because forced expiration causes worsening of airway obstruction owing to higher positive intrathoracic pressures. An increase of 12% *and* 200 mL in the SVC compared with the FVC indicates **air trapping:**

SVC > FVC by *both* 12% and 200 mL

OVDs change the shape of the flow–volume curve. The curve still has a rapid initial peak, but the expiratory flow drops progressively quicker with worsening obstruction. As a result, the expiratory limb of the curve takes on a progressively increasing concavity. Eventually, there is also a decrease in the peak expiratory flow of the initial portion of the curve. In severe disease, there is an initial rapid but reduced peak followed by a precipitous drop in flow and a very gradual taper of the flow to zero (Fig. 2-2).

METHACHOLINE CHALLENGE TESTING

Asthma is defined as reversible obstructive airway disease. Therefore, in individuals suspected of having asthma, multiple PFTs may only demonstrate normal spirometry. In these individuals, bronchial provocation testing is indicated to induce airway constriction and allow for the diagnosis (and further management) of asthma. Individuals

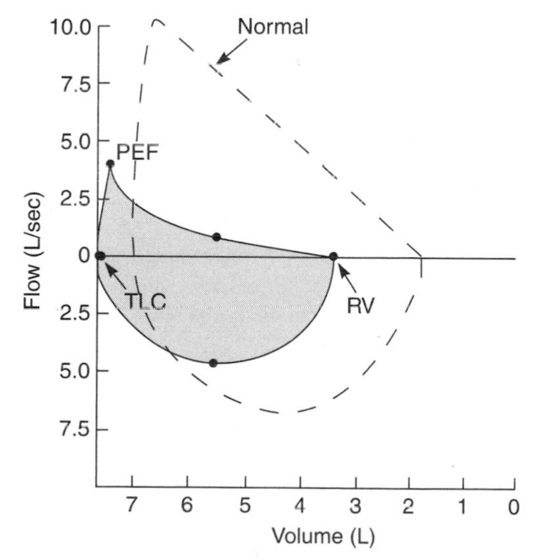

FIG. 2-2. Obstructive lung disease. PEF, peak expiratory flow; RV, residual volume; TLC, total lung capacity. Modified from Beers MH, Berkow R, eds. *The Merck manual of diagnosis and therapy,* 17th ed. Whitehouse Station, NJ: Merck, 1999:526–527.

who should be considered for bronchial provocation testing include those with **chronic cough, wheezing, intermittent dyspnea, workplace-related cough/wheezing/dyspnea, and exercise-associated cough/wheezing.**

The methacholine challenge test is a nonspecific test of airway responsiveness. It allows for a semiquantitative assessment of airway reactivity but gives no insight into the specific stimulus affecting an individual. The advantage of the test is that it has good reproducibility. The disadvantage is that multiple factors can affect the test, including medications (bronchodilators, steroids, antihistamines, beta-agonists, calcium-channel blockers), respiratory infection, and exposures to sensitizers (allergens or chemicals).

The test begins with the administration of a sterile saline aerosol (as a control) followed by the measurement of the FEV_1 after 3–5 mins (as a baseline). Increasing concentrations of methacholine in sterile saline are then administered to the patient at 5-min intervals, and the FEV_1 is measured 3–5 mins after each increase in concentration. The concentrations range from 0.003 mg/mL to 16 mg/mL of methacholine in sterile saline and are increased (roughly doubled each time) until either a positive response is obtained or a maximum concentration is achieved. The results are plotted in graphic form.

A positive test for **reversible** airway obstruction is defined as a **decrease in FEV_1 from baseline of ≥20%.** If the decrease in FEV_1 is <20% once a concentration of 16 mg/mL has been reached, the test is said to be negative:

Decrease in FEV_1 >20% is a positive response to methacholine challenge when it occurs at methacholine concentrations of ≤16 mg/mL.

RESTRICTIVE VENTILATORY DEFECTS

A restrictive ventilatory defect (RVD) is defined as a **pathologic reduction in TLC.** It is assessed by comparing the measured TLC to the predicted TLC as a percent. Values <80% of predicted **define an RVD:**

TLC <80% of predicted (RVD)

The presence of an RVD may be suspected using spirometry when the FVC is reduced in the face of a normal or increased FEV_1:FVC ratio. However, to diagnose an RVD definitively, lung volumes must be obtained to determine the TLC.

As the name implies, there is restriction of outward movement of the lungs and/or chest wall, and as a result, the lungs are at smaller volumes than normal. An RVD is not specific for any pathologic cause of decreased movement. For example, in interstitial pulmonary fibrosis, the restriction is the result of thickening of the alveolar septae and "firming" of the lung parenchyma, whereas in scoliosis, the thoracic deformity and a fixed thoracic cage are the culprit lesions. An RVD can also be caused by removal of lung tissue because this results in a decrease in TLC compared to that predicted.

Once the diagnosis of an **RVD** has been made, the defect needs to be **quantified,** which is done by comparing the measured TLC to the predicted TLC as a percent:

Normal: TLC >80% of predicted
Mild: TLC = 65–80% of predicted
Moderate: TLC = 50–64% of predicted
Severe: TLC <50% of predicted

The shape of the flow–volume loop is essentially unchanged in RVDs. The curve is narrowed, reflecting the smaller lung volumes associated with RVDs (Fig. 2-3). As mentioned before, the shape of the curve is only suggestive of an RVD; lung volumes must be measured to make the diagnosis.

UPPER AIRWAY OBSTRUCTION

The OVDs discussed earlier all represent obstruction at the level of the smaller (more distal) airways. Obstruction of the larger, more proximal airways (trachea and major bronchi) presents differently and is most easily identified on inspection of both the

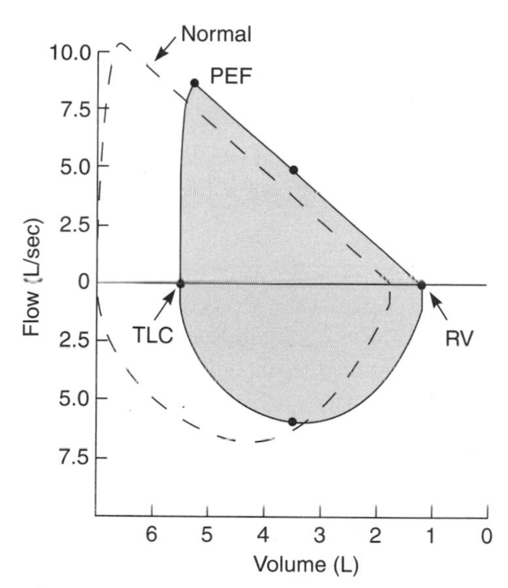

FIG. 2-3. Restrictive lung disease. PEF, peak expiratory flow; RV, residual volume; TLC, total lung capacity. Modified from Beers MH, Berkow R, eds. *The Merck manual of diagnosis and therapy,* 17th ed. Whitehouse Station, NJ: Merck, 1999:526–527.

inspiratory and expiratory limbs of the flow–volume loop. The three forms of upper airway obstruction are

- Fixed obstruction
- Variable intrathoracic obstruction
- Variable extrathoracic obstruction

When an airway contains a fixed obstruction, the cross-sectional area of the obstructed airway does not change throughout the respiratory cycle (hence its characterization as *fixed*). Thus, the obstruction is present during both inspiration and expiration, and both limbs are almost always equally affected. There is characteristic truncation of both limbs with the resulting "box" shape on the flow–volume loop (Fig. 2-4).

When an airway contains a variable obstruction, the obstruction is dependent on both the location of the obstruction (within or external to the thorax) and the phase of the respiratory cycle. The cross-sectional area of the obstructed airway changes during inspiration and expiration such that either the inspiratory *or* the expiratory limb of the flow–volume loop is predominantly affected.

In variable intrathoracic obstruction, the expiratory limb is primarily affected. During forced expiration, the pleural pressure exceeds the tracheal pressure downstream (toward the mouth) of the lesion. As a result, the airway collapses, and the obstruction worsens. During forced inspiration, the pressures are reversed, and the obstruction is relieved. Thus, only the expiratory limb is truncated (Fig. 2-5).

In variable extrathoracic obstruction, the inspiratory limb is primarily affected. During forced inspiration, the atmospheric pressure exceeds the tracheal pressure upstream (toward the alveoli) of the lesion. As a result, the airway collapses, and the obstruction worsens. During forced expiration, the pressures are reversed, and the obstruction is relieved. Thus, only the inspiratory limb is truncated (Fig. 2-6).

DIFFUSING CAPACITY

Diffusing capacity is often measured as part of a PFT. It is performed separately from spirometry and lung volume measurement. It is a surrogate measure of the integrity

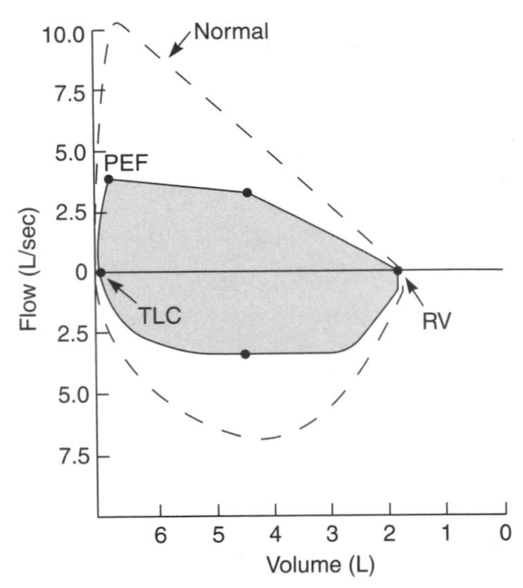

FIG. 2-4. Fixed upper airway obstruction. PEF, peak expiratory flow; RV, residual volume; TLC, total lung capacity. Modified from Beers MH, Berkow R, eds. *The Merck manual of diagnosis and therapy,* 17th ed. Whitehouse Station, NJ: Merck, 1999:526–527.

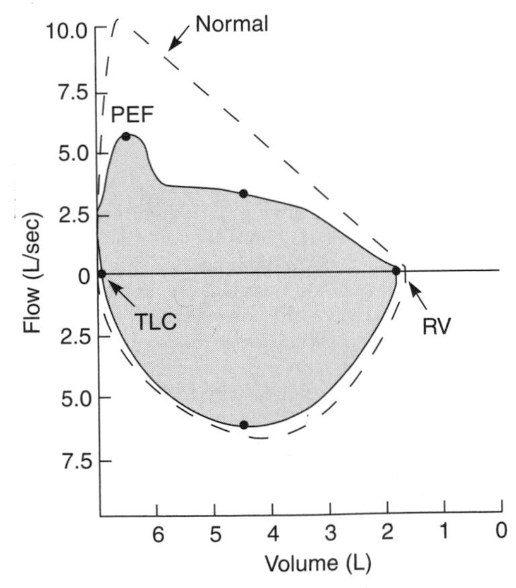

FIG. 2-5. Variable intrathoracic obstruction. PEF, peak expiratory flow; RV, residual volume; TLC, total lung capacity. Modified from Beers MH, Berkow R, eds. *The Merck manual of diagnosis and therapy,* 17th ed. Whitehouse Station, NJ: Merck, 1999:526–527.

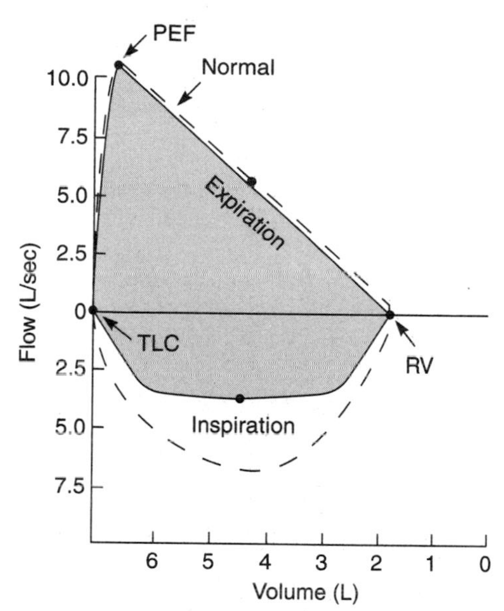

FIG. 2-6. Variable extrathoracic obstruction. PEF, peak expiratory flow; RV, residual volume; TLC, total lung capacity. Modified from Beers MH, Berkow R, eds. *The Merck manual of diagnosis and therapy,* 17th ed. Whitehouse Station, NJ: Merck, 1999:526–527.

of the alveolar–capillary membrane across which gas exchange takes place. The diffusing capacity is a nonspecific measurement and provides only a physiologic assessment of the **efficiency of gas exchange.** Any disease affecting the pulmonary parenchyma or circulation can alter the diffusing capacity.

The gas used to measure the diffusing capacity is carbon monoxide, and the diffusing capacity is expressed as **diffusing capacity for carbon monoxide (DLCO).** The *measured* value is often corrected to eliminate the effects of the individual's Hgb concentration, which may artificially increase (high concentration) or reduce (low concentration) the DLCO. The corrected value is expressed as the **corrected DLCO ($DLCO_C$).** Calculation of $DLCO_C$ is not mandatory but is desirable.

Measured values are compared to predicted values as a percent (the percentile or confidence interval methods may also be used). Percent predicted values for DLCO or $DLCO_C$ between 60% and 120% are considered normal:

DLCO <60% of predicted (low DLCO)
DLCO >120% of predicted (high DLCO)
or
$DLCO_C$ <60% of predicted (low $DLCO_C$)
$DLCO_C$ >120% of predicted (high $DLCO_C$)

The reason for the wide interval is the large amount of variability between different measurements in the same individual at any given time.

CONCLUSION

The following is a suggested method of evaluating PFTs (Fig. 2-7). The algorithm and the discussion in this chapter are far from exhaustive and are simply an introduction to help with the basic evaluation of PFTs. For more detailed information on PFTs, the reader is again referred to a number of excellent texts in the bibliography.

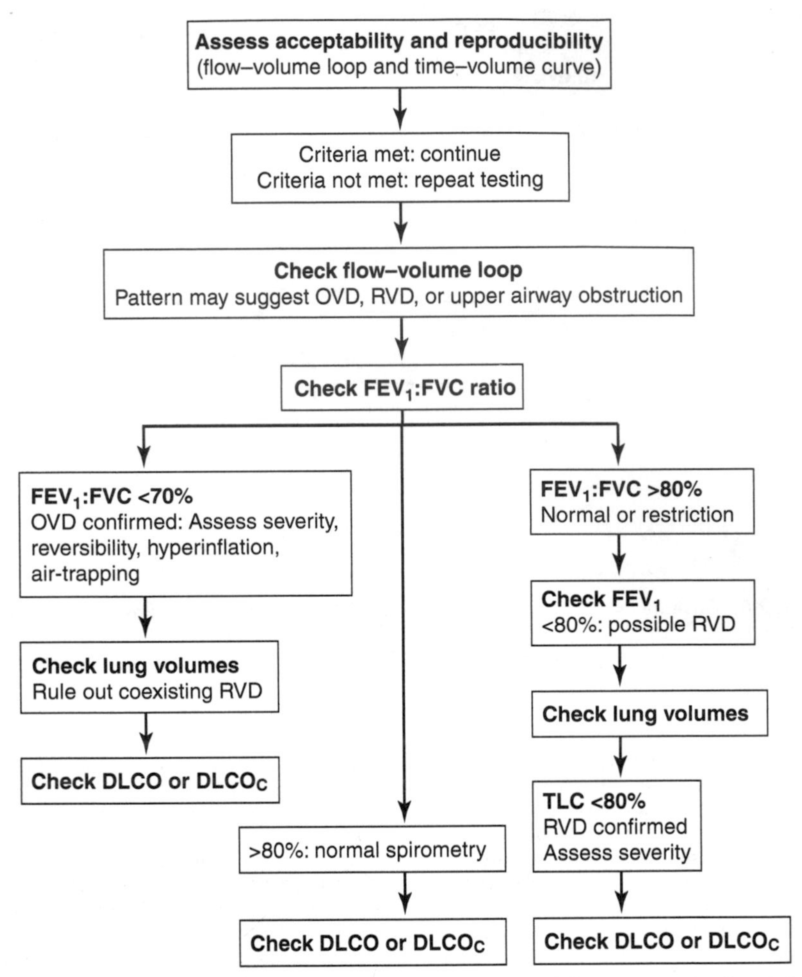

FIG. 2-7. Evaluation of pulmonary function tests. DLCO, diffusing capacity for carbon monoxide; $DLCO_C$, corrected diffusing capacity for carbon monoxide; FVC, forced vital capacity; OVD, obstructive ventilatory defect; RVD, residual volume defect; TLC, total lung capacity.

KEY POINTS TO REMEMBER

- PFTs do not make pathologic diagnoses; they provide physiologic measurements identifying obstructive or restrictive ventilatory defects and in doing so, provide support for the existence of the relevant disease process.
- Normal spirometry is defined by a normal shaped flow–volume loop. A normal flow–volume loop has a rapid peak and a gradual decline in flow back to zero on the expiratory limb. The inspiratory limb should be a nice rounded shape.
- Normal spirometry is also defined by the measured values for the FVC and the FEV in 1 sec.
- The three forms of upper airway obstruction include fixed obstruction, variable intrathoracic obstruction, and variable extrathoracic obstruction.

REFERENCES AND SUGGESTED READINGS

American Thoracic Society. Lung function testing: selection of reference values and interpretive strategies. ATS Statement. *Am Rev Respir Dis* 1991;144:1202–1218.

American Thoracic Society. Standardization of spirometry: 1994 update. ATS Statement. *Am J Respir Crit Care Med* 1995;152:1107–1136.

American Thoracic Society. Guidelines for methacholine and exercise challenge testing—1999. ATS Statement. *Am J Respir Crit Care Med* 2000;161:309–329.

Global Initiative for Chronic Obstructive Lung Disease (GOLD), U.S. Department of Health and Human Services, Public Health Service, National Institutes of Health, National Heart, Lung, and Blood Institutes; 2001.

Gold WM. Pulmonary function testing. In: Murray JF, Nadel JA, et al., eds. *Textbook of respiratory medicine*, 3rd ed. Philadelphia: WB Saunders, 2000:781–882.

Grippi MA, et al. Pulmonary function testing. In: Fishman AP, ed. *Pulmonary diseases and disorders*, 2nd ed. New York: McGraw-Hill, 1988:2469–2522.

Hankinson JL, et al. Spirometric reference values from a sample of the general U.S. population. *Am J Respir Crit Care Med* 1999;159:179–187.

Hargreave FE, et al. Bronchial responsiveness to histamine or methacholine in asthma: measurement and clinical significance. *J Allergy Clin Immunol* 1981; 68:347–355.

Lippmann M. Health significance of pulmonary function responses to irritants. *J Pollut Control Assoc* 1988;38:881–887.

Lippmann M. Health effects of ozone: a critical review. *J Pollut Control Assoc* 1989;39:672–695.

Schwartz JD, et al. Sex and race differences in the development of lung function. *Am Rev Respir Dis* 1988;138:1415–1421.

Steinberg M, Becklake MR. Socio-environmental factors and lung function. *S Afr Med J* 1986;70:270–274.

Wasserman K, Hansen JE, Sue DY, et al. *Principles of exercise testing and interpretation: including pathophysiology and clinical applications*. Vol. 15, 3rd ed. Philadelphia: Lippincott Williams & Wilkins, 1999:556.

3 Exercise Testing

Sujith Kalathiveetil

INTRODUCTION

Exercise testing is a well-established clinical procedure that has been used since the 1960s in the evaluation of exercise intolerance. **Exercise intolerance** results when a person is unable to sustain a work rate for a period sufficient to complete a given task. The interactions of the cardiovascular, pulmonary, and musculoskeletal systems determine the physiologic response to exercise. When a patient presents with complaints of exercise intolerance, exercise testing can be useful in determining the extent to which the three organ systems are involved. Exercise testing is also useful for assessing the response of cardiac and pulmonary diseases to therapy, for obtaining prognostic information in patients with cardiac or pulmonary disease, and in evaluating patients for organ transplantation.

Exercise intolerance may be the result of a number of factors. Generally, patients with exercise intolerance cite one of three reasons for their inability to exercise: **dyspnea, fatigue,** or **pain.**

Exertional dyspnea is the most common complaint of patients with lung parenchymal disease. It is also a common complaint in patients with pulmonary vascular disease, cardiac disease, severe anemia, and obesity. Resting dyspnea is a more ominous symptom that may be due to severe lung disease, unstable angina equivalent, decompensated heart failure, acute pulmonary vascular disease, or neuromuscular disease.

Fatigue is the symptom that stops the normal subject from continuing heavy exercise. The most common cause of early fatigue is deconditioning. Fatigue also occurs in patients with heart disease, lung disease (not as common as in dyspnea), and neuromuscular disease (in whom it is often the predominant symptom).

Pain is a less common complaint. Exertional pain is a common feature of peripheral vascular disease (claudication), angina, and various forms of arthritis. Pain is not usual with isolated pulmonary causes of exercise intolerance, but pulmonary vascular disease or pleural disease can present with exertional chest pain.

Before exercise testing, a careful history may shed light on which organ system(s) is responsible for a patient's symptoms, but it is often difficult for patients to describe which symptom(s) limits their ability to exercise. Furthermore, it can be challenging to assess the severity of exercise intolerance using symptoms alone. Exercise testing can be used to quantify and define the underlying cause of the patient's symptoms.

TEST OVERVIEW

There are six widely accepted exercise tests. These tests, in order of increasing complexity, are

- Stair climbing
- Six-minute walk test
- Shuttle-walk test
- Detection of exercise-induced asthma
- Cardiac stress test (Bruce Protocol)
- Cardiopulmonary exercise test

As they increase in complexity, these tests provide more information but take longer to perform and become more expensive. Thus, selecting the appropriate test is important. In this chapter, we focus on the two most commonly used tests: the 6-minute walk test (6MWT) and the cardiopulmonary exercise test (CPET).

SIX-MINUTE WALK TEST

Overview

The 6MWT is a simple yet useful way of assessing functional exercise capacity. The primary measurement calculated by the test is the distance that the patient can walk in 6 mins [6-min walk distance (6MWD)]. Secondary measurements collected include the patient's blood oxygen saturation and his or her perception of dyspnea with exercise.

Indications

Clinically, the 6MWT is used in three different situations: to assess response to therapy, to assess functional status, and to provide prognostic information about cardiopulmonary disease.

Protocol

Equipment required for performing the 6MWT includes a stopwatch, a mechanical lap counter, two small cones, an oxygen source, a sphygmomanometer, a telephone, a chair, a clipboard with worksheets, and a crash cart. Supplies in the crash cart should include a defibrillator, sublingual nitroglycerine, aspirin, and albuterol.

The 6MWT should be performed indoors along a 30-m (100 ft) hallway with a hard and flat surface. The test should not be performed on a treadmill, an oval/circular track, or an incline. A starting line should be marked with brightly colored tape, and the turn-around point (at 30 m) should be marked with cones.

Patients should wear comfortable clothing and footwear. If patients require supplemental oxygen, it should be administered during the test. Patients requiring a portable oxygen device should push or carry the device themselves during the test to give a more accurate picture of the patient's exercise capacity when at home.

There is no warm-up period before the test. The patient should sit at rest in a chair for at least 10 mins before testing, during which time BP and heart rate (HR) should be measured. If pulse oximetry and dyspnea scoring are to be assessed, they should be measured at baseline and at completion of the 6MWT. Patients should be instructed to walk as far as they can in 6 mins. When they reach the cones, they should turn around and walk back to the starting line, where they will turn around and repeat the procedure. Laps should be counted with a lap counter. Patients are permitted to slow down and stop as necessary.

Standardized phrases should be used during the 6MWT, as words of encouragement can affect the 6MWD. In addition, the patient should walk alone without the examiner, as this can also affect the 6MWD. No more than one patient should perform the 6MWT at a time.

Reasons for immediately stopping a test are chest pain, severe dyspnea, diaphoresis, staggering, ill appearance, or leg cramps. As noted above, a crash cart and telephone should be available at the site of the 6MWT. A physician does not have to be present during testing, but the technician performing the 6MWT should at least be proficient in basic life support.

Contraindications

Absolute contraindications to performing the 6MWT are **myocardial infarction** or **unstable angina** in the last month. Stable exertional angina is not an absolute contraindication, but patients with stable angina should take their antianginal medications before the test.

Relative contraindications include a resting heart rate of >120 bpm, an SBP of >180 mm Hg, and a DBP of >100 mm Hg.

Interpretation

The primary measurement of the 6MWT is the 6MWD. Healthy subjects' 6MWDs range from 500 to 700 m. Different patient characteristics may affect 6MWD. These include stature (taller patients walk farther), gender (male patients tend to walk farther), motivation, and previous testing (patients familiar with the test often perform better).

A low 6MWD is both nondiagnostic and nonspecific. It should lead to further testing of pulmonary function, cardiac function, vascular sufficiency, muscle strength, orthopedic function, cognitive function, and nutritional status, as indicated.

The 6MWD is much more useful in assessing response to therapy. Although there is no gold standard for predicted improvement in 6MWD with intervention, several studies have quantified improvements in the 6MWD after therapy for underlying cardiopulmonary conditions. For example, in COPD patients who receive supplemental oxygen, 6MWD may improve by up to 36%, whereas heart failure patients undergoing cardiac rehabilitation may improve their 6MWD by up to 15%.

Clinical Relevance

An important functional question concerns how improvement in the 6MWD correlates with a perceived difference in exercise tolerance. A study looking at patients with severe COPD showed a perceived improvement in clinical performance at a mean 6MWD increase of 54 m. A similar study in patients with heart failure showed perceived improvement in clinical performance with a mean 6MWD increase of 46 m. Given the range of the 6MWD in these groups of patients, these studies demonstrate a perceived improvement in exercise tolerance when patients achieve an 8–12% increase in their 6MWD.

Conclusion

The 6MWT is a useful exercise test. Its strengths and weaknesses lie in its simplicity. It is quick and inexpensive to perform and makes an excellent initial screening test. It is also very useful in assessing prognosis and therapeutic response in patients with an established diagnosis of cardiopulmonary disease. However, it is also nonspecific in that it does not differentiate which organ system is responsible for exercise intolerance.

CARDIOPULMONARY EXERCISE TEST

Overview

The CPET is much more complex than the 6MWT. The CPET is an integrated exercise test usually performed on a cycle ergometer or treadmill. During the CPET, oxygen uptake ($\dot{V}O_2$), anaerobic threshold (AT), carbon dioxide output ($\dot{V}CO_2$), minute ventilation ($\dot{V}_E$), vital signs, ABG, and 12-lead ECG are monitored. Because of the large amount of data that it provides, the CPET requires more time and considerably more equipment than the 6MWT.

The primary goal of the CPET is to measure peak exercise capacity. Peak exercise capacity is defined as the maximum ability of the cardiovascular system to deliver oxygen to exercising skeletal muscle, and of the exercising muscle to extract oxygen from blood. There are several tests used to measure peak exercise capacity. The two most common methods measure maximal $\dot{V}O_2$ ($\dot{V}O_{2max}$ and peak $\dot{V}O_2$) and AT.

Exercise capacity can be quantified by $\dot{V}O_2$. Breath gas analyzers are used during exercise to obtain these measurements. $\dot{V}O_2$ is measured in liters of oxygen consumed per minute (L/min). This value is sometimes expressed as milliliters per minute and then divided per kilogram (mL/min/kg). The Vo_2 is expressed mathematically as cardiac output multiplied by the arterial-venous oxygen difference:

$$Vo_2 = (SV \times HR) \times (Cao_2 - Cvo_2)$$

where Cao_2 = arterial oxygen saturation, and
Cvo_2 = venous oxygen saturation

Peak Vo_2 refers to the highest Vo_2 achieved during exercise testing. It is a useful index because it has a strong correlation with both cardiac output and skeletal muscle blood flow.

The Vo_{2max} is the point at which no further increase in Vo_2 occurs despite a continued increase in workload. Vo_2, which normally increases linearly with workload, then flattens to a plateau. It is defined mathematically as the maximum cardiac output multiplied by the maximum arterial-venous oxygen difference:

$$Vo_{2max} = (HR_{max} \times SV_{max}) \times (Cao_{2max} - Cvo_{2min})$$

In other words, the Vo_{2max} is the maximal ability of a subject to inspire, transport, and utilize oxygen (Table 3-1). The Vo_{2max} is the gold standard in determining a patient's aerobic capacity. The Vo_{2max} is affected by multiple factors: age, gender, exercise habits, heredity, and (most important) cardiovascular clinical status. It is worth noting that a subject's peak Vo_2 may not be his or her Vo_{2max} (the patient's Vo_2 does not reach a plateau during the CPET). Many subjects can have difficulty achieving Vo_{2max}, as it usually occurs after they have reached their AT.

The AT is another useful index for measuring exercise capacity. The AT is defined as the point at which V_E rises disproportionately to Vo_2. In more practical terms, the AT is the point at which exercise switches from aerobic to anaerobic. When subjects reach their AT, their lactate levels begin to increase. As a result, there is a marked compensatory increase in ventilation. Patients also develop a linear increase in carbon dioxide production. Indeed, Vco_2 begins increasing more rapidly than Vo_2. ABG analysis at this time also shows a drop in serum HCO_3^- levels, as patients develop a metabolic acidosis from lactate production. Owing to increased metabolic demands, subjects have reduced endurance time at exercise intensities beyond the AT. The AT usually occurs at 60–70% of the Vo_{2max}. The AT can be used to distinguish between cardiac and noncardiac (pulmonary and musculoskeletal) causes of exercise intolerance: Subjects who fatigue before reaching their AT are more likely to have a noncardiac etiology for their symptoms. The AT can also be improved (increased) with the addition of supplemental oxygen and exercise training.

TABLE 3-1. NORMAL VALUES OF Vo_{2MAX} WITH AGE AND GENDER

Age (yrs)	Male Vo_{2max} (mL/min/kg)	Female Vo_{2max} (mL/min/kg)
20–29	43 ± 7.2	36 ± 6.9
30–39	42 ± 7.0	34 ± 6.2
40–49	40 ± 7.2	32 ± 6.2
50–59	36 ± 7.1	29 ± 5.4
60–69	33 ± 7.3	27 ± 4.7
70–79	29 ± 7.3	27 ± 5.8

From Fletcher GF, Balady GJ, Amsterdam EA, et al. AHA scientific statement: exercise standards for testing and training. *Circulation* 2001;104:1694–1740, with permission.

TABLE 3-2. CONTRAINDICATIONS TO PERFORMING THE CARDIOPULMONARY EXERCISE TEST

Absolute	Relative
Acute myocardial infarction	Left main coronary stenosis
Unstable angina	Moderate stenotic valvular disease
Uncontrolled arrhythmias	SBP >180, DBP >100, heart rate >120
Electrolyte abnormalities	Tachyarrhythmias or bradyarrhythmias
Symptomatic aortic stenosis	Atrial fibrillation with rapid ventricular rate
High-degree atrioventricular block	Mental impairment
Disability	
Inability to obtain consent	

From Fletcher GF, Balady GJ, Amsterdam EA, et al. AHA scientific statement: exercise standards for testing and training. *Circulation* 2001;104:1694–1740, with permission.

Indications/Contraindications

The CPET provides data regarding the pulmonary, cardiac, peripheral vascular, and skeletal muscle systems during exercise and can aid in identifying the cause of exercise intolerance or exertional dyspnea. The CPET can be used for applications other than evaluating exercise intolerance, including

- Grading severity of heart disease
- Prioritizing patients for heart transplantation
- Preoperative evaluation of surgical risk
- Measuring impairment for disability evaluation
- Assessing effectiveness of treatment
- Screening for the development of disease in high-risk patients
- Graded exercise testing for athletes

A brief history and physical exam should be performed to look for contraindications to the CPET. Because the CPET places the subject under more physical stress than does the 6MWT, there are more contraindications to performing the CPET (Table 3-2). Once again, stable exertional angina is not an absolute contraindication, and patients with stable angina should take their antianginal medications before the CPET.

Protocol

Mandatory equipment for the CPET includes a treadmill or bicycle ergometer, sphygmomanometer, ECG capable of continuous recording, breath gas analyzers capable of measuring breath-by-breath oxygen and carbon dioxide concentrations (i.e., gas exchange analysis), and an ABG analyzer. Other safety equipment used during the 6MWT (oxygen source, telephone, crash cart with an automatic electronic defibrillator, sublingual nitroglycerine, aspirin, and albuterol) should also be present during the CPET.

On the day of the exam, patients should abstain from food and smoking for 3 hrs before the CPET. As in the 6MWT, patients should wear comfortable clothing and footwear. Patients should take their morning medications (especially antianginal medications). The role of holding beta-blockers remains controversial. Although beta-blockers can reduce exercise tolerance, abrupt cessation can lead to withdrawal reactions, which can lead to uncontrolled HTN and/or myocardial ischemia. Some recommend taking beta-blockers at a decreased dose on the day of the test.

A resting 12-lead ECG should be obtained. Before the CPET actually begins, the electrodes are often moved to modified positions so that better waveforms can be recorded during activity. A BP cuff is also placed so that BP measurements can be taken throughout the CPET. Breath gas analyzers should also be placed over the patient's face. A resting ABG is often performed before the test begins. In some patients, an arterial catheter is placed to allow repeated blood gas sampling and invasive BP monitoring during exercise.

The CPET is performed on a bicycle or a treadmill ergometer. An electrically braked cycle, which varies resistance based on pedaling speed, is preferred. The treadmill should have variable speed and grade capability. Both of these modalities offer their own advantages and drawbacks. The cycle ergometer is less expensive, quieter, and causes less upper body motion (allowing better ECG and BP readings). The major drawback to the bicycle ergometer is that patients who are unfamiliar with cycling can develop significant discomfort in their quadriceps muscles, which can lead to fatigue and cause subjects to stop the CPET before they reach their VO_{2max}. The treadmill ergometer adversely affects BP and ECG measurements because of increased upper body motion but may give a more accurate measurement of the VO_{2max} in those who are not accustomed to cycling.

There are multiple protocols used for grading the intensity of the test. All protocols can be divided broadly into two groups: incremental exercise and constant work rate. With incremental protocols, the patient exercises on an ergometer while measurements of gas exchange are made at rest, during 3 mins of low-intensity exercise (warm-up), and then while the work rate is increased each minute or continuously. The patient is encouraged to continue as long as possible. When the patient is no longer able to continue, a 2-min recovery period begins, which returns the patient to low-intensity exercise. In a constant protocol, the work rate is fixed and does not increase with time. If an increase in work rate is desired, a rest period occurs between changes in work rate. It is believed that a constant work rate protocol that increases intensity based on how the patient tolerates each workload is better than the incremental protocol for measuring VO_{2max} and AT. However, it takes longer to perform and may be more likely to result in injury to the patient.

Interpretation

Interpreting the results of the CPET can be complex and challenging owing to the large amount of data generated. In *Principles of Exercise Testing and Interpretation*, Wasserman et al. describe a useful flowchart approach to interpretation. Patients who take the CPET are immediately stratified into three groups based on their measured VO_{2max} and AT: normal peak VO_2, low peak VO_2/normal AT, and low peak VO_2/low AT. Once the patients have been stratified, additional tests are performed to help establish the etiology of their exercise intolerance. We discuss these additional tests and explain how they assist in diagnosis below. This discussion requires explanation of pulmonary, cardiac, and ventilation/perfusion indices.

Pulmonary Indices

There are several indices of pulmonary function during exercise testing. Our discussion focuses on four: breathing reserve (BR), respiratory rate (RR) at peak VO_2, ventilatory equivalent for carbon dioxide, and vital capacity (V_C).

BR represents the body's potential for increasing ventilation at maximum exercise. A low BR is seen in patients with primary lung disease who have ventilatory limitation. The BR is high when cardiovascular or other diseases limit exercise performance.

The **RR** at peak VO_2 can also give insight into the nature of underlying lung disease. Specifically, RR at peak VO_2 helps distinguish restrictive lung disease from obstructive lung disease. As a result of the decreased lung volumes inherent to restriction, there is a compensatory increase in RR during heavy exercise. Thus, the RR at peak VO_2 is dramatically increased in restrictive lung disease (often RR >50 breaths/min). However, in obstructive lung disease, lung volumes are normal to increased. Airway obstruction also prolongs expiration, increasing the time needed to complete a full respiration. The combination of these phenomena results in a smaller increase in RR at peak VO_2.

V_E is the volume of air taken into or expired from the body in 1 min. VCO_2 is defined as the volume of carbon dioxide that is expired from the body in 1 min. The ratio of these two values is known as the ventilatory equivalent for carbon dioxide (V_E/VCO_2).

Normal values of V_E/VCO_2 for middle-aged sedentary men are 29.1 ± 4.3. V_E/VCO_2 can be an index of dead space ventilation and total ventilation. V_E/VCO_2 rises when there is an increase in dead space ventilation and during hyperventilation. Wasserman et al. demonstrate that V_E/VCO_2 initially decreases during early exercise but increases after reaching the AT owing to hyperventilation. However, with problems in pulmonary circulation (resulting in increased dead space), V_E/VCO_2 rises even higher than expected. Thus, an abnormally high V_E/VCO_2 at the AT suggests defects in pulmonary circulation.

V_C is defined as the maximum volume that can be expired after a maximal inspiration. Two possible causes for a higher than expected V_E/VCO_2 at AT are left ventricular failure and intrinsic pulmonary vascular disease (thromboembolic disease, primary pulmonary HTN, and vasculitis). V_C is useful because it allows one to distinguish between these two conditions. In left ventricular failure, pulmonary congestion occurs, and V_C decreases as a result of the altered mechanics of the lung. However, in intrinsic pulmonary vascular disease, there is less change in the mechanics of the lung, and V_C is usually preserved.

Cardiac Indices

Although there are a multitude of cardiac indices that can be used in the CPET, two are particularly important: the ECG and the oxygen pulse.

The **ECG** can be very useful in detecting exercise-induced myocardial ischemia. The three most common ECG findings in myocardial ischemia are ST segment changes, T-wave changes, and exercise-induced arrhythmias.

ST segment changes are the most sensitive and specific ECG findings in myocardial ischemia. ST depression of at least 1 mm that is horizontal or down-sloping is abnormal, as is up-sloping ST depression of at least 2 mm. Down-sloping ST depression that occurs after termination of exercise is also very suggestive of ischemia. ST elevation in a patient with Q waves from a prior myocardial infarction is often a normal finding. However, in a patient without Q waves from a prior myocardial infarction, ST elevation during exercise is a sign of marked transmural myocardial ischemia.

T-wave changes are less specific but still useful in detecting ischemia. The T wave normally decreases in amplitude during early exercise but increases during maximal exercise. One minute after termination of exercise, the T wave usually returns to its baseline morphology. T-wave inversion during exercise is a moderately sensitive but nonspecific marker of myocardial ischemia.

The most common arrhythmia to occur during exercise-induced myocardial ischemia is **premature ventricular contraction.** However, the appearance of premature ventricular contractions is neither sensitive nor specific. **Exercise-induced left bundle branch block** is a very worrisome sign that can be caused by myocardial ischemia. Sustained ventricular tachycardia and ventricular fibrillation can occur in patients with significant coronary artery disease, but fortunately, these rarely occur.

The **oxygen pulse** is defined as VO_2 divided by the HR. In other words, it represents the amount of oxygen extracted by the tissues of the body during each cardiac cycle. In patients with heart disease (due to coronary artery disease, cardiomyopathy, or valvular causes), the oxygen pulse is low and fixed even as the intensity of exercise increases. Normally, stroke volume and heart rate increase to compensate for increased metabolic demands. However, in patients with heart disease, there is not an appropriate rise in stroke volume and/or HR, which restricts the amount of oxygen that can be supplied to peripheral tissues. The consequence of this phenomenon is an oxygen pulse that remains low and nonchanging. Conversely, in conditions in which cardiac function is preserved (such as peripheral vascular disease), stroke volume and HR rise appropriately with increasing metabolic demands. Thus, the oxygen pulse rises with exercise.

Ventilation and Perfusion Indices

There are three indices that are commonly used to assess ventilation and perfusion: dead space/tidal volume ratio (V_D/V_T), alveolar-arterial PO_2 difference [$P(A\text{-}a)O_2$] and the arterial–end-tidal PCO_2 difference [$P(a\text{-}ET)CO_2$].

V_D/V_T is defined as the proportion of the V_T that is made of the physiologic V_D. Thus, it measures the inefficiency of the elimination of carbon dioxide by pulmonary gas exchange. At rest, the physiologic V_D is normally one-third of the breath. During exercise in a normal individual, it is reduced to about one-fifth of the breath. However, in patients with ventilation-perfusion abnormalities, V_D/V_T is increased at rest and fails to decrease with exercise. This finding is often present in patients with primary pulmonary vascular disease, pulmonary vascular disease secondary to obstructive or restrictive lung disease, or heart failure.

$P(A\text{-}a)O_2$ is defined as the difference between PAO_2 and PaO_2. It measures the inefficiency of oxygen uptake by pulmonary gas exchange. Normally, PaO_2 does not decrease during exercise and the $P(A\text{-}a)O_2$ remains at <20 mm Hg. However, in patients with abnormalities in oxygen transport, arterial-exercise hypoxemia develops, resulting in an increased $P(A\text{-}a)O_2$. Conditions that produce an abnormally elevated $P(A\text{-}a)O_2$ include ventilation-perfusion mismatches (airway disease, pulmonary vascular disease, pulmonary fibrosis), diffusion defects (alveolar proteinosis), and right-to-left shunting (patent foramen ovale).

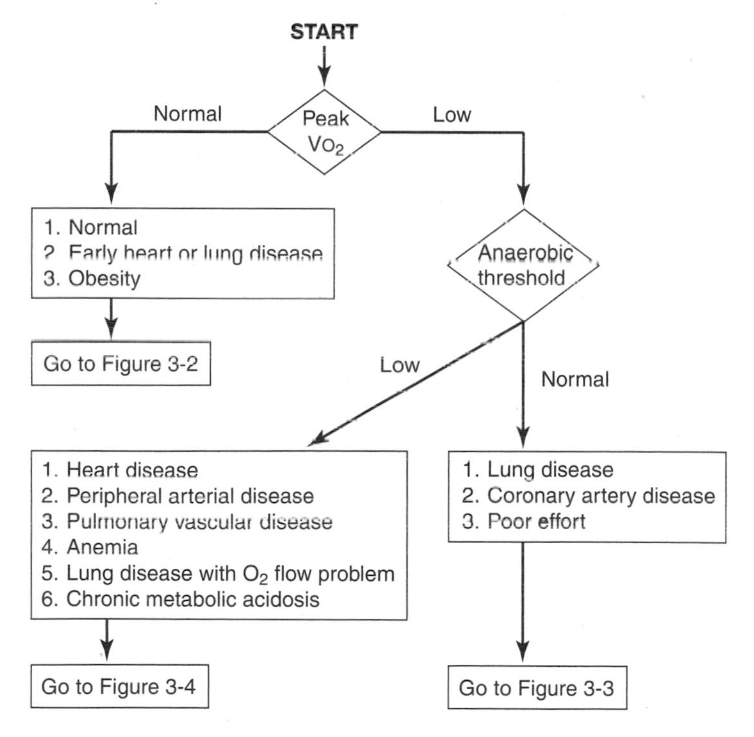

FIG. 3-1. Stratifying based on peak oxygen uptake (VO_2) and anaerobic threshold. Adapted with permission from Wasserman K, Hansen J, Sue D, et al. *Principles of exercise testing and interpretation*, 3rd ed. Philadelphia: Lippincott Williams & Wilkins, 1999:167.

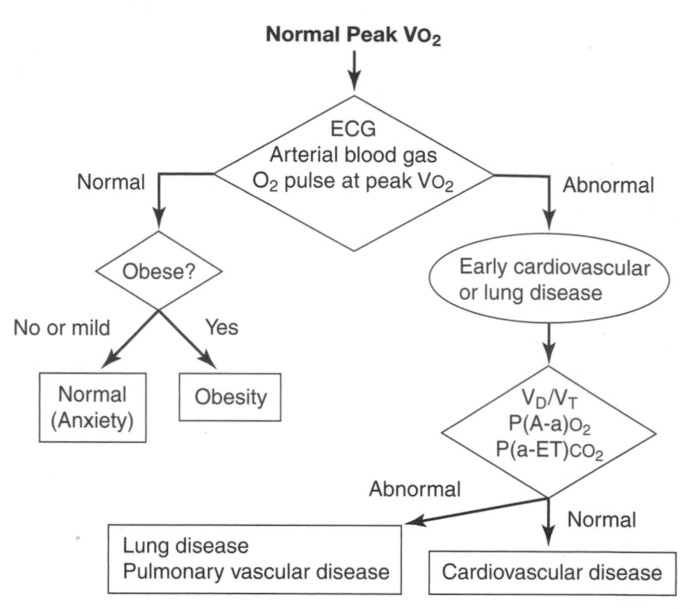

FIG. 3-2. Causes of a normal peak oxygen uptake (VO_2). $P(A-a)O_2$, alveolar-arterial PO_2 difference; $P(a-ET)CO_2$, arterial–end-tidal PCO_2 difference; V_D/V_T, dead space/tidal volume ratio. Adapted with permission from Wasserman K, Hansen J, Sue D, et al. *Principles of exercise testing and interpretation,* 3rd ed. Philadelphia: Lippincott Williams & Wilkins, 1999:168.

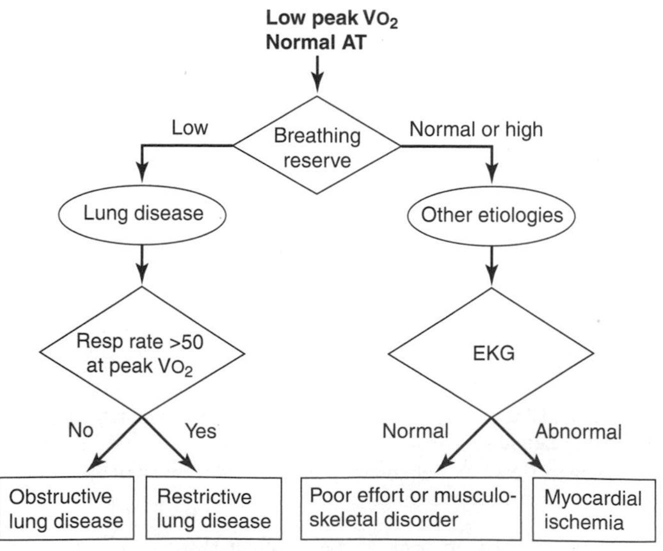

FIG. 3-3. Causes of a low peak oxygen uptake (VO_2) and a normal anaerobic threshold (AT). EKG, electrocardiogram; Resp, respiratory. Adapted with permission from Wasserman K, Hansen J, Sue D, et al. *Principles of exercise testing and interpretation,* 3rd ed. Philadelphia: Lippincott Williams & Wilkins, 1999:170.

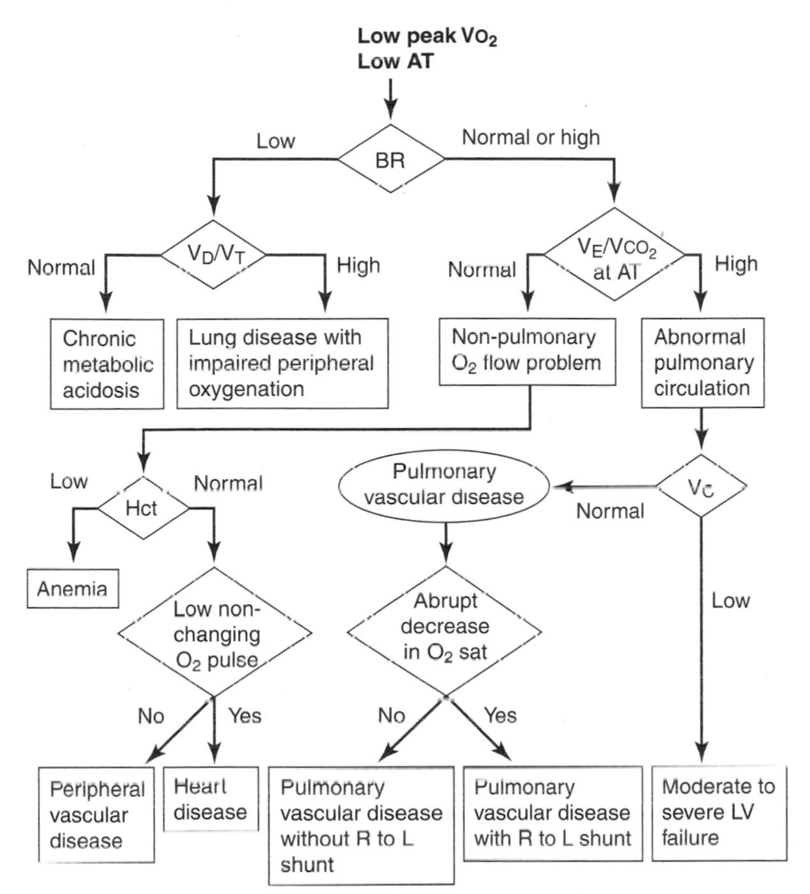

FIG. 3-4. Causes of low peak oxygen uptake (V_{O_2}) and low anaerobic threshold (AT). BR, breathing reserve; L, left; LV, left ventricle; R, right; sat, saturation; V_C, vital capacity; V_D/V_T, dead space/tidal volume ratio; V_E/V_{CO_2}, ventilatory equivalent for carbon dioxide. Adapted with permission from Wasserman K, Hansen J, Sue D, et al. *Principles of exercise testing and interpretation,* 3rd ed. Philadelphia: Lippincott Williams & Wilkins, 1999:172.

The **$P(a\text{-}ET)CO_2$** also measures the inefficiency of the elimination of carbon dioxide. In the healthy lung at rest, $PaCO_2$ is approximately 2 mm Hg greater than end-tidal PCO_2. During exercise, end-tidal PCO_2 increases relative to $PaCO_2$ and actually exceeds it. Thus, $P(a\text{-}ET)CO_2$ is normally positive at rest and negative with exercise. If $P(a\text{-}ET)CO_2$ remains positive during exercise, there is evidence for decreased perfusion to ventilated alveoli, obstructive or restrictive lung disease, or a right-to-left shunt.

By using these concepts, we can diagnose the causes of exercise intolerance. Figs. 3-1 through 3-4 demonstrate how to interpret CPET results.

Conclusion

The CPET is a complex yet useful tool for evaluating exercise capacity. It requires much more equipment than the 6MWT but provides the clinician with information that can identify which organs are affected by disease.

KEY POINTS TO REMEMBER

- The interactions of the cardiovascular, pulmonary, and musculoskeletal systems determine the physiologic response to exercise.
- Generally, patients with exercise intolerance cite one of three reasons for their inability to exercise: dyspnea, fatigue, or pain.
- Exertional dyspnea is the most common complaint of patients with pulmonary parenchymal disease.
- Exertional pain is a common feature of peripheral vascular disease (claudication), angina, and various forms of arthritis. Pulmonary vascular disease and pleural disease may present with exertional chest pain.

REFERENCES AND SUGGESTED READINGS

ACC/AHA guidelines for exercise testing: exercise testing with ventilatory gas analysis 2002 update. Available at: http://www.acc.org/clinical/guidelines/exercise/dirindex.htm. Accessed September 22, 2005.

Borg GA. Psychophysical bases of perceived exertion. *Med Sci Sports Exerc* 1982;14:377–381.

Burdon JGW, Juniper EF, Killian KJ, et al. The perception of breathlessness in asthma. *Am Rev Respir Dis* 1982;126:825–828.

Calahan LP, Mathier MA, Semigran MJ, et al. The six minute walk test predicts peak oxygen uptake and survival in patients with advanced heart failure. *Chest* 1996;110:325.

Cooper KH, Purdy J, White S, et al. Age-fitness adjusted maximal heart rates. *Med Sci Sports* 1977;10:78–86.

Dennis C. Rehabilitation of patients with coronary artery disease. In: Braunwald E, ed. *Heart disease: a textbook of cardiovascular medicine,* 4th ed. Philadelphia: WB Saunders, 1992:1382–1394.

Enright PL. The six-minute walk test. *Respir Care* 2003;48(8):783–785.

Enright PL, Sherrill DL. Reference equations for the six-minute walk in healthy adults. *Am J Respir Crit Care Med* 1998;158:1384–1387.

Fletcher GF, Balady GJ, Amsterdam EA, et al. AHA scientific statement: exercise standards for testing and training. *Circulation* 2001;104:1694–1740.

Gibbons RJ, Balady GJ, Beasley JW, et al. ACC/AHA guidelines for exercise testing: a report of the American College of Cardiology/American Heart Association Task Force on Practice Guidelines. *J Am Coll Cardiol* 1997;30:260–311.

Gibbons WJ, Fruchter N, Sloan S, Levy RD. Reference values for a multiple repetition 6-minute walk test in healthy adults older than 20 years. *J Cardiopulm Rehabil* 2001;21(2):87–93.

Guyatt GH, Pugsley SO, Sullivan MJ, et al. Effect of encouragement on walking test performance. *Thorax* 1984;39:818.

Knox AJ, Morrison JF, Muers MF. Reproducibility of walking test results in chronic obstructive airways disease. *Thorax* 1988;43:388.

Leger LA, Lambert J. A maximal multistage 20 meter shuttle run test to predict VO_2 max. *Eur J Appl Physiol Occup Physiol* 1982;49:1.

McElroy PA, Janicki JS, Weber KT. Cardiopulmonary exercise testing in congestive heart failure. *Am J Cardiol* 1988;62:35A.

Noseda A, Carpiaux J, Prigogine T, Schmerber J. Lung function, maximum and submaximum exercise testing in COPD patients: reproducibility over a long interval. *Lung* 1989;167:247.

Revil SM, Morgan MD, Singh SJ, et al. The endurance shuttle walk: a new field test for the assessment of endurance capacity in chronic obstructive pulmonary disease. *Thorax* 1999;54:213.

Singh SJ, Morgan MDL, Hardman AE, et al. Comparison of oxygen uptake during a conventional treadmill test and the shuttle walking test in chronic airflow limitation. *Eur Respir J* 1994;7:2016.

Singh SJ, Morgan MDL, Scott S, et al. Development of a shuttle walking test of disability in patients with chronic airway obstruction. *Thorax* 1992;47:1019.

Sullivan MJ, Knight JD, Higginbotham MB, Cobb FR. Relation between central and peripheral hemodynamics during exercise in patients with chronic heart failure. Muscle blood flow is reduced with maintenance of arterial perfusion pressure. *Circulation* 1989;80:769.

Wasserman K, Hansen J, Sue D, et al. *Principles of exercise testing and interpretation,* 3rd ed. Philadelphia: Lippincott Williams & Wilkins, 1999.

Wasserman K, VanKessel A, Burton GB. Interaction of physiologic mechanisms during exercise. *J Appl Physiol* 1980:44:97–108.

Weber KT, Janicki JA, eds. *Physiologic principles and clinical applications.* Philadelphia: WB Saunders, 1986:151–167.

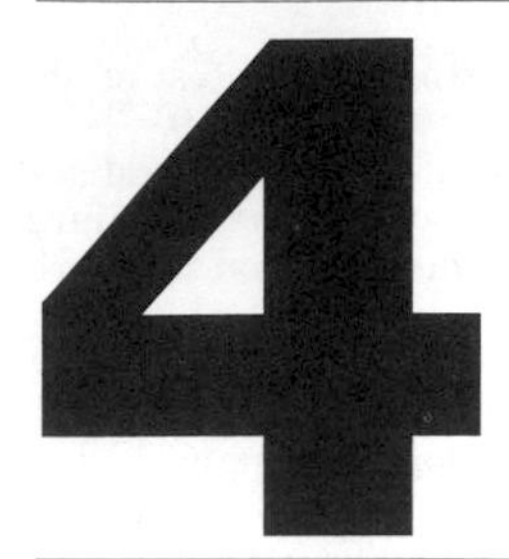

Bronchoscopy

Stephen B. Osmon and
Martin L. Mayse

FIBER-OPTIC BRONCHOSCOPY

Since its creation in the 1960s by Shigeto Ikeda, fiber-optic bronchoscopy (FOB) has grown in use and utility, with approximately 500,000 procedures performed in the United States per year. FOB has become a defining procedure for pulmonologists as well as an indispensable tool for thoracic surgeons, anesthesiologists, and intensivists.

Indications, Contraindications, and Safety

As technology has improved, indications for FOB have increased (Table 4-1). Most contraindications to FOB are relative, and the potential reward must merit the possible risk (Table 4-2). In general, FOB is very safe, with a reported mortality of 0–0.04% with major complications (defined as bleeding, respiratory depression, cardiorespiratory arrest, arrhythmia, and pneumothorax) occurring in <1% of procedures.

Prebronchoscopy Workup

In an American College of Chest Physicians survey, a majority of operators obtain a preprocedure chest radiograph, coagulation studies, and CBC. Less than one-half obtain an ECG, an ABG, electrolytes, or pulmonary function tests. Although nearly impossible to resist, routine preprocedure lab tests are not indicated unless specific concerns exist. Cardiac evaluation in patients with known coronary disease undergoing elective bronchoscopy can be considered because cardiac disease may increase the procedural risk for bronchoscopy. Guidelines have been published by the American College of Physicians and the American College of Cardiology/American Heart Association for preprocedural evaluation of cardiac patients.

Preprocedure Medications

Medications are commonly used before bronchoscopy to facilitate a safe, comfortable, and successful procedure. Commonly, antisialagogues and a mild sedative are given 30 mins before the procedure. During the procedure, topical anesthetics are applied to the airway, and additional sedation and pain medications are given to provide relief from anxiety, pain, and cough.

Antisialagogues are used with the intent of drying secretions, reducing vasovagal response, and increasing the efficacy of topical anesthetics. Common side effects of antisialagogues include tachycardia, hypotension, arrhythmias, urinary retention, angle-closure glaucoma, and decreased GI motility. There are no convincing data indicating that antisialagogues are efficacious, and because of the side effects, they are not recommended on a routine basis. If an antisialagogue is used at our institution, atropine, 0.4 mg IM, is usually the drug of choice.

Most operators use a balanced combination of medications that provide amnesia, anxiolysis, depressed cough response, and analgesia to the airways. As a general rule, drugs with a quick onset, short half-life, and minimal side effects are used. The selection of drugs used is often determined by physician preference, the patient's previous response and allergies, and institutional practices.

TABLE 4-1. INDICATIONS FOR FIBER-OPTIC BRONCHOSCOPY

Inspection of the upper aerodigestive tract, larynx, vocal cords, and related structures

Inspection of the major conductive airways

Evaluation/diagnosis/management of vocal paralysis, unresolved hoarseness, chronic cough, wheezing, etiology of pneumonia, persistent infiltrates, disrupted bronchial tree after trauma, thermal/chemical inhalation injury, tracheoesophageal fistula, epiglottitis, tumors, laryngeal polyps, tracheobronchial stenosis, foreign bodies, hemoptysis, atelectasis, cysts, and abscesses

Procurement of distal bronchial or alveolar fluid, endo- or transbronchial tissue, or lymph node tissue

Assisting in intubation and extubation

Evaluation of the position/patency of an ETT/tracheostomy tube

Intralesional injection of drugs

Brachytherapy

Assisting percutaneous tracheostomy

Stent placement

Surveillance for rejection after lung transplant

Many operators give medications in the preoperative holding area 30–45 mins before the procedure. Various combinations of benzodiazepines, opiate narcotics, antisialagogues, and antihistamines can be used for their individual properties. Little is published on the drug combinations, procedure success, and patient satisfaction.

TABLE 4-2. CONTRAINDICATIONS TO BRONCHOSCOPY

Absolute
- Life-threatening arrhythmias
- Uncorrectable hypoxia or shock

Relative
- Recent myocardial infarction
- Unstable angina
- Cardiac arrhythmias
- Refractory hypoxemia
- Uncorrected bleeding diathesis[a]
- Pulmonary HTN[a]
- Uremia[a] (creatinine >3 mg/dL)
- Thrombocytopenia[a]
- Superior vena cava syndrome[a]
- Unstable neck or temporomandibular joint disease[b]
- Uncooperative patient

[a]Biopsy may be contraindicated.
[b]Contraindicated for rigid bronchoscopy.

Benzodiazepines play the central role in providing amnesia and anxiolysis. IV midazolam is useful during the procedure because of its fast onset of action and short half-life. Boluses of 0.5–2 mg are given q2–5mins until the desired level of sedation is generated. Lorazepam (2 mg) has been used as a preprocedure medication with improved patient satisfaction (due to retrograde amnesia) at 24 hrs vs placebo.

Flumazenil, a competitive inhibitor of the GABA receptor, can be used to reverse the sedative effects of benzodiazepines. Its use should be limited to reversing serious benzodiazepine overdosing. Flumazenil has a short half-life, and resedation can occur. Close observation is mandatory after its use.

Narcotics decrease the laryngeal reflexes and cough response and provide some anxiolysis. They can also cause undesired nausea and dysphoria. IV fentanyl is commonly used and given in small 25–50 mg boluses q2–5mins. The usual range of effective dosing is 50–300 mg. Meperidine has been used as a preprocedure and intraprocedure narcotic, but due to its active metabolites, long half-life, and increased risk of seizures, its use is discouraged.

Naloxone is used to reverse narcotic sedation through direct competitive inhibition. Its duration of action is shorter than that of most narcotics, and repeated doses or a continuous drip may be required. Naloxone should only be used in cases of significant narcotic overdose, and close observation for resedation is mandatory.

Topical anesthesia to the upper aerodigestive tract, glottic area, and bronchial tree can be accomplished by the application of lidocaine, benzocaine, tetracaine, or cocaine. Lidocaine is the most commonly used topical anesthetic for FOB because it has a fast onset of action, is relatively short acting, and has a wide therapeutic window. Safety for lidocaine is well established for doses <7 mg/kg. The amount of lidocaine in a 1% solution is 10 mg/cc. Our institutional practice is to use 5 cc of 2% lidocaine nebulized and breathed by the patient, followed by 5 cc of 2% lidocaine sprayed blindly at the glottic opening during inspiration before significant sedation is administered. During bronchoscopy and under direct vision, additional 2-cc aliquots are sprayed through the cords, dripped on the carina, and sprayed down each mainstem bronchus. For our average procedure, we use 10 cc of 2% and 6–10 cc of 1% lidocaine (for a total lidocaine dose of ≤ 300 mg). Operators must be aware of methemoglobinemia when using topical anesthetics, even in small amounts. Although rare, methemoglobinemia can cause death. When methemoglobinemia occurs, it can be reversed by IV administration of methylene blue.

Propofol is a sedative-hypnotic drug with rapid onset and very short duration of action that gives dose-dependent sedation by continuous infusion. The recovery time after an infusion is only minutes. Propofol takes experience to titrate to avoid the most common side effect—hypotension.

Clonidine attenuates stress-induced sympathetic responses to pain, may decrease myocardial ischemia, and decreases anesthetic requirements. Oral doses of 150–300 mg may be given, but higher dosing can cause increased risk for hypotension.

Monitoring

The operator is the proverbial "captain of the ship" and is ultimately responsible for the overall care and safety of the patient during bronchoscopy. Trained personnel are mandatory for achieving the goals of a safe and successful procedure. Assistants observe the patient, record vital signs, give medications, handle specimens, and assist the operator during bronchoscopy. A minimal requirement is one assistant in addition to the operator, but we routinely have two or more trained respiratory technicians to assist on outpatient bronchoscopy. For ICU patients, one trained assistant and/or the patient's nurse is sufficient. One assistant monitors and records vital signs, draws up and records medications, and places specimens in receptacles. The other assistant directly observes the clinical response of the patient, monitors vital signs, gives medications, and handles specimens with the operator. Having well-trained personnel allows the operator to concentrate on the technical aspects of the procedure to accomplish the preprocedure goals.

Equipment for monitoring and supporting the patient should include continuous pulse oximetry and ECG, vascular access, supplemental oxygen, suction, automated

BP cuff (manual cuff pressures are acceptable but not preferred), and all necessary equipment for intubating, CPR, vascular access, and decompression of a pneumothorax. Additional equipment may be necessary depending on the clinical situation. These may include (among others) a fluoroscopy arm, dual-lumen ETTs, and bronchial blockers for severe bleeding.

Technique

The most common position of the patient is supine, in a bed, with the operator standing at the patient's head and using a transoral approach. For outpatient FOB, many operators use a chair (which can recline if necessary) and a transnasal approach while standing in front of the patient.

After the appropriate monitoring equipment is in place, the eyes are protected, and anesthesia and sedation are obtained, the bronchoscope can be passed through the nose or mouth with or without an ETT or through a tracheostomy. For the oral approach, a bite block is used to avoid bite damage to the bronchoscope. Our preferred approach is to use an ETT for all bronchoscopies, which best suits our patient population, length of procedure, and interventions used.

During insertion of the bronchoscope, the operator should note abnormalities of the nasal passageway, epiglottis, arytenoids, base of the tongue, and false and true vocal cords. Inspiratory and vocalization maneuvers can be used to test for normal movements of the cords and arytenoids. Under direct vision, a small amount of lidocaine is sprayed on and through the vocal cords. Entry into the trachea is obtained, the airway is secured, and lidocaine is sprayed on the carina and down each mainstem bronchus. A systematic inspection is carried out before any procedures.

For patients on positive pressure ventilation, special attention to the ventilator setup during the procedure is required. Even with an 8-mm ETT in place, an adult bronchoscope significantly decreases the cross-sectional area of the tube and increases airway resistance. If an ETT <8 mm is used, a pediatric bronchoscope may be needed. The increased airway resistance can significantly increase positive end-expiratory pressure, contributing to hemodynamic instability, barotrauma, or pneumothorax. During the procedure, patients are placed on 100% oxygen; positive end-expiratory pressure is minimized; ventilator flow, tidal volume, and rate are reduced; and peak airway alarms raised. After the procedure, the ventilator can usually be returned to the preprocedure settings.

Postprocedure paperwork needs to be completed, including a note in the chart (regardless of dictation) indicating findings, interventions, drugs used, estimated blood loss, fluids given, specimens taken, and any special considerations or monitoring required. Patients are monitored closely until stable. A postprocedure chest x-ray may be needed.

RIGID BRONCHOSCOPY

Gustav Killian performed the first rigid bronchoscopy in 1897 when he used a Mikulicz-type esophagoscope with direct visualization to remove a pork bone from the bronchus of a 63-yr-old farmer. Over the subsequent 70 yrs, the indications for rigid bronchoscopy expanded beyond foreign body removal, and the rigid bronchoscope became an important tool in the practice of both medicine and surgery. However, with the recent development of new techniques and tools for use in conjunction with FOB (such as the neodymium:yttrium-aluminum-garnet laser, electrocautery, argon plasma coagulation, cryotherapy, wire mesh stents, bronchoplasty, and balloon catheters), flexible bronchoscopy began to replace the rigid bronchoscope as the main instrument for therapeutic bronchoscopy. By 1995, rigid bronchoscopy was referred to as "the forgotten art."

Indications

An estimated 170,000 new lung cancers are diagnosed in the United States annually. Surgical resection with intent to cure is possible for <25% of these patients, and lung cancer recurs in as many as 70% of patients following resection. With poor initial resectability and high recurrence rates, it is estimated that almost 30% of all patients with lung cancer will develop symptomatic airway obstruction requiring treatment.

Given the special features of the rigid bronchoscope, there are several indications for which the rigid bronchoscope remains superior to the flexible bronchoscope. These indications are largely therapeutic in nature. Among them, the most common is relief of neoplastic airway obstruction. This use is highlighted by the 15-yr experience of Cavaliere and Ardigo from 1982 to 1997, in which relief of airway obstruction secondary to tumor was the indication for 74% of their rigid bronchoscopic procedures.

Treatment of symptomatic airway obstruction remains one of the main indications for rigid bronchoscopy. Other indications include, but are not limited to, control of hemoptysis, relief of tracheal stenosis, removal of obstructing tracheobronchial neoplasms, lung biopsy, and pediatric bronchoscopic procedures. Of note, foreign body aspiration is relatively uncommon in adults, as demonstrated by the removal of only 60 foreign bodies by Prakash at the Mayo Clinic over a 33-yr period.

Equipment

The rigid bronchoscope is composed of a barrel and a handpiece, the features of which give the rigid bronchoscope its utility as a therapeutic instrument. The barrel has several important features: It is rigid, has a large diameter, is perforated distally, and has a beveled tip. These features allow the operator to manipulate tissue with the tip of the barrel, perform mechanical dilation of the airway, receive tactile feedback on the consistency of tissue, and pass a telescope and multiple tools into the airway while providing ventilation to the patient. However, these same features make it impossible to use in patients with an unstable cervical spine or maxillofacial trauma (both absolute contraindications) and limit the ability of the bronchoscope to access the upper airways. The distal perforations of the bronchial barrel allow for ventilation of a lone lung even when the tip of the barrel is positioned in the opposite main bronchus.

The handpiece has several important features: It has one or more side arms and an open end. One side arm is provided on all bronchoscopes for the instillation of gases. A second side arm is often provided and can be used for the insertion of flexible tools, such as a suction catheter or laser fiber. The end of the handpiece opposite the barrel and closest to the operator is open to allow passage of rigid tools such as a light guide, a telescope, forceps, or a large-bore suction catheter. This open end can be used to provide positive pressure ventilation.

The greatest advantage of the rigid bronchoscope over the flexible bronchoscope is its ability to obtain and maintain a patent airway, not only in the proximal trachea but in the distal trachea and main bronchi as well. This airway control is made possible by the open design and larger diameter of the barrel.

Special Techniques

Therapeutic bronchoscopy for relief of neoplastic airway obstruction often combines several techniques. Whereas some bronchoscopy techniques are possible using a flexible bronchoscope, others are only possible (or at the very least greatly eased) by the use of the rigid bronchoscope. In addition to the general benefits offered by the large diameter and open barrel of the rigid bronchoscope (facilitating the passage of multiple instruments, large-diameter suction, and simultaneous ventilation), the rigid bronchoscope also facilitates placement of certain stents, is capable of rigid dilation, and can perform a rigid "core-out" of lesions. Furthermore, it is possible to secure a patient's distal trachea or main bronchi by advancing the barrel of the bronchoscope beyond an airway obstruction that may be present in these locations, thus ensuring a patent airway during the procedure.

Stent Placement

Currently, there are a wide variety of stents available for use. The most commonly used include self-expanding wire mesh stents, silicone stents, and hybrid stents (essentially a silicone stent reinforced with metal struts). Each type has advantages and disadvantages.

Self-expanding wire mesh stents can be deployed easily with the flexible or rigid bronchoscope and are less likely to become dislodged; however, they tend to induce more tissue reaction and are subsequently difficult to remove. Silicone stents prevent tumor ingrowth, tend to induce less tissue reaction, and are relatively easy to remove; however, they are more likely to become dislodged and are very difficult to place with a flexible bronchoscope. Hybrid stents prevent tumor ingrowth, are highly resistant to compressive forces, and are less likely to become dislodged; however, they are difficult to place with the flexible bronchoscope and are difficult to remove. When the clinical situation warrants a silicone or hybrid stent, insertion is facilitated by the rigid bronchoscope.

Bougie and Rigid Dilation

There are several dilation techniques that are possible only with the rigid bronchoscope. Bougie dilation involves the passage of a rigid dilator (a device that looks like a chili pepper on a stick) through an airway obstruction. Rigid dilation can be performed by advancing rigid bronchoscopes with progressively larger diameter barrels through the airway obstruction or by advancing a rigid bronchoscope with a relatively large-diameter barrel through the obstruction with a gentle corkscrew or rocking motion. These methods can be used to open a stenotic airway or push a neoplastic obstruction to one side of a lumen. The corkscrew technique is useful because it opens an occluded airway very quickly.

Rigid core-out is perhaps the quickest way to debulk a large airway obstruction. Before using this technique, it is necessary to ensure a patent airway distal to the obstruction. In addition, the lesion should be unlikely to bleed excessively (the lesion should either be avascular and nonfriable or able to be coagulated with a laser or electrocautery probe). The rigid bronchoscope is advanced toward and into the lesion along the axis of the obstruction airway. As the bronchoscope is advanced, it is important to monitor for bleeding and to ensure that the barrel of the bronchoscope remains within the anatomic confines of the airway. As the bronchoscope is advanced farther into the lesion, the leading edge of the barrel shears tissue away from the lesion, and a core of tissue is formed within the lumen of the barrel. After this core of tissue is removed, the bronchoscope can be advanced past the obstruction.

SAFETY

Of the 5049 therapeutic bronchoscopies (91% performed with a rigid bronchoscope) reported by Cavaliere and Ardigo, death occurred in 0.3% (15 of 5049), and serious complications occurred in 2.4% (119 of 5049). Serious complications included hemorrhage >250 cc, pneumothorax, mediastinal emphysema, respiratory failure, cardiac arrest, myocardial infarction, and pulmonary embolism. This rate of mortality and serious complications is similar to that of diagnostic flexible bronchoscopy.

SUMMARY

The main benefits of the flexible bronchoscope are its wide availability, its ability to be performed with topical anesthesia and conscious sedation, and its ability to access distal airways and the upper lobes of the lung. The main disadvantages are its relatively small working channel and the fact that it partially obstructs the patient's airway when in place.

The main benefits of the rigid bronchoscope are its large working channel, open barrel, and ability to secure a patent airway and facilitate ventilation. The main disadvantages of the rigid bronchoscope are the limited number of experienced operators, the need for general anesthesia, and its inability to access the distal and upper lobe airways.

KEY POINTS TO REMEMBER

- Cardiac evaluation in patients with known coronary disease undergoing elective bronchoscopy can be considered, since cardiac disease may increase the procedural risk for bronchoscopy.

- Commonly, antisialagogues and a mild sedative are given 30 mins before the procedure. During the procedure, topical anesthetics are applied to the airway and additional sedation and pain medications are given.
- The most common position of the patient during the procedure is supine, with the operator standing at the patient's head and using a transoral approach.
- Treatment of symptomatic airway obstruction remains one of the main indications for rigid bronchoscopy.
- The greatest advantage of the rigid bronchoscope over the flexible bronchoscope is its ability to obtain and maintain airway patency, not only in the proximal trachea, but in the distal trachea and main bronchi as well.

REFERENCES AND SUGGESTED READINGS

American Cancer Society. What are the key statistics for lung cancer? 2002. Available at: http://www.cancer.org. Accessed September 22, 2005.

Benumof J. Removal of tracheobronchial foreign bodies. In: *Anesthesia for thoracic surgery*. Philadelphia: WB Saunders, 1987:399–401.

Bulpa PA, Dive AM, Mertens L, et al. Combined bronchoalveolar lavage and transbronchial lung biopsy: safety and yield in ventilated patients. *Eur Respir J* 2003:21:489–494.

Cavaliere S, Ardigo M. Endoscopic relief of airway obstruction. *Ann Thorac Surg* 1990;50(1):163–164.

Cavaliere S, Foccoli P, Farina PL. Nd:YAG laser bronchoscopy. A five-year experience with 1,396 applications in 1,000 patients. *Chest* 1988;94(1):15–21.

Credle WF Jr, Smiddy JF, Elliott RC. Complications of fiberoptic bronchoscopy. *Am Rev Respir Dis* 1974;109:67–72.

Eagle KA, et al. Guidelines for perioperative cardiovascular evaluation for noncardiac surgery. *Circulation* 1996;93:1278–1317.

Ernst A, Silvestri GA, Johnstone D. Interventional pulmonary procedures. *Chest* 2003;123:1693–1717.

Grønnebech H, Johansson G, Smedebøl M, et al. Glycopyrrolate vs. atropine during anaesthesia for laryngoscopy and bronchoscopy. *Acta Anaesthesiol Scand* 1993;37:454–457.

Guidelines for assessing and managing the perioperative risk from coronary artery disease associated with major noncardiac surgery. *Ann Intern Med* 1997;127:309–312.

Jaggar SI, Haxby E. Sedation, anaesthesia and monitoring for bronchoscopy. *Paediatr Respir Rev* 2002;3(4):321–327.

Kupeli E, Mehta AC. Therapeutic bronchoscopy in lung cancer. Laser therapy, electrocautery, brachytherapy, stents, and photodynamic therapy. *Clin Chest Med* 2002;23(1):241–256.

Matot I, Kramer MR. Sedation in outpatient bronchoscopy *Respir Med* 2000:94:1145–1153.

Natalini G, Fassini P, Seramondi V, et al. Remifentanil vs. fentanyl during interventional rigid bronchoscopy under general anaesthesia and spontaneous assisted ventilation. *Eur J Anaesthesiol* 1999;16(9):605–609.

O'Brien JD, Ettinger NA, Shevlin D, Kollef MH. Safety and yield of transbronchial biopsy in mechanically ventilated patients. *Crit Care Med* 1997;25(3):440–446.

Ovassapian A. The flexible bronchoscope: a tool for anesthesiologists. *Clin Chest Med* 2001;22(2):281–299.

Pasternak LR. Preoperative laboratory testing: general issues and considerations. *Anesthesiol Clin North Am* 2004;22(1):13–25.

Prakash UB. Current indications for bronchoscopy. *Contemp Intern Med* 1992;4(10):13–18.

Pue CA, Pacht ER. Complications of fiberoptic bronchoscopy at a university hospital. *Chest* 1995;107:430–432.

Raoof S, Mehta AC. Therapeutic flexible bronchoscopy. *Chest Surg Clin N Am* 2001;11(4): 657–690.

Suratt PM, Smiddy JF, Gruber B. Deaths and complications associated with fiberoptic bronchoscopy. *Chest* 1976;69:747–751.

Wain JC. Rigid bronchoscopy: the value of a venerable procedure. *Chest Surg Clin N Am* 2001;11(4):691–699.

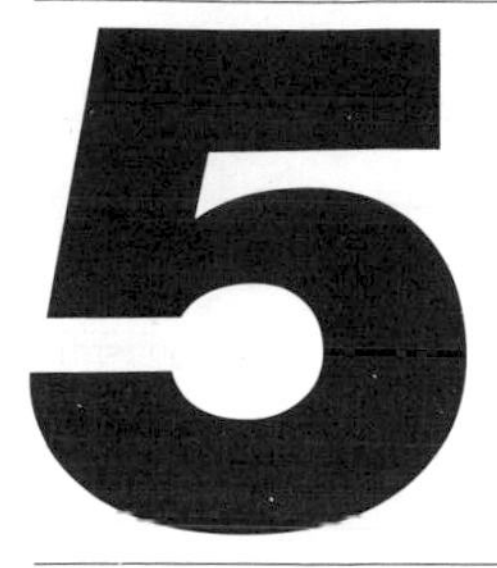

Oxygen Delivery Devices

Ting-hsu Chen

RESPIRATORY FAILURE

Respiratory failure comprises a set of disorders resulting in abnormalities of oxygenation or ventilation severe enough to impair or threaten the function of vital organs. ABG criteria defining respiratory failure are not absolute but are arbitrarily set at **Pao_2 <60 mm Hg and $Paco_2$ >50 mm Hg.**

Acute hypercapnic respiratory failure occurs with sudden carbon dioxide retention ($Paco_2$ >50 mm Hg) producing a respiratory acidosis (pH <7.35). Acute hypoxic respiratory failure occurs when normal gas exchange is impaired, resulting in hypoxemia [PaO_2 <60 or arterial oxygen saturation (SaO_2) <90%] (Table 5-1).

Chronic respiratory failure is characterized by a gradual decline in overall functional status most commonly brought on by chronic obstructive lung disease. Other etiologies include neuromuscular diseases such as amyotrophic lateral sclerosis, multiple sclerosis, myasthenia gravis, Guillain-Barré syndrome, cystic fibrosis, or alpha-1-antitrypsin deficiency.

Diagnosis

Although profound hypoxemia can be asymptomatic, the most frequent presenting sign of hypoxemia is dyspnea. Other manifestations of hypoxemia include cyanosis, restlessness, confusion, anxiety, delirium, tachypnea, tachycardia, HTN, cardiac arrhythmias, and tremor. Hypercapnia can present as dyspnea and headache. Other manifestations of hypercapnia include peripheral and conjunctival hyperemia, HTN, tachycardia, tachypnea, impaired consciousness, papilledema, and asterixis. All of these clinical signs are both insensitive and nonspecific.

Treatment

Treatment of acute respiratory failure revolves around treatment of the underlying cause as well as general and respiratory supportive care. The therapeutic goal is to ensure adequate oxygenation of vital organs. The inspired oxygen concentration should be the lowest value that results in **adequate Pao_2 (Sao_2 >90%).** Higher arterial oxygen tensions are of no proven benefit and may cause hypoventilation with chronic hypercapnia (i.e., COPD), although treatment should never be withheld for fear of respiratory depression.

An important distinction must be made between adequate blood oxygenation and tissue oxygenation. There is a poor correlation between arterial hypoxemia and tissue hypoxia. **Improvement in arterial oxygenation may not provide a subsequent improvement in tissue oxygen availability** owing to a drop in cardiac output or systemic vasoconstriction. A profound decrease in tissue oxygenation is defined as shock.

One of the most common types of respiratory failure is acute exacerbation of COPD. Traditional teaching expounds that hypercapnia arises from suppression of the hypoxic ventilatory drive and results in oxygen being inappropriately withheld from some patients. In COPD, hypercapnia secondary to oxygen therapy arises primarily from worsening ventilation-perfusion mismatch owing to attenuation of hypoxic pulmonary vasoconstriction, which essentially increases the dead space/tidal

TABLE 5-1. CAUSES OF ACUTE RESPIRATORY FAILURE

Hypoxic
- Shunt (cardiogenic and noncardiogenic pulmonary edema), near-drowning, reperfusion injury
- Ventilation-perfusion mismatch (COPD, interstitial lung disease, pulmonary embolism)
- Low inspired oxygen (high altitudes, smoke inhalation)
- Hypoventilation (elevated $Paco_2$)
- Diffusion impairment (interstitial lung disease)
- Low mixed venous oxygenation (increased oxygen consumption, congestive heart failure)

Hypercapnic
- Increased carbon dioxide production (fever, sepsis, seizure, excessive carbohydrates)
- Increased dead space (widened alveolar-arterial gradient: COPD, asthma, cystic fibrosis, pulmonary fibrosis, scoliosis)
- Decreased minute ventilation (normal alveolar-arterial gradient: CNS disorders, Guillain-Barré, botulism, myasthenia gravis, amyotrophic lateral sclerosis, polymyositis, muscular dystrophy, myxedema, upper airway obstruction)

Mixed
- Postsurgical (atelectasis, pain, postanesthesia respiratory depression, phrenic nerve injury)

volume (V_T) ratio. Lesser components include a decreased binding affinity of carbon dioxide to hemoglobin (Haldane effect) and decreased minute ventilation.

Appropriate oxygen delivery generally involves slowly increasing the inspired oxygen concentration with monitoring of both Pao_2 and $Paco_2$. This evaluation is most effectively performed with a Venturi mask to allow close regulation of the fraction of inspired oxygen (Fio_2) to a goal Pao_2 of 60–70 mm Hg or a Sao_2 of 88–90%. Noninvasive positive pressure ventilation may help avoid the need for intubation and decrease morbidity. It is important to realize that in most patients with acute-on-chronic respiratory failure, there exists a compensated chronic respiratory acidosis with only a small derangement of arterial pH even with profound hypercapnia. These patients are at much greater risk from hypoxemia than hypercapnia.

However, hypercapnia with significant acidemia (pH <7.20) or a significantly decreased level of consciousness in which the patient's ability to protect the airway becomes suspect is an indication for intubation and mechanical ventilation.

Oxygen should never be removed from a patient to avoid intubation. Rapid removal of oxygen can produce a drastic fall in Pao_2 to below the original levels and development of hypoxemia more rapidly than resolution of hypercapnia, which results in tissue hypoxia and potentially worsened acidemia.

OXYGEN DELIVERY DEVICES FOR HYPOXIC RESPIRATORY FAILURE

For conscious, spontaneously breathing patients, supplemental oxygen is one of the most important initial treatments for acute hypoxic respiratory failure. The selection of the appropriate noninvasive delivery system depends on the stability of the patient, availability of devices, and level of respiratory support required. For the critically ill or unstable patient, a planned, controlled intubation is always more desirable than emergent intubation. Predefined criteria for intubation and mechanical ventilation are broad and nonspecific. They include a number of physiologic criteria that generally define profound respiratory failure (Table 5-2). However, even considering intubation in a patient may be reason enough to perform the procedure.

TABLE 5-2. INDICATIONS FOR INTUBATION AND MECHANICAL VENTILATION

Diminished arterial oxygenation	
PaO_2	<55 mm Hg
$PaO_2/PaCO_2$	<0.15
Alveolar-arterial gradient (FIO_2 – 1.0)	>450
Diminished ventilatory reserve	
Respiratory rate	>35 breaths/min
Rise in $PaCO_2$	>10 mm Hg
Minute ventilation	>10 L/min
Negative inspiratory force	< -25 cm H_2O
Tidal volume	<5 mL/kg
Vital capacity	<10 mL/kg

Adapted from Luce JM. Ventilator management in the intensive care unit. In: Andreoli T, ed. *Cecil's essentials of medicine*, 5th ed. Philadelphia: WB Saunders, 2001.

The two classes of oxygen delivery devices for hypoxic respiratory failure include low-flow (nasal cannula, face masks) and high-flow (Venturi masks). **Low-flow** devices provide a variable FIO_2 based on the size of the oxygen reservoir, the rate at which the reservoir is filled, and the ventilatory pattern of the patient. **High-flow** devices provide a constant FIO_2 by delivering a higher flow rate of oxygen than the patient's peak inspiratory flow rate or by providing a fixed proportion of room air.

Nasal Cannulas

Nasal cannulas are low-flow systems that provide insufficient gas to supply an entire inspired V_T. They are appropriate in patients with minimal or no respiratory distress or those who are unable to tolerate a face mask. The benefits include allowing the patient to eat, drink, and speak. Their main disadvantage is that the exact FIO_2 is unknown because it is influenced by the patient's spontaneous inspiratory flow rate.

A large part of each breath is composed of ambient (room air) gas. The inspired FIO_2 depends on oxygen flow and spontaneous V_T. For every liter per minute, the oxygen concentration increases by approximately 4%. With a normal V_T, the common flow rates of 1–6 L/min provide an FIO_2 of 24–44%. Routine humidification of oxygen may provide little or no benefit in reducing the drying effects of nasal cannula oxygen on the nose and throat, especially with flow rates >5 L/min.

Reservoir Cannula (Oxymizer)

There are two types of reservoir cannulas commonly available: an oxygen-conserving nasal cannula with a reservoir situated below the nose, and an oxygen-conserving pendant with a reservoir situated on the patient's chest. The cannulas trap the initial portion of expired gas from the conducting airways that contains a higher percentage of oxygen. The reservoirs also receive a continuous flow of oxygen from the wall source or tank, resulting in a higher FIO_2 during the next inspiration and allowing for the total flow rate to be reduced. This is especially useful for home oxygen delivery in patients with COPD. Oxymizers may also be appropriate for inpatient treatment of patients who require a higher FIO_2 than a nasal cannula can provide and who are also resistant to wearing a face mask.

Face Masks and Venturi Masks

Face masks provide a means of delivering a higher FIO_2 than can be achieved via oxygen cannula. Two types exist: those with and those without an oxygen reservoir. To

TABLE 5-3. EXAMPLE OF VENTURI MASK SPECIFICATIONS

Entrainment port color	FIO_2
Blue	24
Yellow	28
White	31
Green	35
Pink	40
Orange	50

avoid accumulation of expired air in the mask, the oxygen flow rate should be >5 L/min. Face masks generally provide a FIO_2 of 40–60%. Advanced cardiac life support recommendations indicate flow rates between 8 and 10 L/min.

A **Venturi mask** is a high-flow system delivering a more accurate oxygen concentration. Oxygen passes through a narrow orifice under pressure into a larger tube, creating subatmospheric pressure that draws room air into the system by creating a shearing force known as *viscous drag*. Oxygen concentration is adjusted by changing the size of the orifice (entrainment ports) and oxygen flow. The entrainment port sections of a Venturi mask are often color coded for convenience (Table 5-3); however, colors and concentrations are not standardized and may differ between manufacturers. The maximum FIO_2 achievable is 50%. This type of mask provides a constant FIO_2 independent of changes in oxygen flow rate or inspiratory flow rate. It is commonly used in chronic hypercarbia (i.e., COPD), in which there is a concern for inducing worsening hypercapnia and acute respiratory acidosis with oxygen therapy. It allows for an easy step-wise increase or decrease in FIO_2 as oxygen flow is titrated to PaO_2 and $PaCO_2$. The main disadvantage is that the FIO_2 provided by these masks is limited and may be insufficient in some patients.

Nonrebreather face masks consist of a face mask that provides a constant flow of oxygen into an attached reservoir, resulting in an FIO_2 >60% at 6 L/min. Each liter per minute of flow added >6 L/min increases inspired oxygen concentration by 10%. Placed correctly, the oxygen concentration can reach almost 100%. This type of mask is most appropriate for spontaneously breathing patients who require the highest possible oxygen concentration but who cannot be intubated immediately (because of an intact gag reflex, clenched teeth, or head trauma) or those who refuse intubation. The disadvantages of nonrebreather masks include oxygen toxicity, the inability to feed patients owing to the tight seal required, limitation of speech, patient discomfort, and the inability to provide aerosolized treatments.

Partial rebreather masks allow exhaled air to enter the reservoir, although this air is mainly that from the conducting airways and is high in oxygen. FIO_2 achievable by these masks is approximately 70%.

Oxygen Concentrators

Oxygen concentrators are electrically powered home oxygen delivery devices commonly used with a cannula. Most use molecular sieve beds to filter and concentrate oxygen molecules from the ambient air, generating oxygen concentrations of 90–98%. Maximum flows of 3–5 L/min can be reached, although FIO_2 decreases as flow increases. Concentrators are the most cost-effective type of stationary oxygen delivery system. A backup oxygen cylinder should always be provided.

OXYGEN DELIVERY DEVICES FOR HYPERCAPNIC RESPIRATORY FAILURE

Continuous positive airway pressure (CPAP) may be administered with tight-fitting nasal pillows or a nonrebreathing mask with pressure-limited valves. It is indicated for patients who are conscious, stable, and able to protect their airway. Many patients cannot tolerate CPAP because of persistent hypoxemia, hemodynamic instability, and feelings of claustrophobia or aerophagia. A common indication is nighttime use for patients with obstructive sleep apnea. The initial setting is usually 3–5 cm H_2O of CPAP while monitoring PaO_2 or SaO_2. It may be increased in steps of 3–5 cm H_2O to 10–15 cm H_2O. Nasal pillows may become uncomfortable at high flow rates because air is blown directly into the nose (see Chap. 6, Noninvasive Ventilation, for more detail).

Bilevel positive airway pressure (BiPAP) provides inspiratory support to decrease a patient's work of breathing. It may be delivered via the same types of masks and nasal pillows as CPAP. The expiratory support improves gas exchange by preventing alveolar collapse. It is used for patients with neuromuscular disease, COPD, or postoperative respiratory insufficiency, or for patients in whom intubation is not possible or permitted. Common initial settings include an inspiratory positive airway pressure of 5–10 cm H_2O and expiratory positive airway pressure of 4–5 cm H_2O. Pressure support (both inspiratory positive airway pressure and expiratory positive airway pressure) can be titrated in increments of 3–5 cm H_2O using the respiratory rate and arterial oxygenation as guides (see Chap. 6, Noninvasive Ventilation, for more detail).

The benefits of noninvasive ventilation include decreased rates of intubation, decreased mortality (likely from reduction of nosocomial pneumonia), decreased ICU length of stay, and decreased hospital length of stay. Contraindications for use include an uncooperative patient; respiratory arrest; hemodynamic or cardiovascular instability; facial burns; head trauma; recent facial, esophageal, or gastric surgery; high aspiration risk; a profound decrease in mental status resulting in an inability to protect the airway; or fixed anatomic defects of the nasopharynx.

OXYGEN DELIVERY DEVICES FOR UNSTABLE PATIENTS

A **bag-valve device** consists of a self-inflating bag with a nonrebreathing valve. It may be used with a mask or ETT in individuals with depressed or absent ventilatory drive as a bridge to intubation or mechanical ventilation or reversal from general anesthesia or conscious sedation. A bag volume of 1600 mL is generally adequate for most adults to ensure adequate lung inflation. In the unintubated patient, it may be difficult for a single individual to provide an adequate V_T of 10–15 mL/kg with a mask while maintaining an effective seal and patent airway.

MECHANICAL VENTILATION

A full discussion of mechanical ventilation extends beyond the scope of a pulmonary consult book. The two most common modes of ventilation are assist-control ventilation and synchronized intermittent mandatory ventilation.

Assist-control (AC) ventilation senses a patient's inspiratory effort above a certain sensitivity threshold and delivers a fixed V_T with each sensed inspiration. The backup rate, V_T, flow rate, FIO_2, and amount of positive end-expiratory pressure are commonly set.

Synchronized intermittent mandatory ventilation (SIMV) allows the patient to breathe spontaneously (usually with additional pressure support) over a backup intermittent mandatory ventilation rate that delivers a full V_T at preset intervals and is timed with the patient's sensed inspiratory efforts.

In pressure-control ventilation (PCV), the delivered volume and minute ventilation are not assured because they are highly dependent on lung mechanics as well as resistance from the ETT.

KEY POINTS TO REMEMBER

- ABG criteria defining respiratory failure are not absolute but are arbitrarily set at PaO_2 <60 mm Hg and $PaCO_2$ >50 mm Hg.
- Chronic respiratory failure is characterized by a gradual decline in overall functional status most commonly brought on by chronic obstructive lung disease.

- The therapeutic goal is to ensure adequate oxygenation of vital organs. The inspired oxygen concentration should be the lowest value that results in adequate arterial saturation (SaO_2 >90%).

REFERENCES AND SUGGESTED READINGS

Ahya S, Flood K, Paranjothi S. *The Washington manual of medical therapeutics,* 30th ed. Philadelphia: Lippincott Williams & Wilkins, 2001.

Andreoli T. *Cecil's essentials of medicine,* 5th ed. Philadelphia: WB Saunders, 2001.

Bach JR, Brougher P, Hess DR, et. al. Consensus conference: noninvasive positive pressure ventilation. *Respir Care* 1997;42:361.

Campbell EJ, Baker MD, Crites-Silver P. Subjective effects of humidification of oxygen for delivery by nasal cannula. *Chest* 1988;93(2):289–293.

Cummins R. *Advanced cardiac life support.* Dallas, TX: American Heart Association, 1997.

Marino P. *The ICU book*, 2nd ed. Philadelphia: Lippincott Williams & Wilkins, 1998.

Tierney L, McPhee SJ, Papadakis MA, eds. *Current medical diagnosis & treatment,* 40th ed. New York: McGraw-Hill, 2001.

Waldau T, Larsen VH, Bonde J. Evaluation of five oxygen delivery devices in spontaneously breathing subjects by oxygraphy. *Anaesthesia* 1998;53(3):256–263.

Weg JG, Haas CF. Long-term oxygen therapy for COPD. *Postgrad Med* 1998;103(4):143–144.

Noninvasive Ventilation

Randy Sasich

INTRODUCTION

Noninvasive ventilation (NIV) or **noninvasive positive pressure ventilation** refers to the use of a mask or similar device to provide ventilatory support. This proposed definition is broad and could correctly include external negative pressure devices (e.g., the "iron lung" that is historically associated with paralysis from polio) and rocking beds an effective means to ventilate a patient with bilateral diaphragmatic paralysis. NIV by definition excludes any modality that bypasses the upper airway, such as laryngeal masks, endotracheal intubation, or tracheostomy. For the purposes of this chapter, NIV refers to mechanical ventilatory support delivered through a face mask, nasal mask, or similar device. (*Please note that all studies referred to within the text are contained within the complete reference list at the end of the chapter.*)

VENTILATORY MODES

Invasive mechanical ventilation and NIV share many of the same physiologic principles. Additionally, the modes of ventilatory support provided (i.e., the way in which the ventilator triggers, delivers, and ends the breath) are similar to invasive mechanical ventilation. One caveat is that there is no standardization between manufacturers regarding mode terminology, and subsequently, different hospitals and different training programs may use different terms. Two of the most commonly encountered modes, bilevel positive airway pressure (BiPAP) and continuous positive airway pressure (CPAP), are described in some detail below.

PHYSIOLOGY

Continuous Positive Airway Pressure

CPAP maintains a set positive pressure throughout the respiratory cycle during both inhalation and exhalation efforts and thus is not ventilatory support in a strict physiologic sense. A common way to think of CPAP is as a pressure "stenting open" the upper airway. This concept helps explain the utility of CPAP in disorders such as obstructive sleep apnea but does not explain why a treatment that does not provide ventilatory support can be of use in the patient who is suffering from hypoxemic or hypercapnic respiratory failure.

In **hypoxemic respiratory failure,** CPAP improves oxygenation in two ways. In the alveolar gas equation $PAO_2 = FIO_2\,(P_B - 47) - 1.2\,(PaCO_2)$, if P_B is barometric pressure (or in our case, the pressure delivered from the ventilator through the mask), an increase in the mean airway pressure throughout the respiratory cycle for a given fraction of inspired oxygen (FIO_2) will increase the partial pressure of inspiratory oxygen and therefore oxygen tension in the alveoli (PAO_2). Second, similar to its correlate in invasive mechanical ventilation, extrinsic positive end-expiratory pressure ($PEEP_e$), it recruits the underventilated or collapsed lung, probably by preventing alveolar collapse during exhalation.

The utility of CPAP in **hypercapnic respiratory failure** is slightly less intuitive and requires an understanding of intrinsic positive end-expiratory pressure ($PEEP_i$). In the hyperinflated patient (exemplified by the emphysematous patient in a COPD exacerbation), airflow obstruction, compounded by the decreased elastic recoil of the lungs, leads to a prolongation of expiration. Inspiration occurs in this patient before expiration can complete alveolar emptying, and dynamic hyperinflation ensues. The patient begins the next breath in this cycle at a functional residual capacity (FRC) higher than the more mechanically efficient normal FRC. A vicious cycle of ineffective ventilation and increasing work of breathing causes the buildup of carbon dioxide and worsening acidemia that typifies hypercapnic respiratory failure. The positive elastic recoil pressure left behind in this hyperinflated patient at the end of expiration is termed $PEEP_i$.

It seems counterintuitive at first that giving the patient additional pressure in the form of **CPAP** would be beneficial. Delivering $PEEP_e$ in the form of CPAP in fact lessens the work of breathing. A $PEEP_i$ level of 10 cm H_2O is present in most COPD patients with acute respiratory failure, and this pressure must be overcome on the initiation of inhalation before air can enter the lungs. Because the spontaneously breathing patient effects respiration by generating negative pleural pressures to draw in air, the residual $PEEP_i$ creates an added work of breathing—that is, the initial 10 cm H_2O of pleural pressure the patient generates effectively gets the patient only back to baseline when applied against the 10 cm H_2O of $PEEP_i$ left behind. By adding 10 cm H_2O of $PEEP_e$ or CPAP, the work of breathing is lessened as the $PEEP_i$ is effectively negated and any degree of negative pleural pressure created by a respiratory effort produces airflow. In intubated patients with acute respiratory failure, $PEEP_e$ has been demonstrated to reduce the work of breathing by 50%. The same principle applies to the noninvasively ventilated patient.

Bilevel Positive Airway Pressure

BiPAP is simply CPAP with a second level of pressure support added. Pressure support or pressure support ventilation is a commonly used mode during invasive mechanical ventilation and may be a more familiar term in reference to its use during trials of liberation from mechanical ventilation in the ICU setting. It refers to a set pressure that is delivered to the patient only during inspiration. In practical terms, the use of BiPAP requires the operator to set two variables after placing a nasal or face mask on the patient. The first, inspiratory positive airway pressure (IPAP), is the pressure support portion of BiPAP and is measured in cm H_2O. This portion is the ventilatory pressure support the patient receives when either the machine or the patient initiates a breath. The second variable, expiratory positive airway pressure (EPAP), also measured in cm H_2O, is the CPAP component of BiPAP, the pressure against which the patient exhales at the termination of inhalation.

Common **initial settings** are often referred to by the EPAP followed by the IPAP—e.g., "five and twelve." The greater the difference between the EPAP and the IPAP, the greater the theoretical ventilatory support the patient receives. It should be recognized, however, that progressively higher levels of EPAP and IPAP are not usually well tolerated by the patient, and as with any initiation of NIV, the patient should be observed closely to see if effective patient–ventilator synchrony occurs. Conversely, the smaller the difference between the inspiratory and expiratory pressures, the closer one is to approaching a functional CPAP modality. Obviously, setting both the EPAP and the IPAP to the same level—e.g., 8 cm H_2O—provides a continuous 8-cm H_2O pressure to the patient and effectively delivers a CPAP of 8.

SPECIFIC INDICATIONS

NIV has been studied in a variety of specific clinical presentations of acute respiratory failure. In general, NIV is most effective in patients with COPD with a respiratory acidosis, patients with hypercapnic respiratory failure secondary to chest wall deformity or neuromuscular disease, and patients with cardiogenic pulmonary edema. NIV has a more controversial role in the treatment of acute hypoxemic respiratory failure (that most commonly occurs in pneumonia) and in the treatment of acute asthma.

Chronic Obstructive Pulmonary Disease

There is a substantial and growing body of evidence favoring NIV as the initial respiratory support modality in the setting of acute COPD exacerbation. The majority of studies have shown improvements in clinical parameters such as pH, PCO_2, and respiratory rate, and most have shown lower intubation rates in addition to a lower mortality when compared to standard therapy.

The largest study examined 236 patients in a multicenter randomized controlled trial and compared BiPAP via nasal or face mask with standard therapy. The authors found that the use of NIV reduced the need for intubation. In-hospital mortality was significantly reduced in the NIV group when compared to the standard therapy group. NIV should be considered in patients with acute exacerbations of COPD in whom a respiratory acidosis persists (pH <7.35) despite maximum medical therapy.

Chest Wall Deformity and Neuromuscular Disease

NIV can be an appropriate first-line choice in patients with acute and acute-on-chronic respiratory failure. In a study comparing 14 patients with acute respiratory failure of neuromuscular origin with 14 matched historical control patients who had received endotracheal intubation, the authors found a lower intrahospital mortality and a significantly shortened stay in the ICU for the NIV-treated group.

One randomized controlled trial exists supporting the use of CPAP in patients with isolated chest trauma. Patients had more than two rib fractures and hypoxemia. CPAP and regional anesthesia were compared with intubation followed by intermittent positive pressure ventilation and PEEP. The CPAP group had fewer mean ICU days and fewer hospital days. Patients with greater than moderate lung injury, as defined by a PaO_2 of <60 mm Hg on an FIO_2 of ≥ 40% were excluded from the study, and the injury severity score was higher in the intubated group.

NIV is indicated in acute or acute-on-chronic hypercapnic respiratory failure due to chest wall deformity or neuromuscular disease. CPAP should be used in patients with chest wall trauma who remain hypoxemic despite regional anesthesia and high-flow oxygen.

Cardiogenic Pulmonary Edema

CPAP and noninvasive positive pressure ventilation both unload the respiratory muscles in respiratory failure caused by heart failure and pulmonary edema and improve cardiac performance by reducing right and left ventricular preload and mean transmural filling pressures. Multiple trials have been conducted, and most have shown a decreased need for intubation in the noninvasively treated group. One study showed improvement in multiple physiologic variables such as heart rate, oxygenation, and BP but no difference in mortality or intubation rate. A subgroup analysis, however, showed a reduced risk of intubation for patients who were hypercapnic at baseline. Notably, one study comparing CPAP to NIV was prematurely terminated owing to increased myocardial infarction in the NIV group, but there may have been a greater number of patients with chest pain in the NIV arm. A more recent study comparing CPAP to BiPAP in acute cardiogenic pulmonary edema and acidosis concluded that patients treated with CPAP were more likely to survive to discharge compared to those in the BiPAP group. It is important to remember that noninvasive methods of respiratory support should not be used in hemodynamically unstable patients or in those with ongoing cardiac ischemia. Current recommendations are to use CPAP in hypoxemic patients with cardiogenic pulmonary edema who remain hypoxemic despite maximal medical therapy.

Acute Hypoxemic Respiratory Failure and Pneumonia

The use of NIV in hypoxemic respiratory failure is less clear than in the above disorders. One study reported a prospective randomized controlled trial of 56 patients with severe community-acquired pneumonia and hypoxemic acute respiratory failure who received either NIV or conventional treatment. The group receiving NIV had a decreased need for endotracheal intubation and decreased mean duration of ICU stay. There was no difference in hospital mortality. Another study, however, found no difference in endotracheal intubation rates in patients with acute hypoxemic respiratory failure when NIV was compared to conventional therapy. Subgroup analysis showed that all patients with pneumonia who were randomized to receive NIV eventually required intubation.

CPAP has been studied in nonhypercapnic respiratory failure, with the results showing that it is ineffective and potentially dangerous. The results of a randomized controlled trial of 123 patients, 51 of whom had pneumonia, showed no difference in intubation rates, length of ICU stay, or mortality. There were more adverse effects in the CPAP group, including four cardiopulmonary arrests, presumably secondary to delayed intubation.

The current recommendation is that NIV can be used as an alternative to endotracheal intubation in acute hypoxemic respiratory failure secondary to pneumonia if the patient becomes hypercapnic.

Asthma

There is only a single reported case series studying NIV in status asthmaticus. The study reported the successful use of NIV in 17 cases with a mean pH of 7.25. Only two patients in this series required intubation.

Current recommendations are not for routine use of NIV in acute asthma until more data are available.

INITIATION OF NONINVASIVE VENTILATION

Once the determination is made that a patient requires ventilatory assistance, the decision must be made about whether NIV or intubation is the appropriate therapy. Success of NIV is most likely to be achieved in patients with a high $PaCO_2$ (pH range of 7.25–7.35) with a low alveolar-arterial oxygen gradient, patients who are cooperative and have a good level of consciousness, and those who show improvement in pH, $PaCO_2$, and respiratory rate after 1 hr of NIV.

None of the studies examining the above indications was without NIV failure. Because failure of NIV can result in a delay in intubation—a situation that can cause increased morbidity and mortality—it is important to identify absolute and relative contraindications to the initial choice of NIV (Table 6-1).

NIV should only be initiated in locations in which the supporting staff have appropriate experience in this treatment and are immediately available. In practice, this tends to restrict NIV to ICUs or a designated respiratory ward. Certain situations such as severe acidosis (pH <7.30) or a lack of improvement in clinical state and blood gas values make the immediate availability of intubation and critical care a necessity. Table 6-2 contains recommendations for initial settings when using BiPAP in acute hypercapnic respiratory failure due to COPD exacerbation.

FIO_2 is an additional variable in the initial setup of CPAP or BiPAP. Adjusting the FIO_2 in older noninvasive ventilators requires changing the flow rate in L/min of 100%

TABLE 6-1. CONTRAINDICATIONS TO NONINVASIVE VENTILATION

Cardiac or respiratory arrest
Nonrespiratory organ failure (e.g., hemodynamic instability, unstable angina, severe GI bleeding, severe encephalopathy)
Life-threatening hypoxemia
Facial surgery or trauma/burns
Fixed upper-airway obstruction
Inability to protect the airway and/or high risk of aspiration (e.g., vomiting)
Inability to clear secretions
Undrained pneumothorax

Adapted from Vianello A, Bevilacqua M, Arcaro G, et al. Non-invasive ventilatory approach to treatment of acute respiratory failure in neuromuscular disorders. A comparison with endotracheal intubation. *Intensive Care Med* 2000;26:384–390; and Mehta S, Hill NS. Noninvasive ventilation. *Am J Respir Crit Care Med* 2001;163:540–577.

TABLE 6-2. TYPICAL INITIAL VENTILATOR SETTINGS FOR BILEVEL POSITIVE AIRWAY PRESSURE IN A PATIENT WITH ACUTE HYPERCAPNIC RESPIRATORY FAILURE DUE TO COPD

Mode	Spontaneous/timed
Expiratory positive airway pressure	4–5 cm H_2O
Inspiratory positive airway pressure	12–15 cm H_2O (to be increased as tolerated to 20 cm H_2O)
Triggers	Maximum sensitivity
Back up rate	15 breaths/min
Back up inspiration:expiration ratio	1:3

Adapted from British Thoracic Society Standards of Care Committee. Non-invasive ventilation in acute respiratory failure. *Thorax* 2002;57:192–211.

oxygen delivered proximally into the ventilation circuit or directly into the mask mixed with entrained room air. The pressure on the face from an adjustment of flow rates >6 L/min often becomes progressively more uncomfortable to the patient, and dyssynchrony with the ventilator may worsen ventilation and subsequently worsen hypoxemia, obviating any benefit of an increased FIO_2. Newer ventilators largely overcome this drawback by providing an oxygen mixer that allows for titration of FIO_2 before its entry into the circuit without adjusting the flow rate. This setup is subsequently more comfortable for the patient and more beneficial for ventilation.

CONCLUSION

NIV can be an effective means of treating acute respiratory failure when used selectively and can lower the morbidity and mortality associated with endotracheal intubation. NIV is most likely to succeed in patients with hypercapnic respiratory failure, respiratory failure secondary to chest wall deformities or neuromuscular disease, and patients with cardiogenic pulmonary edema. NIV is least likely to succeed in patients with severe hypoxemic respiratory failure without hypercapnia, such as patients with lobar pneumonia. ABG values and clinical parameters usually improve within the first 1–2 hrs if NIV is going to succeed. Significant improvement or stabilization should definitely be seen in the first 4–6 hrs. NIV is inappropriate in patients with noncardiogenic pulmonary edema or acute respiratory distress syndrome. Pay close attention to patients after initiation of NIV for synchrony with the ventilator, and check ABGs within the first hour after initiation. Do not hesitate to intubate the patient if NIV is failing. Delay in intubation is a significant cause of rapid clinical deterioration and significant morbidity and mortality.

KEY POINTS TO REMEMBER

- NIV (or NIPPV or NPPV) refers to the use of a mask or similar device to provide ventilatory support.
- CPAP maintains a set positive pressure throughout the respiratory cycle during both inhalation and exhalation efforts and thus is not ventilatory support in a strict physiologic sense.
- BiPAP is simply CPAP with a second "level" of pressure support added. The use of BiPAP requires the operator to set two variables: IPAP and EPAP.
- Success of NIV is most likely to be achieved in patients with an elevated $PaCO_2$ and a low A-a oxygen gradient, patients who are cooperative and have a good level of consciousness, and those who show improvement in pH, $PaCO_2$, and respiratory rate after 1 hr of NIV.
- Initiation of NIV should only be done in locations where the supporting staff have appropriate experience in this treatment and are immediately available.

REFERENCES AND SUGGESTED READINGS

Bollinger CT, Van Eeden SF. Treatment of multiple rib fractures. Randomized controlled trial comparing ventilatory with nonventilatory management. *Chest* 1990;97:943–948.

Bott J, Carroll MP, Conway JH, et al. Randomized controlled trial of nasal ventilation in acute ventilatory failure due to chronic obstructive airways disease. *Lancet* 1993; 341:1555–1557.

British Thoracic Society Standards of Care Committee. Non-invasive ventilation in acute respiratory failure. *Thorax* 2002;57:192–211.

Brochard L, Mancebo J, Wysocki M, et al. Noninvasive ventilation for acute exacerbations of chronic obstructive pulmonary disease. *N Engl J Med* 1995;333:817–822.

Broseghini C, Brandolese R, Poggi R, et al. Respiratory mechanics during the first day of mechanical ventilation in patients with pulmonary edema and chronic airway obstruction. *Am Rev Respir Dis* 1988;138:355–361.

Celikel T, Sungur M, Ceyhan B, et al. Comparison of non-invasive positive pressure ventilation with standard medical therapy in hypercapnic acute respiratory failure. *Chest* 1998;114:1636–1642.

Chadda K, Annane D, Hart N, et al. Cardiac and respiratory effects of continuous positive airway pressure and noninvasive ventilation in acute cardiac pulmonary edema. *Crit Care Med* 2002;30(11):2457–2461.

Confalonieri M, Potena A, Carbone G, et al. Acute respiratory failure in patients with severe community-acquired pneumonia. A prospective randomized evaluation of noninvasive ventilation. *Am J Respir Crit Care Med* 1999;160:1585–1591.

Crane SD, Elliott MW, Gilligan P, et al. Randomised controlled comparison of continuous positive pressure, bilevel non-invasive ventilation, and standard treatment in emergency department patients with acute cardiogenic pulmonary edema. *Emerg Med J* 2004;21:155–161.

Delclaux C, L'Her E, Alberti C, et al. Treatment of acute hypoxemic nonhypercapnic respiratory insufficiency with continuous positive airway pressure delivered by a face mask: a randomized controlled trial. *JAMA* 2000;284:2352–2360.

Kramer N, Meyer TJ, Meharg J, et al. Randomized, prospective trial of noninvasive positive pressure ventilation in acute respiratory failure. *Am J Respir Crit Care Med* 1995;151:1799–1806.

Lenique F, Habis M, Lofaso F, et al. Ventilatory and hemodynamic effects of continuous positive airway pressure in left heart failure. *Am J Respir Crit Care Med* 1997;155(2):500–505.

Meduir GU, Cook TR, Turner RE, et al. Noninvasive positive pressure ventilation in patients in status asthmaticus. *Chest* 1996;110:767–774.

Mehta S, Hill NS. Noninvasive ventilation. *Am J Respir Crit Care Med* 2001;163:540–577.

Mehta S, Jay GD, Woolard RH, et al. Randomized, prospective trial of bilevel versus continuous positive airway pressure in acute pulmonary edema. *Crit Care Med* 1997;25:620–628.

Murciano D, Aubier M, Bussi S, et al. Comparison of esophageal, tracheal, and mouth occlusion pressure in patients with chronic obstructive pulmonary disease during acute respiratory failure. *Am Rev Respir Dis* 1982;126:837–841.

Nava S, Carbone G, DiBattista N, et al. Noninvasive ventilation in cardiogenic pulmonary edema. *Am J Respir Crit Care Med* 2003;168:1432–1437.

Petrof BJ, Legaré M, Goldberg P, et al. Continuous positive airway pressure reduces work of breathing and dyspnea during weaning from mechanical ventilation in severe chronic obstructive pulmonary disease. *Am Rev Respir Dis* 1990;141:281–289.

Plant PK, Owen JL, Elliott MW. Early use of non-invasive ventilation for acute exacerbations of chronic obstructive pulmonary disease on general respiratory wards: a multicenter randomized controlled trial. *Lancet* 2000;355:1931–1935.

Vianello A, Bevilacqua M, Arcaro G, et al. Non-invasive ventilatory approach to treatment of acute respiratory failure in neuromuscular disorders. A comparison with endotracheal intubation. *Intensive Care Med* 2000;26:384–390.

Wysocki M, Tric L, Wolff MA, et al. Noninvasive pressure support ventilation in patients with acute respiratory failure. A randomized comparison with conventional therapy. *Chest* 1995;107:761–768.

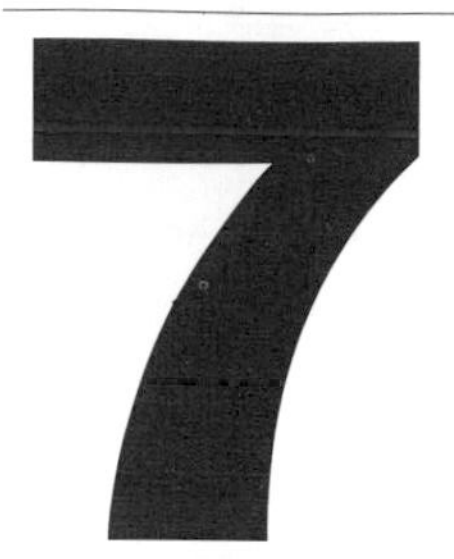

Singultus

Christine Yeh

INTRODUCTION

Singultus, more commonly known as **hiccups,** is a pervasive problem. Hiccups spare no population and have been observed in human beings from preterm infants to adults. Hiccups also occur in other mammals. Hiccups appear to serve no particular function and may be remnants of a primitive reflex.

Hiccups are often classified by the duration of the episodes. **Hiccup bouts** are acute episodes that terminate within 48 hrs. Hiccups lasting >48 hrs but <1 mo are identified as **persistent hiccups,** and those unfortunate enough to be afflicted with hiccups for >1 mo are identified as having **intractable hiccups.**

The frequency of hiccups numbers between 4 and 60 hiccups/min. Increased frequency of hiccups is noted with falls in $PaCO_2$. Transient hiccups tend to occur at night, and intractable hiccups tend to predominate in men. Although the majority of hiccups are benign, chronic hiccups may portend more ominous pathology.

PATHOPHYSIOLOGY

Hiccups are believed to result from the stimulation of a **hiccup reflex arc** that involves both central and peripheral components. The afferent limb is composed of the phrenic nerve, vagus nerve, and sympathetic chain from T6 to T12. The efferent limb includes multiple brainstem and midbrain areas interacting with the motor fibers of the phrenic nerve. Within cervical spinous processes C3–C5, a central connection between afferent and efferent limbs exists. These interactions then manifest as repetitive, involuntary contractions of intercostal and diaphragmatic muscles with glottic closure resulting in the familiar "hiccup." Irritation in any component of this reflex arc may result in hiccups. Hiccups more commonly involve unilateral diaphragmatic contraction.

ETIOLOGY

The multiple components of the hiccup reflex arc allow for broad susceptibility to structural, inflammatory, infectious, or metabolic disturbances. More than 100 causes of hiccups have been described (Table 7-1).

Benign transient hiccups are believed to arise from such common occurrences as gastric distention, aerophagia, tobacco use, sudden excitement or stress, or sudden changes in environmental or internal temperatures.

Chronic hiccups are often pathologic in nature and can be broadly classified into organic, psychogenic, medication induced, and miscellaneous origins. Central processes include any disruption of the brainstem or midbrain areas. Peripheral nervous system etiologies include those that irritate the vagus or phrenic nerves anywhere along their courses, including their cranial (vagus), cervical, thoracic, or abdominal portions.

TABLE 7-1. CAUSES OF HICCUPS

Organic

Central

Vascular: ischemic/hemorrhagic strokes, arteriovenous malformations, head trauma lesions, vasculitis

Infections: encephalitis/meningitis, brain abscess, neurosyphilis

Structural: mass lesions

Peripheral

Meningeal/pharyngeal afferents: meningitis/laryngitis/abscess, goiters/cysts/tumors

Auricular afferents: foreign body

Thoracic afferents: chest trauma, neoplasm of lung, lymphadenopathy, myocardial infarction, pulmonary edema, pericarditis/pleuritis/esophagitis, aortic aneurysm, asthma/bronchitis/pneumonia, esophagitis/stricture/hernia, achalasia

Abdominal afferents: gastric distention, gastritis/hepatitis, peptic ulcers, pancreatic/biliary disease, bowel obstruction, appendicitis, inflammatory bowel disease, intraabdominal surgery, genitourinary disorders, direct diaphragmatic irritation

Psychogenic: stress/excitement, conversion/grief reactions, anorexia nervosa, malingering

Medications: steroids, barbiturates, benzodiazepines, alpha-blockers, dopaminergic agonists, antibiotics, nonsteroidal antiinflammatory

Miscellaneous: idiopathic, toxic/metabolic causes, alcohol, tobacco, sepsis, electrolyte abnormalities (sodium/calcium/potassium), uremia, diabetes mellitus

EVALUATION

A detailed **history** and physical exam are critical to clarifying the etiology of hiccups. The onset, severity, and duration of hiccups are useful details. For example, hiccups occurring during sleep often point to an organic cause. A careful review of systems allows further assessment of the clinical impact of hiccups. Chronic persistent hiccups have been associated with such complications as malnutrition, fatigue, dehydration, cardiac arrhythmias, and insomnia. Social history also provides helpful diagnostic clues, as excessive alcohol and tobacco use can cause hiccups. Medications need to be discussed, as a number of medicines are known to precipitate hiccups (see Table 7-1).

The **physical exam** allows further investigation into the cause of the patient's hiccups. A thorough exam of the head and neck allows for a search for masses, foreign bodies, or evidence of infection, which may be culprits in inducing hiccups. Lymphadenopathy may cause compression of neural structures and merit more intensive investigation for underlying pathologies. Given the extensive number of thoracic causes of hiccups, the chest exam is also crucial to identifying the underlying diagnosis and can shed light on underlying processes such as pneumonia or asthma. The physical exam should also include a careful neurologic assessment, because strokes and various neurologic disorders such as multiple sclerosis can often manifest with hiccups.

No one **lab study** can diagnose hiccups. However, based on suspected etiologies from the history and physical exam, specific lab studies may be helpful. Specific tests such as serum alcohol or electrolyte levels can exclude metabolic and toxic causes of persistent hiccups. The chest radiograph can be helpful for ruling out cardiac, pulmonary, and mediastinal sources of peripheral nerve irritation. More specialized tests such as electroencephalogram, MRI, and endoscopy may be performed based on clinical findings.

MANAGEMENT

When persistent hiccups adversely affect a patient's quality of life, treatment is absolutely indicated. Given the numerous etiologies of hiccups, treatment should first be directed at rectifying the specific cause as determined by history, physical exam, and testing. The number of therapies directed at the resolution of hiccups far surpasses the numerous etiologies behind the process itself.

Anecdotal evidence for **nonpharmacologic therapies** directed at hiccups abounds. These therapies are aimed at manipulating phrenic and vagal nerve activity and include respiratory maneuvers, nasopharyngeal stimulation, and methods to decrease gastric distention. Such ancient remedies include sneezing, inducing unexpected fright, swallowing granulated sugar, carotid massage, Valsalva maneuvers, supraorbital pressure, holding one's breath, or other various maneuvers to manipulate $PaCO_2$. Targeted **pharmacologic therapy** is aimed at inhibition of stimulated points in the hiccup reflex arc, largely effecting blockade through inhibitory neurotransmitters. Most pharmacologic therapies have been evaluated in case studies rather than in controlled clinical trials. Idiopathic chronic hiccups have been treated with such pharmacologic agents as GABA and dopamine antagonists (baclofen, chlorpromazine, haloperidol, metoclopramide); anticonvulsants (valproic acid, carbamazepine, phenytoin); and numerous miscellaneous agents (nifedipine, sertraline, anesthetics, gastric acid suppressors). In a small number of case studies, gabapentin has been reported as successful therapy in refractory hiccups.

Hiccups usually respond rapidly to therapy if the therapy is to be effective. However, multiple agents may be initiated before a successful drug is found. In cases refractory to both conservative (nonpharmacologic) and pharmacologic therapy, surgical manipulation of either the phrenic or vagal nerves may need to be considered.

CONCLUSION

Hiccups are a pervasive problem that usually represent nothing more than a benign nuisance. However, chronic hiccups may be the manifestation of underlying pathology that merits further investigation. Multiple therapies for the treatment of hiccups exist, but the morbidity associated with each case merits careful assessment to evaluate the risks and benefits of treatment.

KEY POINTS TO REMEMBER

- Hiccup bouts last <48 hrs. Persistent hiccups last >48 hrs but <1 mo. Intractable hiccups last >1 mo.
- Hiccups are thought to result from the stimulation of a "hiccup reflex arc," which involves both central and peripheral components.
- Hiccups occurring during sleep often point to an organic cause.
- Treatment should first be directed at rectifying the specific cause as determined by history, physical exam, and testing.

REFERENCES AND SUGGESTED READINGS

Friedman NL. Hiccups: a treatment review. *Pharmacotherapy* 1996;16(6):986–995.

Kolodzik PW, Eilers MA. Hiccups (singultus): review and approach to management. *Ann Emerg Med* 1991;20(5):565–573.

Launois S, et al. Hiccups in adults: an overview. *Eur Respir J* 1993;6(4):563–575.

Lewis JH. Hiccups: causes and cures. *J Clin Gastroenterol* 1985;7(6):539–552.

Rousseau P. Hiccups. *South Med J* 1995;88(2):175–181.

Smith HS, Busracamwongs A. Management of hiccups in the palliative care population. *Am J Hosp Palliat Care* 2003;20(2):149–154.

Thompson DF, Landry JP. Drug-induced hiccups. *Ann Pharmacother* 1997;31(3):367–369.

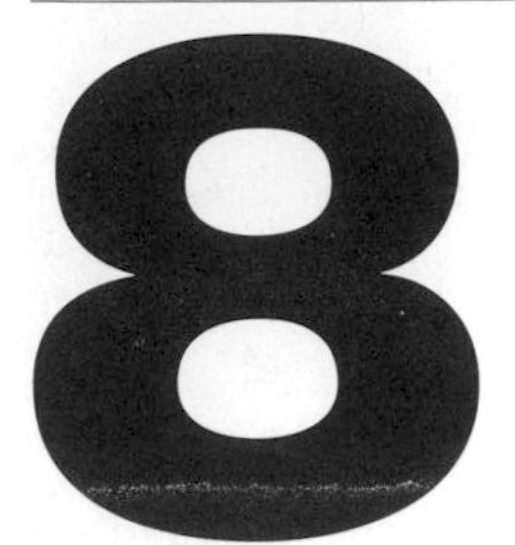

Cough

Faye Lialios

INTRODUCTION

Cough is one of the most common symptoms for which outpatient care is sought. It is responsible for an estimated 30 million physician visits and can account for up to 38% of an outpatient pulmonary practice. As such, it is not surprising that the cost of treating acute cough exceeds $1 billion annually. This figure does not include the cost of diagnostic testing and the complications associated with chronic cough, such as exhaustion, headache, hoarseness, urinary incontinence, and musculoskeletal pain. Because of the adverse effects on the quality of patients' lives, a systematic approach is essential to the management of cough in adults.

ACUITY

The duration of the cough at the time of presentation determines the spectrum of likely causes. An **acute** cough is defined as lasting **<3 wks,** whereas cough is considered **chronic** if it persists for ≥**3 wks.**

PATHOGENESIS

Cough receptors exist in the epithelium of the upper and lower respiratory tracts, pericardium, stomach, esophagus, and diaphragm. Afferent receptors are located within the sensory distribution of the trigeminal, glossopharyngeal, superior laryngeal, and vagus nerves. Efferent receptors located in the recurrent laryngeal and spinal nerves respond to signals from a **"cough center"** in the medulla. Irritation of the cough receptors by smoke, dust, or fumes leads to stimulation of a complex reflex arc. Once stimulated, an impulse is sent to the cough center. After a series of muscle contractions, an increase in intrathoracic pressures develops, leading to increased airflow through the trachea. These shearing forces help to eliminate mucus and foreign materials.

ACUTE COUGH

Viral infections of the upper respiratory tract are the most common cause of acute cough. Rhinoviruses, coronaviruses, and respiratory syncytial virus are the pathogens most frequently associated with common cold symptoms. Less frequent viruses include influenza, parainfluenza, and adenoviruses. Clinical features of the common cold include rhinorrhea, sneezing, irritation of the throat, lacrimation, and nasal obstruction. Fever may or may not be a presenting symptom. Cough typically presents on day four or five. Diagnostic testing such as a chest radiograph in this setting is usually negative and therefore of low yield in the general population. However, in the elderly or immunocompromised, further diagnostic testing is beneficial to rule out pneumonia, left ventricular dysfunction, or other insidious infection. **Viral or bacterial rhinosinusitis** can result in postnasal drainage and acute cough. Viral rhinosinusitis can often not be clinically distinguished from bacterial sinusitis. Viral rhinosinusitis can be managed symptomatically with antihistamines and decongestants.

Allergic rhinitis is an IgE-mediated syndrome characterized by paroxysms of sneezing, nasal congestion, and irritation of the eyes and nose. Cough is frequently an associated symptom and is often improved by using nonsedating antihistamines and avoiding offending allergens. Postnasal drainage is probably the mechanism leading to cough and may be a prominent symptom when cough is severe.

Exacerbations of COPD may result from smoking, air pollutants, allergens, and viral infections. *Streptococcus pneumoniae, Haemophilus influenzae,* and *Moraxella catarrhalis* are among the most common bacterial pathogens isolated in COPD exacerbations and are therefore the most frequently treated. Antibiotics are frequently prescribed if the acute cough is accompanied by worsening shortness of breath, increased sputum production, or change in character of the sputum.

***Bordetella pertussis* infection** is a less common cause of acute cough in adults, although it should be suspected in the presence of a barking cough, which may be accompanied by posttussive vomiting. It should also be suspected in the face of a recent outbreak in the community or if there is a history of contact with a known case. Any patient with a paroxysmal cough should be evaluated for pertussis with a sputum culture or nasopharyngeal swab for *B. pertussis* PCR.

CHRONIC COUGH

Chronic cough can be divided into conditions that are associated with cigarette smoke and those that are not. Although cough that lasts >3 wks may be caused by many diseases, most cases are attributable to one of a handful of diagnoses. One study found postnasal drip, asthma, and gastroesophageal reflux responsible for 90% of cases of chronic cough in nonsmokers.

Postnasal drip is the most common cause of persistent cough in nonsmokers. Symptoms of postnasal drip include frequent nasal discharge and throat clearing. Often, patients complain of a nasal discharge dripping into the back of the throat. However, postnasal drip may be silent, leaving a practitioner with nonspecific symptoms to guide treatment. Therefore, when there is a lack of alternative cause of a patient's cough, empiric therapy for postnasal drip should be attempted before further extensive workups for other etiologies.

Asthma is the second most common cause of chronic cough in adults and the most common cause in children. The clinical spectrum of symptoms includes recurrent episodes of wheezing, chest tightness, breathlessness, and cough, particularly at night and/or in the early morning. It may also be the sole manifestation of a form of asthma known as *cough variant asthma*.

Gastroesophageal reflux (GERD) is often reported to be the third most common cause of chronic cough. Patients often present complaining of heartburn or sour taste in the mouth, but they may lack these symptoms. Prolonged esophageal pH monitoring is generally considered the gold standard study for confirmation of GERD.

Chronic bronchitis from cigarette smoking is by far the most common cause of chronic cough. It is defined as ≥ 3 mos of cough with sputum production for ≥ 2 consecutive yrs in the absence of any other lung disease. Patients have usually been smoking >20 cigarettes per day for >20 yrs. An acute chest illness, such as a superimposed bacterial infection, often prompts smokers to visit their physician. Dyspnea on exertion may or may not be present.

ACE inhibitors are associated with cough in 3–20% of treated patients. Although the exact mechanism is unknown, it is believed that the accumulation of bradykinin may stimulate afferent nerve fibers in the airway. Supporting this theory is the lack of cough in patients treated with angiotensin II receptor antagonists, which do not increase kinin levels. The cough associated with these medications usually begins within 1 wk of initiating therapy but may be delayed for up to 6 mos. It typically resolves within 1–4 days of discontinuing therapy. Beta-blockers may cause cough in patients with reversible airway hyperresponsiveness, such as asthmatics and certain patients with COPD.

Bronchiectasis occurs less frequently than the above causes. In some studies, bronchiectasis is responsible for chronic cough in approximately 4% of patients. Bronchiectasis is the result of severe, repeated, or persistent airway inflammation leading to progressive airway damage. Bronchiectasis may be focal, or it may be more diffuse. Most patients produce chronic sputum that is mucopurulent and becomes frankly purulent during an infectious exacerbation.

Eosinophilic bronchitis is increasingly recognized as a cause of chronic cough. Although not as frequent as asthma, it should be evaluated in patients who demonstrate atopic features, elevated sputum eosinophils, and active airway inflammation. Although similar characteristics are seen in patients with cough-variant asthma, patients with eosinophilic bronchitis do not have airway hyperresponsiveness.

Rarer causes include interstitial lung diseases, lung cancers, and lesions that compromise the upper airway, including arteriovenous malformations and retrotracheal masses. Although practitioners are frequently concerned about missing lung cancer as a cause of chronic cough, it is an infrequent presentation of occult bronchogenic carcinoma. Other rare causes include tracheobronchomalacia, TB, tracheal diverticuli, occult cystic fibrosis, recurrent aspiration, hyperthyroidism, carcinoid syndrome, and psychogenic cough. Psychogenic cough is always a diagnosis of exclusion and occurs less frequently in adults than in children. Many patients with this condition do not cough during sleep, are not awakened by cough, and do not cough when otherwise occupied (working or playing).

EVALUATION

History

A complete history provides important clues in the patient presenting with cough complaints. Important clues include the onset, frequency, and severity of the cough, and coexisting symptoms (fever, weight loss, dyspnea, night sweats). Patients should be questioned on medications, especially beta-blockers and ACE inhibitors, environmental exposures, and respiratory tract infections within the past 3 mos. It is important to establish TB risk factors. Ascertain when the last PPD skin test was completed.

Medical history should focus on underlying medical illnesses that may predispose a patient to aspiration, congestive heart failure, and interstitial lung disease. Social history should include a detailed history of tobacco and alcohol use. A detailed occupational history should be obtained, including past and present exposure to asbestos, silica, coal dust, and fumes. Family history should include information regarding asthma and cystic fibrosis.

Sputum Production

For patients with chronic bronchitis, sputum production is usually insidious. It is often worse in the morning, and the appearance is whitish to gray. During exacerbations, the sputum may become more profuse and more purulent. Cigarette smokers are used to the productive cough and are less likely to present to their physician unless there is a change in their respiratory status or the character of their sputum.

Postnasal Drip

The absence of symptoms does not exclude the diagnosis of postnasal drip. These patients may have "silent" postnasal drip and still have a favorable response to combination therapy with an antihistamine and/or a decongestant.

Gastroesophageal Reflux Disease

The patient may complain of heartburn, regurgitation, or dysphagia. Although these symptoms are seen in the majority of patients, they may be absent in up to 75% of cases.

Asthma

The classic triad of cough, shortness of breath, and wheezing does not occur in every patient. Chronic cough as the sole presenting symptom is seen in an estimated 24% of patients.

Physical Exam

The patient should be observed for signs of labored breathing. Palpate the frontal and maxillary sinuses for tenderness. Evaluate the auditory canal and tympanic membranes. Irritation of the external canal by impacted foreign bodies or cerumen can lead to a chronic dry cough. Examine the nose for boggy turbinates, mucopurulent secretions, and polyps. A cobblestone appearance to the oropharynx suggests postnasal drip. Auscultate the lung for wheezes and crackles. Inspect the extremities for clubbing, which may occur with interstitial lung disease or cystic fibrosis. Note the presence or absence of lower extremity edema.

Diagnostic Tests

The differential diagnosis may be narrowed down by a careful review of the patient's history and physical exam. Focusing on the three most common causes of chronic cough—postnasal drip, asthma, and GERD—is helpful in limiting the need for extensive evaluation.

Chest X-Ray

Chest x-ray can be useful for establishing an initial diagnosis and for guiding trials of empiric therapy. A normal radiograph in an immunocompetent patient makes a diagnosis such as bronchogenic carcinoma, sarcoidosis, tuberculosis, or bronchiectasis less likely.

Sinus CT Scan

Limited sinus CT is the usual test of choice in selected cases with suspected sinus disease. Plain films of the sinuses are not generally recommended. A CT scan should be obtained if a patient has not responded to one or two courses of appropriate antibiotic therapy for sinusitis, which occurs in about 10% of treated patients. Nasal endoscopy is generally not indicated except in cases in which resistant or unusual organisms are suspected.

Pulmonary Function Tests

Methacholine challenge testing should be performed in patients with a history and physical exam suggestive of asthma. A negative test result essentially eliminates cough-variant asthma as the cause of chronic cough. In patients with a positive response to methacholine challenge, a lack of improvement with bronchodilators indicates a false-positive test, and further workup should be initiated.

Gastrointestinal Evaluation

Diagnostic testing for suspected gastroesophageal disease is not routinely recommended. An abnormal barium swallow may demonstrate cough induced by gastroesophageal reflux. However, this study is negative in the majority of patients. Although 24-hr esophageal pH monitoring is the single most sensitive and specific test for reflux disease, it is inconvenient for patients and not widely available. When postnasal drip and asthma have been ruled out, a 4-wk trial of antireflux therapy can be initiated. In the face of an inadequate response to a proton pump inhibitor, pH monitoring may be performed. The study should be performed while the patient is on antireflux therapy to document the efficacy of the medication.

Further Testing

If the history, physical exam, lab tests, and x-ray data do not provide a diagnosis, referral to a cough specialist can be considered. A high-resolution chest CT can be performed to rule out rare causes of chronic cough such as bronchiectasis or interstitial lung disease. If the high-resolution CT is negative, then more invasive studies can be considered. A bronchoscopy with or without biopsy may be indicated. Echocardiography can be performed to rule out left ventricular dysfunction. Other tests that may be performed include a sweat test for cystic fibrosis and quantitative Igs to evaluate for rare immunodeficiencies.

TREATMENT

The first step in the management of a patient with a chronic cough is establishing an etiology. If a systematic approach to the evaluation of persistent cough has been completed, treatment aimed at the underlying disorder is successful in >95% of patients.

Chronic Bronchitis

Chronic bronchitis is managed with smoking cessation and bronchodilators (see Chap. 10, Chronic Obstructive Pulmonary Disease). Cough improves or disappears in >94% of patients with cessation of smoking. In patients who continue to smoke, medical therapy may still be helpful.

Postnasal Drip

Postnasal drip may be due to allergic, perennial nonallergic, or vasomotor rhinitis. Removal of the offending environmental precipitant (if possible) is the treatment of choice. Nasal steroids (e.g., fluticasone nasal spray, two sprays per nostril daily) are also helpful. Nonspecific therapy for any form of rhinitis includes antihistamines and topical decongestants in combination, and ipratropium nasal spray (0.03% nasal solution, 2 sprays each nostril bid or tid). First-generation antihistamines (e.g., diphenhydramine, chlorpheniramine) have been shown to be more effective in the treatment of cough than the newer, nonsedating agents. Improvement should start within 7 days.

Asthma

The treatment of cough-variant asthma is identical to that of atopic asthma. Inhaled bronchodilators and/or inhaled corticosteroids (see Chap. 9, Asthma) are the mainstays of therapy. A short course of oral prednisone (0.5 mg/kg/day for 1–2 wks) may be used with the initiation of inhaled therapy to decrease airway hyperreactivity.

Gastroesophageal Reflux Disease

GERD is treated with both behavioral modification and medication. Patients should avoid eating for 3 hrs before bedtime and, specifically, avoid reflux-inducing foods (fatty foods, chocolate, and alcohol). Patients should elevate the head of the bed with foam wedges or use a mechanized bed. Treatment with a proton pump inhibitor (omeprazole, 40 mg PO bid) should be instituted, especially in patients who do not respond to behavioral therapy or those with severe symptoms. Patients should be advised that it may take up to 6 mos to achieve an optimal response. Patients refractory to conservative measures have been treated with laparoscopic fundoplication.

Sinusitis

Most mild cases of sinusitis respond to topical or oral decongestants. For more severe or recurrent infections, an antihistamine in combination with a decongestant may be more effective. For bacterial sinusitis, an appropriate antibiotic (amoxicillin-clavulanate, 500 mg PO tid, or clarithromycin, 500 mg PO bid) can be prescribed for 10–14 days.

Medication-Induced Cough

Discontinuation of the offending ACE inhibitors or beta-blockers often results in relief of symptoms within 1–4 days but may take up to 4 wks. Substitution of another drug in the same class is unlikely to be effective. Alternatives such as angiotensin II receptor antagonists that are not complicated by cough may be useful substitutes. When a patient's condition necessitates an ACE inhibitor, oral sulindac or indomethacin or inhaled cromolyn sodium may provide relief.

Eosinophilic Bronchitis

Eosinophilic bronchitis is most often treated with a trial of inhaled corticosteroids. In on study, inhaled budesonide, 400 μg twice daily for 4 weeks, markedly improved airway inflammation and cough sensitivity in patients with eosinophillic bronchitis. The optimal duration of therapy is not clear, however.

Bronchiectasis

Antibiotics directed against the most frequently encountered pathogens, *H. influenzae, Pseudomonas aeruginosa,* and *S. pneumoniae*, help to reduce cough and sputum production. Patients generally require a minimum of 7 days of therapy.

Interstitial Lung Disease

Treatment is directed at the underlying disease.

Lung Cancer

For non–small-cell lung cancer, resection, if possible, is the treatment of choice. Treatment for small-cell lung cancer and most non–small-cell cancers involves chemotherapy and/or radiation therapy.

Congestive Heart Failure

Therapy is directed at the underlying disorder.

Psychogenic Cough

Removal of psychologic stressors and behavior modification therapy are probably the best therapy for psychogenic cough. Antitussives have little or no proven role in the therapy of psychogenic cough.

Cough of Unknown Etiology

Nonspecific therapy may be useful in those circumstances in which no cause of cough can be found. There are a number of agents that are believed to suppress cough through action on the central medullary cough center. Codeine (codeine sulfate, 10–20 mg PO q4–6h) is the traditional narcotic agent used for cough suppression. Dextromethorphan is the most common nonnarcotic agent used for treating cough. Studies comparing these two agents have been limited and have yielded variable results with respect to efficacy.

KEY POINTS TO REMEMBER

- An acute cough is defined as lasting <3 wks, whereas a chronic cough is one that lasts 3 wks or longer.
- Cough receptors exist in the epithelium of the upper and lower respiratory tracts, pericardium, stomach, esophagus, and diaphragm. Afferent receptors are located within the sensory distribution of the trigeminal, glossopharyngeal, superior pharyngeal, and vagus nerves.
- Irritation of the cough receptors leads to stimulation of a complex reflex arc.
- Viral infections of the upper respiratory tract are the most common cause of acute cough.
- Postnasal drip is the most common cause of persistent cough in nonsmokers.
- The first step in the management of a patient with a chronic cough is establishing an etiology.

REFERENCES AND SUGGESTED READINGS

Brightling CE, Ward R, et al. Airway inflammation, airway responsiveness and cough before and after inhaled budesonide in patients with eosinophilic bronchitis. *Eur Respir J* 2000;15:682–686.

Irwin RS, Boulet L-P, Cloutier MM, et al. Managing cough as a defense mechanism and as a symptom: a consensus panel report of the American College of Chest Physicians. *Chest* 1998;114[Suppl]:133S–181S.

Irwin RS, Curley FJ, French CL. Chronic cough. The spectrum and frequency of causes, key components of the diagnostic evaluation, and outcome of specific therapy. *Am Rev Respir Dis* 1990;141:640–647.

Irwin RS, French CL, Curley FJ, et al. Chronic cough due to gastroesophageal reflux. Clinical, diagnostic, and pathogenetic aspects. *Chest* 1993;104:1511–1517.

Irwin RS, French CL, Smyrinos NA, Curley FJ. Interpretation of positive results of a methacholine inhalation challenge and one week of inhaled bronchodilator use in diagnosing and treating cough-variant asthma. *Arch Intern Med* 1997;157:1981–1987.

Irwin RS, Madison JM. Symptom research on chronic cough: a historical perspective. *Ann Intern Med* 2001;134(9 pt 2):809–814.

Pratter MR, Bartter T, Akers S, DuBois J. An algorithmic approach to chronic cough. *Ann Intern Med* 1993;119:977–983.

Stein MT, Harper G, Chen J. Persistent cough in an adolescent. *Pediatrics* 2001;107:959–965.

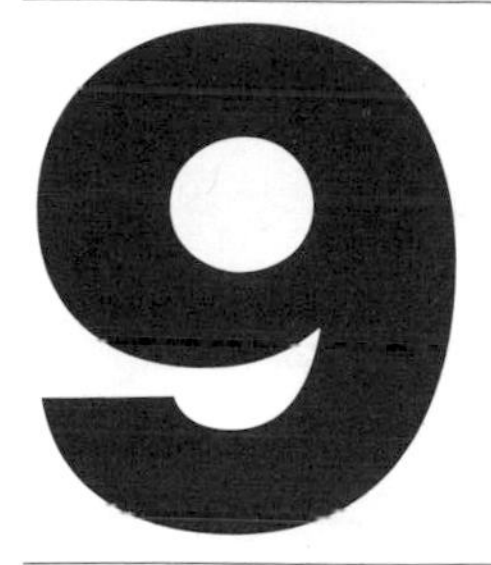

Asthma

Adrian Shifren, Lance Cohen, and Mario Castro

INTRODUCTION

Asthma is a disease of the airways characterized by airway inflammation and increased responsiveness (hyperreactivity) to a wide variety of stimuli (triggers). This hyperreactivity leads to obstruction of the airways, the severity of which may be widely variable in the same individual. As a consequence, patients have paroxysms of cough, dyspnea, chest tightness, and wheezing. Other conditions may present with wheezing and must be considered, especially in patients who are unresponsive to therapy (Table 9-1).

Asthma is an episodic disease, with acute exacerbations and attacks interspersed with symptom-free periods. Asthma attacks are episodes of shortness of breath or wheezing that last minutes to hours. Patients may be completely symptom free between attacks. Typically, attacks are triggered by acute exposure to irritants (e.g., smoke) or allergens. Asthma exacerbations occur when airway reactivity is increased and lung function becomes unstable. During an exacerbation, attacks occur more easily and are more severe and persistent. Exacerbations are associated with factors that increase airway hyperreactivity, such as viral infections, allergens, and occupational exposures.

DIAGNOSIS

Pulmonary function tests (PFTs) are essential for diagnosing asthma. In patients with asthma, PFTs demonstrate an **obstructive pattern,** the hallmark of which is a decrease in expiratory flow rates. Patients experience a reduction in the forced expiratory volume over 1 sec (FEV_1) and a proportionally smaller reduction in the forced vital capacity (FVC). These reductions produce a decreased FEV_1/FVC ratio (generally <0.70). With mild obstructive disease that involves only the small airways, the FEV_1/FVC ratio may be normal, and the only abnormality may be a decrease in airflow at midlung volumes (forced expiratory flow, 25–75%). Patients with lung hyperinflation have an increased residual volume and increased residual volume–total lung capacity ratio. The flow–volume loop demonstrates a decreased flow rate for any lung volume and is useful to rule out other causes of dyspnea, such as upper airway obstruction or restrictive lung disease.

The clinical diagnosis of asthma is supported by an obstructive pattern that improves after bronchodilator therapy. Improvement is defined as an **increase in FEV_1 of >12% and 200 cc after 2–3 puffs of a short-acting bronchodilator.** In patients with chronic, severe asthma with airway remodeling, the airflow obstruction may no longer be completely reversible. In these patients, an alternative method of establishing the maximal degree of airway reversibility is to repeat the spirometry after a course of oral corticosteroids (usually 40 mg/day PO in adults for 10 days).

Lack of demonstrable airway obstruction or reactivity still does not rule out a diagnosis of asthma. In cases in which the spirometry is normal, the diagnosis can be substantiated by showing heightened airway responsiveness to a **methacholine** or **histamine** challenge. A chest radiograph should be obtained to eliminate other causes of dyspnea, cough, or wheezing in patients being evaluated for asthma.

ACUTE ASTHMA ATTACKS

History

A number of historical data have been associated with severe asthma attacks. These include a previous history of mechanical ventilation, recurrent need for oral cortico-

TABLE 9-1. CONDITIONS THAT MAY MIMIC ASTHMA

Upper airway obstruction
Tumor
Epiglottitis
Vocal cord dysfunction
Obstructive sleep apnea
Tracheomalacia
Endobronchial lesion
Foreign body
Congestive heart failure
Gastroesophageal reflux
Sinusitis
Adverse drug reaction
Aspirin
Beta-adrenergic antagonist
ACE inhibitors
Inhaled pentamidine
Allergic bronchopulmonary aspergillosis
Hyperventilation with panic attacks

steroids, hospitalization within the past year, the use of more than two canisters per month of inhaled short-acting bronchodilator, and seizures related to asthma attacks.

Physical Exam

An initial rapid assessment should be performed to identify those patients who need immediate intervention. The presence or intensity of wheezing is an unreliable indicator of the severity of an attack. Certain clinical findings may help to identify patients having severe asthma attacks. A pulsus paradoxus >25 mm Hg, use of accessory muscles of inspiration (scalenus anterior, sternocleidomastoid), nasal alar flaring, inability to talk in full sentences, tachycardia >110 bpm, and tachypnea >28 breaths/min all indicate severe airflow obstruction.

Patients with depressed mental status require intubation. Subcutaneous emphysema should alert the examiner to the presence of a pneumothorax or pneumomediastinum. Impending respiratory muscle fatigue may cause a depressed respiratory effort and paradoxical diaphragmatic movement. However, these findings are not sensitive indicators of severe attacks, and up to 50% of patients with severe airflow obstruction do not manifest any of these findings.

Evaluation

Peak Flow Assessment

The best method for assessment of the severity of an asthma attack is the use of a peak flow meter. Normal values differ with size and age, but a peak flow rate <200 L/min indicates severe obstruction for most adult patients. Peak flow results, if repeated over time, are an effective tool in assessment of a patient's response to therapy.

Arterial Blood Gas

Peak expiratory flow (PEF) is a poor predictor of hypoxemia, and a transcutaneous oximeter is needed to ensure that the patient's oxygen saturation remains >90%. Supplemental oxygen may be required to maintain adequate oxygen saturation.

Initially, most patients with an acute asthma attack have a **low $Paco_2$** secondary to an increased respiratory drive. Thus, an *elevated* or even *normal* $PaCO_2$ indicates that the respiratory system cannot respond adequately to the output of the respiratory center because of a combination of severe airway obstruction, increased dead space ventilation, or respiratory muscle fatigue. Respiratory failure can then develop rapidly.

Peak flow measurements provide a useful screening tool for the presence of hypercapnia. Hypercapnia typically begins to occur when the PEF is <25% of normal. Thus, ABG measurements in acute asthma are indicated in patients with persistent dyspnea whose PEF remains <25% of normal after initial treatment.

Chest X-Ray

The most common abnormality seen on chest x-ray during an asthma attack is hyperinflation. Other abnormal findings such as pneumothorax, pneumomediastinum, pneumonia, or atelectasis are infrequent and occur in approximately 2% of chest radiographs obtained from patients presenting to the ER with an asthma exacerbation. Obtaining chest x-rays should therefore be limited to patients with suspected complications or significant comorbidities.

TREATMENT

The primary goal of therapy in an asthma attack is the rapid reversal of airflow obstruction and the correction, if necessary, of hypercapnia or hypoxemia. Airflow obstruction is most rapidly alleviated by the repeated administration of inhaled beta agonists and early institution of systemic corticosteroids.

Inhaled Beta Agonists

Inhaled beta agonists are the mainstay of bronchodilator therapy. Initial care is albuterol (Proventil, Ventolin), 2.5 mg by continuous flow (updraft) nebulization q20mins until improvement is obtained or toxicity noted. Alternatively, it can be given by MDI at 6–12 puffs in a similar dosing interval. An MDI plus a spacer allows lower doses of beta agonist to be used and is as effective as nebulized beta agonist when performed under direct supervision to ensure proper inhalation technique. For critically ill patients, continuous nebulization of albuterol, approximately 10–15 mg over 1 hr, may be used.

Ipratropium

Ipratropium (Atrovent; 0.5 mg by updraft nebulization q2h until improvement is obtained), an anticholinergic agent, can be used in combination with beta agonist therapy in patients unresponsive to initial therapy. Other special circumstances in which parasympatholytic therapy may be of benefit include treatment of patients with COPD with an asthmatic (reactive airways) component, patients whose asthma has been triggered by ingestion of a beta-blocker, and patients using MAOI therapy who may experience increased sympathomimetic toxicity owing to impaired drug metabolism.

Theophylline/Aminophylline

IV theophylline or aminophylline in combination with a beta agonist results in no further bronchodilation than that with a beta agonist alone. There is an increase in overall toxicity without added benefit. Thus, the routine use of methylxanthines in the management of acute asthma attacks is not recommended.

Magnesium Sulfate

The use of IV magnesium sulfate, 2 g infused over 20 mins, remains an experimental therapy. There are no conclusive data that it has any additive effect beyond that achieved with conventional treatment with beta agonists and systemic corticosteroids. It is thus not recommended for the routine management of an asthma attack.

Corticosteroids

Systemic corticosteroids speed the resolution of asthma exacerbations and should be administered to all patients with moderate or severe exacerbations of their disease. The ideal dose of corticosteroid needed to speed recovery and limit symptoms is poorly defined. Methylprednisolone, 40–60 mg IV q6h, is the drug of choice for IV therapy. Oral corticosteroids are as effective (when the patient is able to take medicine by mouth) if given in equivalent doses, such as prednisone, 60 mg PO q6–8h. Tapering high-dose corticosteroids should not take place until objective evidence of clinical improvement is observed (usually 36–48 hrs). Patients initially on IV therapy should be switched to an oral corticosteroid. A 7- to 14-day tapering dosage of prednisone is usually prescribed in combination with an inhaled corticosteroid that has been instituted at the beginning of the tapering schedule.

Antibiotics

Antibiotics have been shown to be of no benefit when administered routinely for acute asthma attacks. Antibiotics can only be recommended as needed for treatment of comorbid conditions such as pneumonia or bacterial sinusitis.

Epinephrine

In rare settings, aqueous epinephrine (0.3 mL of a 1:1000 solution SC q20mins) for up to three doses may be used. ECG monitoring is necessary for its administration. Epinephrine should be avoided in patients with underlying coronary artery disease.

Heliox

Heliox is a blend of helium and oxygen that has a lower density than air. It seems to be most promising for patients with respiratory acidosis and a short duration of symptoms, and it may be helpful in avoiding mechanical ventilation. It is not currently recommended as routine therapy for asthma attacks.

Indications for Hospitalization and Level of Care

The response of a patient to initial treatment (60–90 mins after three treatments with a short-acting bronchodilator) is a better predictor of the need for hospitalization than is the initial severity of an attack. Patients who experience prompt resolution of their symptoms with a peak flow that returns to >70% of predicted can be discharged from the ER. It is important to note that bronchospasm may recur within the next 72 hrs. It is thus essential that the patient be well educated before discharge, including providing a detailed asthma action plan and teaching how to follow peak flows and administer short-acting bronchodilators for recurrence of symptoms. The patient should also be given a physician referral for follow-up within 1 wk of discharge.

Patients with poor response to initial therapy should be considered for hospital admission. Generally, **admission** is recommended when the *peak flow is <50% of predicted.* However, the decision to hospitalize a patient needs to be individualized. Patients who should be strongly considered for admission include those with recent hospitalizations for asthma attacks, those with failure of aggressive outpatient management (using oral corticosteroids), and those with a previous life-threatening attack.

Consideration for **admission to an ICU** should be given to patients with evidence of *fatigue, drowsiness, or confusion; use of accessory muscles of respiration; hypercapnia or marked hypoxemia; or peak flows <150 L/min.*

Mechanical Ventilation

It is important to recognize deterioration in a patient with severe asthma despite intensive initial therapy, as respiratory failure can occur rapidly and be catastrophic. The conditions mentioned as criteria for ICU admission often weigh in favor of mechanical ventilation.

Noninvasive Positive Pressure Ventilation

There is a relatively high morbidity and mortality among asthma patients who undergo invasive mechanical ventilation. It has been shown recently that **noninvasive positive pressure ventilation (NIPPV)** is useful for improving alveolar ventilation, decreasing work of breathing, and reducing the need for intubation in a selected group of patients with severe asthma. NIPPV should only be performed in an ICU setting by physicians experienced with noninvasive ventilation. In addition, heliox may be used in conjunction with NIPPV to assist further in avoiding invasive ventilation.

Invasive Positive Pressure Mechanical Ventilation

With positive pressure mechanical ventilation, pleural pressure abruptly becomes positive throughout the respiratory cycle. This change may impede venous return, leading to a fall in cardiac output with resulting hypotension. Hypotension may also be caused by lung hyperinflation owing to incomplete expiration of the machine-delivered tidal volumes, resulting in so-called intrinsic positive end-expiratory pressure. Strategies to minimize intrinsic positive end-expiratory pressure during mechanical ventilation include reduced respiratory rates and tidal volumes (which may result in permissive hypercapnia), avoidance of ventilator-applied extrinsic positive end-expiratory pressure, and increased inspiratory airflow rates so as to maximize the duration of expiration. These maneuvers help limit hemodynamic instability and minimize barotrauma.

Discharge Planning

Before hospital discharge, there is a crucial need for careful review of the patient's understanding of the principles of asthma self-management. These include the use of an asthma action plan, how to measure peak flows, how to administer medical therapy and the functions of each therapeutic agent, when to call a physician, and when to proceed directly to an ER. It is essential that the patient have a follow-up appointment within 1 wk of discharge.

DAILY ASTHMA MANAGEMENT

The goals of daily management are (a) control of symptoms while maintaining normal activity and pulmonary function, (b) prevention of exacerbations, and (c) minimization of medication toxicity. Successful management requires patient education, measurement of airflow obstruction, and a medication plan for both daily therapy and exacerbations.

Asthma Action Plan

The asthma action plan is a **written daily management plan** that teaches patients how to avoid factors that aggravate their disease, how to manage their daily medications, and how to recognize and deal with acute exacerbations.

Patients should be taught the consequences of ongoing exposure to chronic irritants or allergens, and the rationale for avoiding the factors that aggravate their disease should be explained. The number of factors increasing airway responsiveness is immense, and each patient should learn to recognize which factors are responsible for their disease. These include (but are not limited to) dust mites, cockroaches, pet dander, viral upper respiratory tract infections, sinusitis, postnasal drainage, gastroesophageal reflux, tobacco and wood smoke, cold air, exercise, aspirin, and other NSAIDs.

PEF monitoring provides an objective measurement of airflow obstruction and should be used in patients with moderate to severe persistent asthma. PEFs should be measured in the early morning before taking a bronchodilator. The personal best PEF (the highest PEF obtained when the disease is under control) is identified by reviewing the patient's diary on follow-up visits. The PEF should be rechecked when symptoms escalate or in the setting of an asthma trigger. This evaluation should be incorporated into the asthma action plan, setting 80–100% of personal best PEF as the "green" zone, 50–80% as the "yellow" zone, and <50% as the "red" zone. In addition, it is useful for patients to monitor PEFs during times in which medications are changed. Recent evidence suggests that an asthma action plan based on symptoms alone is as effective as a PEF-based plan.

Medical management involves both chronic control and control of acute exacerbations. Typical management includes daily use of antiinflammatory, disease-modifying medications for long-term control and intermittent use of short-acting bronchodilators for quick relief. The National Asthma Education and Prevention Program consensus report (http://www.nhlbi.nih.gov/guidelines/asthma/asthgdln.pdf) classified asthma into four different steps: (a) mild intermittent, (b) mild persistent, (c) moderate persistent, and (d) severe persistent. The goal of this stepwise approach is to gain control of symptoms as quickly as possible by assigning the patient to the most severe step in which any one feature of their asthma occurs. Therapy is started at a level higher than the patient's severity to gain control of the disease and then decreased in follow-up once control has been achieved. Therapy is reviewed q1–6mos to see whether stepwise reduction is possible.

MEDICATIONS

Inhaled Corticosteroids

Inhaled corticosteroids are safe and effective for the treatment of chronic asthma. If delivered by an MDI, corticosteriods should be administered with a spacing device, and patients should rinse their mouth with water after each administration to minimize the possibility of oral candidiasis and hoarseness. The dosing of corticosteroids in asthma is determined both by the severity of the asthma and the potency of the steroid preparation. For comprehensive steroid dosing guidelines, the reader is referred to http://www.nhlbi.nih.gov/guidelines/asthma/asthgdln.pdf, pages 88 and 89. The dose is increased as necessary according to the patients' symptoms, PEF, and asthma severity. In patients with frequent $beta_2$-adrenergic agonist use or other signs of poor control, the dose is increased by 50–100% until symptoms are controlled. If symptoms are severe, there is nighttime awakening, or if the patient has a PEF <65% of predicted, a short course of oral corticosteroid (prednisone, 40–60 mg/day PO for 5–7 days) may be necessary to regain control of the disease. Attempts should be made to decrease the dose of inhaled corticosteroid by 25% q2–3mos to the lowest possible dose needed to maintain control, because systemic absorption can occur in patients using prolonged high doses of inhaled corticosteroids.

Leukotriene Antagonists

Montelukast (10 mg PO/day) and zafirlukast (20 mg PO bid) are oral leukotriene receptor antagonists. They provide effective control of mild persistent asthma in the majority of patients but are not as effective as corticosteroids in improving asthma outcomes. Leukotriene antagonists should be considered in patients with aspirin-induced asthma, in cases of exercise-induced asthma, in asthmatics with allergic rhinitis, and in individuals who cannot master the use of an inhaler.

Methylxanthines

Theophylline is a mild bronchodilator and, in sustained-release form, may be a useful adjuvant therapy in persistent asthma, especially for controlling nocturnal symptoms. It is essential that serum concentrations of theophylline be monitored on a regular basis because it has a narrow therapeutic range and significant toxicities. Theophylline dosing depends on the preparation used, as the absorption and metabolism can be variable. The formulation selected should be capable of maintaining stable serum concentrations when taken no more often than twice daily. Starting doses are usually around 10 mg/kg/day. Serum concentrations of 5–15 μg/mL are recommended, and routine serum concentration montitoring is essential due to significant toxicities, narrow therapeutic range, and individual differences in drug metabolism. Theophylline has multiple potential interactions with other medications, especially antibiotics, which should be kept in mind when prescribing for patients on theophylline therapy.

Long-Acting Beta-Adrenergic Agonists

Long-acting beta-adrenergic agonists such as salmeterol (2 puffs bid), added to low- or medium-dose inhaled corticosteroids, have been shown to improve lung function and symptoms in asthmatics. Evidence also shows that their addition can also help reduce the necessary dose of inhaled corticosteroids in patients with moderate persistent asthma. The benefits of adding long-acting beta-adrenergic agonists to corticosteroid therapy are more substantial than those achieved by leukotriene antagonists, theophylline, or increased doses of inhaled corticosteroid. Combination therapy with an inhaled corticosteroid and a long-acting beta-agonist (fluticasone/salmeterol) is currently available and may improve patient adherence. Combination therapy should be considered in all patients with moderate and severe persistent asthma.

Additional Medications

Medications such as methotrexate, cyclosporin, tacrolimus, and troleandomycin have been studied and may be useful in some patients. These medications should only be prescribed in patients who have been evaluated by an asthma specialist.

KEY POINTS TO REMEMBER

- Asthma exacerbations occur when airway reactivity is increased and lung function becomes unstable. During an exacerbation, attacks occur more easily and are more severe and persistent.
- Exacerbations are associated with factors that increase airway hyperreactivity, such as viral infections, allergens, and occupational exposures.
- Indications of severe airflow obstructions include a pulsus paradoxus >25 mm Hg, use of accessory muscles of inspiration (scalenus anterior, sternocleidomastoid), nasal alar flaring, not being able to speak in full sentences, tachycardia >110 beats/min, and tachypnea >28 breaths/min.
- The most common abnormality seen on chest x-ray during an asthma attack is hyperinflation.

REFERENCES AND SUGGESTED READINGS

Agency for Healthcare Review and Quality Management of chronic asthma. AHRQ publication 01-E044. AHRQ publication 01-E044. Available at: http://www.ahrq.gov/clinic/epcsums/asthmasum.pdf. Accessed September 26, 2005.

Fernandez MM. Non-invasive mechanical ventilation in status asthmaticus. *Intensive Care Med* 2001;27:486–492.

Green SM, Rothrock SG. Intravenous magnesium for acute asthma: failure to decrease emergency treatment duration or need for hospitalization. *Ann Emerg Med* 1992;21:260.

Jani A, Shifren A, Grayson M, Castro M. Allergy and immunology. In: Green GB, Schaiff, RA (eds). *The Washington manual of medical therapeutics,* 31st ed. Philadelphia: Lippincott Williams & Wilkins, 2004.

Leatherman JW, Ravenscroft SA. Low measured auto-positive end-expiratory pressure during mechanical ventilation in patients with severe asthma: hidden auto-positive end-expiratory pressure. *Crit Care Med* 1996;24:541.

Mansel JK, Stogner SW, Petrini MF, Norman JR. Mechanical ventilation in patients with acute severe asthma. *Am J Med* 1990;89:42.

Murphy S, Sheffer AL, Pauwels RA. National Asthma Education and Prevention Program: highlights of the expert panel report II: guidelines for the diagnosis and management of asthma. NIH publication no. 97-4051. Bethesda, MD: National Heart, Lung, and Blood Institute, 1997.

National Heart Lung and Blood Institute. Guidelines for the diagnosis and management of asthma. National Asthma Education Program/Expert Panel Report. Publication no. 02-5075. Bethesda, MD: National Institutes of Health, 2002.

Tsai TW, Gallagher EJ, Lombardi G, et al. Guidelines for the selective ordering of admission chest radiography in adult obstructive airway disease. *Ann Emerg Med* 1993;22:1854.

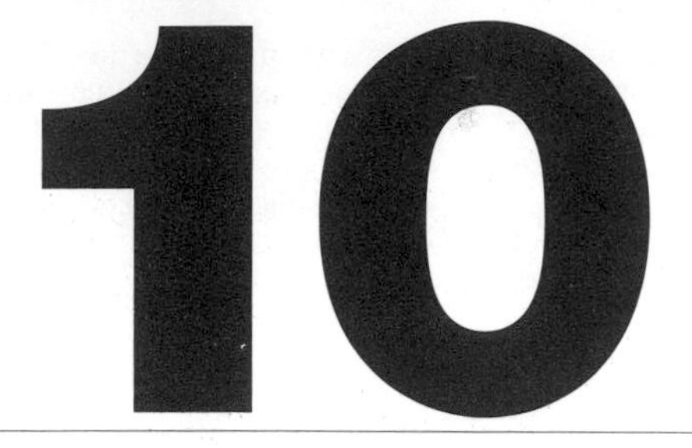

Chronic Obstructive Pulmonary Disease

Adrian Shifren,
Jeanie Park, and
Roger D. Yusen

INTRODUCTION

COPD is a progressive condition characterized by chronic airflow limitation that is not fully reversible. The term COPD refers primarily to the entities of emphysema and chronic bronchitis. **Emphysema** is defined pathologically as nonuniform enlargement of the distal airspaces with destruction of the acini, loss of lung elasticity, and absence of any fibrotic changes. **Chronic bronchitis** is defined clinically as cough productive of at least 2 tbsp of sputum on most days of 3 consecutive mos in 2 consecutive yrs, in the absence of other lung diseases. Although asthma, cystic fibrosis, bronchiectasis, bronchiolitis, and sarcoidosis are associated with expiratory airflow obstruction, they do not fall within the classification of COPD. The diagnosis should be considered in any patient with cough, sputum production, and/or dyspnea, and a history of exposure to risk factors for COPD. Classically, chronic bronchitis accounts for 85% of COPD cases, with the remaining 15% of COPD patients having emphysema. Some patients with COPD exhibit manifestations of both emphysema and chronic bronchitis. The chronic progression of expiratory airflow obstruction is punctuated by episodic worsening in the cough, dyspnea, and sputum production that characterize the condition. These episodes are known as *acute exacerbations* of COPD.

EPIDEMIOLOGY

In the United States, approximately 16 million persons suffer from COPD. These patients account for 500,000 hospitalizations and 18 billion dollars in direct health care costs per year. Currently, 110,000 deaths per year are attributable to COPD, making it the fourth leading cause of death in the United States after heart disease, cancer, and stroke. COPD is the only major cause of death increasing in incidence owing to its high incidence in the elderly, a portion of the American population that has dramatically increased over the last few years.

RISK FACTORS

The most important risk factor for the development of COPD is **cigarette smoking,** which is associated with 85–90% of all cases. Smokers exhibit a substantially greater rate of annual decline in forced expiratory volume in 1 sec (FEV_1) than the normal age-related decline of 15–30 mL/yr. Cigar and pipe smokers are also at increased risk of developing COPD, albeit less than cigarette smokers. However, only a minority (~15%) of smokers develop clinically significant COPD, suggesting that genetic predisposition and other environmental factors may be required for the development of lung injury.

Less than 1% of COPD cases are linked to **alpha$_1$-antitrypsin deficiency,** a known genetic factor associated with premature development of emphysema that is greatly accelerated by smoking. Alpha$_1$-antitrypsin inhibits neutrophil-derived elastase, an enzyme responsible for the destruction of lung parenchyma in emphysema. Patients with alpha$_1$-antitrypsin deficiency carry a genetic polymorphism leading to decreased alpha$_1$-antitrypsin serum levels, which in homozygous individuals may be <10% of normal. Alpha$_1$-antitrypsin deficiency should be considered in a patient with emphysema who has (a) a minimal smoking history, (b) early onset COPD (<45 yrs), (c) a family history of lung disease, or (d) a predominance of lower lobe emphysema on chest x-ray or CT scan.

Other risk factors for COPD include **occupational exposures** to dusts and chemicals; pollution (indoor and outdoor), especially the combustion products of biomass fuels; severe respiratory infections in childhood; and poor socioeconomic status (which predisposes the patient to the preceding factors).

MANAGEMENT OF ACUTE EXACERBATIONS

Triggers

Most acute exacerbations are believed to be caused by **viral infections** (e.g., influenza and adenovirus), although bacterial infection (e.g., *Haemophilus influenzae*, *Streptococcus pneumoniae*, *Moraxella catarrhalis*, and *Mycoplasma pneumoniae*), air pollution, and temperature changes may also trigger worsening of disease in selected patients. In more than one-third of cases, the cause is never elucidated. The differential diagnosis for respiratory decompensation in a patient with COPD should include pneumothorax, pneumonia, congestive heart failure, volume overload, cardiac ischemia, oversedation, and pulmonary embolism.

Initial Assessment

Acute exacerbations of COPD are diagnosed clinically based on one or more of the following three findings: (a) **increased dyspnea compared to baseline,** (b) **an increase in cough and sputum production,** and (c) **an increase in sputum purulence.**

The first step taken when encountering a patient with an acute exacerbation should be a quick assessment to **determine the need for hospitalization.** Patients with severe baseline disease, older age, and significant comorbidities should be admitted to the hospital for further management and observation. In addition, patients exhibiting new physical findings such as cyanosis or peripheral edema, those with new or worsened hypoxemia or hypercapnia, and those who do not respond to initial medical management in the ER should also be admitted. ICU-level treatment may occasionally be needed (Table 10-1).

Initial assessment should also include a **chest radiograph, ABG, ECG, and basic lab tests** if indicated. Results of chest radiographs taken on admission for COPD exacerbations have been shown to change management in one-fourth of admitted patients, mostly owing to pulmonary infiltrates. An ABG is more helpful than oximetry because measurement of oxyhemoglobin saturation with a pulse oximeter does not provide information on $PaCO_2$. ABGs can differentiate between acute and chronic hypercapnia, and an acute respiratory acidosis may indicate a need for assisted ventilation. An ECG can help distinguish a COPD exacerbation from worsening respiratory status owing to cardiac disease (arrhythmias or myocardial ischemia). Spirometric assessment at the time of acute exacerbation is not recommended because the results do not correlate with the severity of hypoxemia or hypercarbia. In general, however, a peak expiratory flow <100 L/min indicates the presence of severe airflow limitation.

TABLE 10-1. INDICATIONS FOR ICU ADMISSION

Inadequate relief of severe dyspnea after initial therapy
Confusion, coma, lethargy
Persistent or worsening hypercapnia ($PaCO_2$ >70 mm Hg)
Persistent or worsening hypoxemia (PaO_2 <50 mm Hg)
Severe or worsening respiratory acidosis (pH <7.30)
Lack of response to supplemental oxygen and/or noninvasive positive pressure ventilation

Oxygen

Oxygen should be administered to achieve a PaO_2 of ≥ 55–60 mm Hg (89% oxyhemoglobin saturation on pulse oximetry). Hypercapnia is a potential hazard of oxygen administration in patients with baseline hypercapnia, and an ABG should be checked 30 mins after starting oxygen therapy. Adequate oxygenation must be maintained, however, despite the presence of preexisting hypercapnia. An increased or new requirement for supplemental oxygen may indicate the presence of a complicating condition—for example, pulmonary embolism, pneumonia, pneumothorax, or right-to-left shunt.

Bronchodilators

Bronchodilators are first-line therapy for symptomatic management of COPD exacerbations. Fourteen randomized controlled trials have demonstrated that short-acting $beta_2$-agonists and anticholinergic agents are equally effective at rapidly improving symptoms during acute COPD exacerbations. Other studies have shown that combination therapy using a $beta_2$-agonist and an anticholinergic agent has added benefits including reducing the number of hospital days and a greater increase in FEV_1 than that obtained with either agent alone. Combination therapy may also have a more rapid onset of action, a longer duration of action, and fewer side effects (owing to smaller doses of each individual agent).

Supervised use of an MDI with a spacer device is as effective as drug delivery by a nebulizer in most patients. Long-acting agents, such as salmeterol and tiotropium, have no known role in the management of acute exacerbations of COPD at this time.

Short-Acting Inhaled Beta-Agonists

Short-acting inhaled $beta_2$-adrenergic agonists such as albuterol have a reduced duration of action in acute exacerbations of COPD. Albuterol may be administered q30–60mins as tolerated. Subsequent treatments can be decreased to 2–4 puffs q4h as the acute exacerbation begins to resolve. All $beta_2$-adrenergic agonists may cause tremor, nervousness, tachycardia, and tachyarrhythmias.

Short-Acting Inhaled Anticholinergics

Short-acting inhaled anticholinergic agents such as ipratropium may be dosed at 4–6 puffs q4–6h for a COPD exacerbation. Ipratropium is generally well tolerated and tends to reduce the risk of hypoxemia and produce fewer of the other side effects characteristic of $beta_2$-adrenergic agents. Anticholinergic agents may cause dry mouth, dry eyes, and bladder outlet obstruction, or exacerbate acute angle glaucoma.

Corticosteroids

Systemic administration of corticosteroids is recommended during acute exacerbations of COPD requiring hospitalization. Corticosteroids have been shown to minimize recovery time, decrease hospital length of stay, reduce the incidence of relapse, and restore lung function to premorbid levels more rapidly than does placebo.

The dosing and length of treatment for systemic corticosteroid therapy are not well standardized. In the largest trial to date, methylprednisolone, 125 mg IV q6h, was given for the first 3 days, followed by oral prednisone, 40–60 mg PO qd, for the following 2 wks. No significant difference in outcomes could be demonstrated for patients receiving 2 wks vs 8 wks of oral steroid treatment. The most common adverse effect of systemic corticosteroid administration is hyperglycemia.

The role of systemic corticosteroids for acute exacerbations treated as an outpatient is controversial. Short courses of oral steroids in patients with moderate to severe COPD can improve the outcomes of patients with COPD exacerbations discharged from the emergency department. Inhaled steroids currently do not have a role in the treatment of acute COPD exacerbations.

Methylxanthines

The role of parenteral or oral methylxanthines (e.g., theophylline) during an acute exacerbation is unclear. They are considered third-line agents, given their narrow therapeutic window and potential for severe side effects, and are therefore used in severe exacerbations that are refractory to treatment with beta$_2$-agonists and anticholinergics. Traditional therapeutic levels range from 10–20 μg/mL. However, most of the potential bronchodilation is believed to occur at lower levels, and the current recommended goal levels are 10 ± 2 μg/mL.

Minor side effects of methylxanthines commonly occur at levels <20 μg/mL and include tremors, insomnia, irritability, nausea, and GI disturbances. Major side effects usually occur at levels >35 μg/mL and are more common with the IV form of the drug. These include vomiting, supraventricular tachyarrhythmias, ventricular arrhythmias, hypotension, and seizures. Various medications and medical conditions, including cimetidine, calcium channel blockers, quinolones, erythromycin, liver disease, cor pulmonale, and pregnancy, increase the likelihood of toxicity by decreasing methylxanthine clearance. Patients are typically started on 10 mg/kg/day of oral theophylline with the dose titrated up slowly to achieve the desired serum levels.

Antibiotics

Controversy surrounds the role of antimicrobial therapy for COPD exacerbations. The most commonly implicated bacterial pathogens are *S. pneumoniae, H. influenzae,* and *M. catarrhalis.* Current methods do not reliably differentiate bacteria-caused exacerbations from those produced by viruses. Antibiotics are beneficial in patients with severe exacerbations and those with severe underlying disease at baseline. Most of the randomized, controlled trials have used 3- to 14-day courses of tetracycline, amoxicillin, and trimethoprim-sulfamethoxazole. However, most of these trials were performed before the emergence of resistant organisms. Because of rampant antibiotic resistance, particularly in *S. pneumoniae*, broader spectrum antibiotic coverage is commonly recommended for acute exacerbations. Reasonable choices include azithromycin (500 mg PO on day 1 and 250 mg PO on days 2–5), or clarithromycin (500 mg PO bid), levofloxacin (500 mg PO qd), or gatifloxacin (400 mg PO qd), all for 7–10 days.

Noninvasive Positive Pressure Ventilation

Noninvasive positive pressure ventilation (NIPPV) is useful for improving oxygenation, decreasing hypercapnia, and avoiding invasive mechanical ventilation patients with COPD exacerbations and acute respiratory failure. Studies have shown that NIPPV is successful in 80–85% of appropriate cases and decreases the length of hospitalization. In addition, NIPPV may decrease mortality. Further studies are needed to determine which patients would benefit most from NIPPV (Table 10-2).

LONG-TERM MANAGEMENT

General

Long-term management of COPD should aim to relieve symptoms, decrease the frequency and severity of acute exacerbations, slow the progression of disease, prevent morbidity, prolong survival, and minimize the side effects of therapy. Although multiple nonsurgical therapies have been studied, only smoking cessation and the correction of hypoxemia with supplemental oxygen have been shown to improve survival in randomized controlled trials.

Smoking Cessation

Smoking cessation should be discussed with all smokers during every office visit (see Chap. 11, Smoking Cessation, for details). This simple and cost-effective intervention is the most effective way to reduce the risk of developing COPD and the rate of decline

TABLE 10-2. CRITERIA FOR NONINVASIVE POSITIVE PRESSURE VENTILATION

Inclusion criteria (two of the following)
Dyspnea with use of accessory muscles and paradoxical chest wall motion
pH 7.30–7.35 and $PaCO_2$ 45–60 mm Hg
Respiratory rate >25
Exclusion criteria (one of the following)
Altered mental status
Respiratory arrest
Cardiovascular instability
High aspiration risk
Recent facial or gastroesophageal surgery
Nasopharyngeal abnormalities
Extreme obesity

in lung function. Standard interventions include providing pharmacotherapy, counseling, and smoking cessation materials to patients. Nicotine replacement therapies, available in multiple forms (gum, patch, inhaler, nasal spray, tablet, lozenge), have been shown to increase abstinence and reduce relapses. Bupropion and nortriptyline are antidepressants that, in combination with smoking cessation counseling, increase long-term abstinence rates. These pharmocotherapies should be offered to assist all patients willing to quit smoking in the absence of specific contraindications.

Oxygen Therapy

Long-term outpatient oxygen therapy (>15 hrs/day) has been shown to **decrease mortality** and **improve physical and mental function** in hypoxemic patients with COPD. A baseline ABG should be performed routinely in all patients with an FEV_1 <40% or clinical signs suggesting respiratory and/or right heart failure. The decision to initiate oxygen therapy should be based on a room air resting ABG (the gold standard for determining the need for supplemental oxygen). Oxygen therapy is indicated for any patient with a $PaO_2 \leq 55$ mm Hg or $SaO_2 \leq 88\%$. If a patient has a PaO_2 of 56–59 mm Hg or $SaO_2 \leq 89\%$, and evidence of pulmonary HTN, polycythemia (Hct of >55%), or heart failure, oxygen therapy is also indicated (Table 10-3). After attaining stability, patients receiving long-term oxygen therapy should undergo routine reevaluation no less than once a year.

Desaturation is more common during sleep in patients with COPD, and patients requiring supplemental oxygen during exertion often need it during sleep, too. While the exact amount required nocturnally might be measured with pulse oximetry, it is

TABLE 10-3. INDICATIONS FOR LONG-TERM OXYGEN ADMINISTRATION

Continuous administration
Resting state $PaO_2 \leq 55$ mm Hg or arterial oxygen saturation (SaO_2) $\leq 88\%$
Resting PaO_2 of 56–59 mm Hg or $SaO_2 \leq 89\%$, if patient has polycythemia (Hct $\geq 55\%$) or evidence of cor pulmonale
Noncontinuous administration (criteria for oxygen supplementation at rest not met)
$PaO_2 \leq 55$ mm Hg or $SaO_2 \leq 88\%$ during low-level exertion
$PaO_2 \leq 55$ mm Hg or $SaO_2 \leq 88\%$ during sleep

reasonable to set the oxygen to be delivered during sleep as 1 L greater than that required during rest when awake.

Oxygen delivery via continuous flow, dual-prong nasal cannula serves virtually all patients regardless of activity level. Patients rarely require higher concentrations of oxygen, and in these cases, the use of a reservoir system with an oxymizer or high-flow nasal cannula may be most cost-effective. In all cases, whenever an oxygen prescription is written, it should state the delivery system required (liquid or compressed gas), the delivery device required (e.g., nasal cannula), and the required oxygen flow rates (liters/minute) for rest, sleep, and exercise.

Pulmonary Rehabilitation

Pulmonary rehabilitation (as defined by the American Thoracic Society) is a multidisciplinary program of care for patients with chronic respiratory impairment that is individually tailored and designed to optimize physical and social performance and autonomy. Pulmonary rehabilitation improves exercise tolerance and dyspnea and may improve quality of life and decrease the frequency of exacerbations in patients with COPD.

Patients with COPD who should be referred to a comprehensive rehabilitation program include those who have severe dyspnea despite optimal medical management, have reduced exercise tolerance, and experience a restriction in activities.

Comprehensive assessment is necessary for the development of the care plan for the individual. Patients should undergo assessment of knowledge base and learning needs, baseline exercise capacity, respiratory muscle strength, activities of daily living, health status, cognitive function, emotional and mood state, and nutritional status/body composition. The components of a comprehensive program include medical therapies, oxygen, an exercise program, education and psychosocial/behavioral intervention, and outcome assessment. A cautious approach toward exercise is required for patients with conditions such as coronary artery disease or pulmonary HTN, and a baseline cardiopulmonary exercise test can help to identify higher-risk individuals.

Exercise training is the foundation of pulmonary rehabilitation, and an exercise program may return a patient to a more functional and satisfactory life. Malnutrition, especially undernutrition, commonly occurs in patients with marked COPD and is associated with increased mortality. Patients may therefore benefit from nutritional counseling and the use of nutritional supplements. Psychosocial and behavioral intervention may assist patients in coping with the depression, anxiety, anger, and fear related to having a chronic illness.

Inhaled Bronchodilators

Bronchodilators control symptoms, increase exercise tolerance, and decrease the frequency and severity of exacerbations. They are considered to be the primary medical treatment for COPD. Both scheduled and on-demand bronchodilators should be prescribed. MDIs are preferred over nebulizers for outpatient management.

Anticholinergic Agents

The American Thoracic Society promotes anticholinergic agents as first-line treatment for those requiring scheduled bronchodilators. Ipratropium is as effective as initial bronchodilator therapy. It has a longer duration of action and less toxicity than available beta$_2$-adrenergic agonists. The usual dosage of 2 puffs q4–6h can be doubled or tripled to achieve maximal bronchodilation. Ipratropium can also improve nocturnal oxyhemoglobin saturation and sleep quality in patients with moderate to severe COPD. Tiotropium (a long-acting anticholinergic agent) has been shown to be superior to salmeterol as a once-daily maintenance treatment.

Beta-Agonists

Beta-agonists are considered first-line therapy comparable to anticholinergic agents by the European Respiratory Society and the British Thoracic Society. Typical starting dosages of albuterol, 2 puffs q4–6h, can be titrated up as needed for symptomatic relief. Interestingly, on-demand use of beta$_2$-adrenergic agonists appears not to differ from scheduled use with respect to decline in lung function, bronchial hyperresponsiveness, and number of exacerbations. Long-acting beta$_2$-adrenergic agonists (salmeterol or formoterol) can improve respiratory symptoms, increase morning peak expiratory flows, and decrease the use of rescue bronchodilator therapy. Oral formulations of beta-agonists should be avoided, as they provide similar efficacy to inhaled agents with a higher risk of toxic side effects.

Combination Therapy

Combination therapy with a beta$_2$-agonist and an anticholinergic provides a greater benefit in terms of symptoms and bronchodilation (FEV_1) than does either agent alone. It also provides the added convenience of having both drugs in a single MDI. Combination short-acting therapy (e.g., Combivent 2–4 puffs q6h) is recommended for patients with moderate to severe disease. Patients often benefit from the use of combination short-acting therapy with a simultaneous long-acting therapy.

Inhaled Corticosteroids

Inhaled glucocorticoids produce a response in only a minority of outpatients with stable COPD. The long-term administration of inhaled steroids should be reserved for patients demonstrating objective bronchodilator responsiveness on spirometry and those with an FEV_1 <50% and frequent exacerbations requiring treatment with oral corticosteroids or antibiotics. In patients who have **objective bronchodilator reversibility** on pulmonary function testing, a trial of inhaled steroids should be given for 6 wks. An increase (after therapy) in FEV_1 of >200 mL *and* >12% above the postbronchodilator FEV_1 on the original spirometry denotes steroid responsiveness.

Although inhaled maintenance corticosteroid therapy increases the FEV_1 and decreases the frequency and severity of exacerbations in patients with moderate to severe disease, steroids have not been shown to slow the progression of disease. Inhaled steroids should be administered after bronchodilator treatment, and patients should rinse the mouth and spit after each use to avoid thrush and hoarseness. Potential side effects, especially with high-dose therapy, are the same as those with systemic steroid therapy. Long-term treatment with oral steroids is generally not recommended in COPD patients.

Methylxanthines

Long-acting methylxanthines have been shown to be effective for the long-term management of COPD in two large randomized trials. They may also improve the overnight decline in lung function and morning respiratory symptoms when dosed at night. The risks of toxicity, however, must be weighed against the benefits. A prudent starting dose of a long-acting theophylline for an average-sized patient is 200 mg PO q12h, with the usual therapeutic dose being between 400 and 900 mg/day. Serum levels should be checked 1–2 wks after each dose adjustment, aiming for a level of 10 ± 2 μg/mL, and also monitored twice yearly. Continued inhalation of tobacco smoke lowers theophylline levels, whereas withdrawal of theophylline may lead to exacerbations of right heart failure. Clinicians should be aware of multiple potential drug interactions.

Vaccines

Vaccination against the influenza virus decreases morbidity and mortality and should be administered annually to all COPD patients. Consensus has not been reached regarding the administration of the pneumococcal vaccine. However, most physicians favor a one-time dose of the vaccine for COPD patients aged >50 yrs. In addition, a single revaccination can be given if the patient received the vaccine >5 yrs earlier and was aged <65 yrs at the time of primary vaccination.

Other Pharmacologic Therapies

Mucolytics, antioxidant agents, and vasodilators have not been shown to be of benefit in COPD. Nedocromil and leukotriene modifiers, used frequently for the treatment of asthma, have not been adequately tested for the treatment of COPD and are therefore not recommended at this time. In addition, antitussives are contraindicated in COPD because of the protective role of coughing in clearing secretions.

Surgical Therapy

Surgical options for the treatment of COPD include bullectomy, lung volume reduction surgery (LVRS), and lung transplantation.

In carefully selected patients with giant bullous disease, bullectomy may improve lung function and decrease symptoms. Generally, patients with a single large bullus occupying approximately 50% of the hemithorax and an FEV_1 of approximately 50% are the best candidates for bullectomy. A thoracic CT scan is useful for determining the extent of emphysema in the nonbullous portions of the lungs that remain behind after surgery.

LVRS performed by experienced surgeons in carefully selected patients decreases symptoms and improves functioning and quality of life. In patients with predominantly upper-lobe disease and poor exercise capacity, LVRS may improve survival. Target areas for resection consist of focal areas of emphysematous lung that are accessible to surgical resection. Poor candidates for LVRS include patients with an $FEV_1 \leq 20\%$, and either a very low DLCO or homogeneously distributed disease (without target areas).

Lung transplantation has emerged as a therapeutic option to improve quality of life and overall function for patients with end-stage COPD, although it may not improve survival. Patients with an $FEV_1 < 25\%$, $Pao_2 < 55$ mm Hg, $Paco_2 > 50$ mm Hg, and secondary pulmonary HTN should be referred for evaluation for lung transplantation. Lung transplantation is typically not an option for elderly patients or those with significant comorbidities.

KEY POINTS TO REMEMBER

- COPD is a progressive condition characterized by chronic airflow limitation that is not fully reversible. The term *COPD* refers primarily to the entities of emphysema and chronic bronchitis.
- The most important risk factor for the development of COPD is cigarette smoking, which is associated with 85–90% of all cases.
- The differential diagnosis for respiratory decompensation in a patient with COPD should include pneumothorax, pneumonia, congestive heart failure, volume overload, cardiac ischemia, oversedation, and pulmonary embolism.
- Patients with COPD who should be referred to a comprehensive rehabilitation program include those who have severe dyspnea despite optimal medical management, have reduced exercise tolerance, and experience a restriction in activities.

REFERENCES AND SUGGESTED READINGS

American Thoracic Society. Standards for the diagnosis and care of patients with chronic obstructive pulmonary disease. *Am J Respir Crit Care Med* 1995;152[Suppl]:S77–S121.

American Thoracic Society. Statement on pulmonary rehabilitation. *Am J Respir Crit Care Med* 1999;159:1666–1682.

Bach PB, Brown C, Gelfand SE, McCrory DC. Management of acute exacerbations of chronic obstructive pulmonary disease: a summary and appraisal of published evidence. *Ann Intern Med* 2001;134:600–620.

Barnes J. Chronic obstructive pulmonary disease. *N Engl J Med* 2000;343(4):269–280.

Brochard L, Mancebo J, Wysocki M, et al. Noninvasive ventilation for acute exacerbations of chronic obstructive pulmonary disease. *N Engl J Med* 1995;333:817–822.

Chaouat A, Weitzenblum E, Krieger J, et al. Association of chronic obstructive pulmonary disease and sleep apnea syndrome. *Am J Respir Crit Care Med* 1995;151:82–86.

Cottrell JJ, Openbrier D, Lave JR, et al. Home oxygen therapy. A comparison of 2- versus 6-month patient reevaluation. *Chest* 1995;107:358–361.

The Department of Veterans Affairs Cooperative Study Group. Effect of systemic glucocorticoids on exacerbations of chronic obstructive pulmonary disease. *N Engl J Med* 1999;340:1941–1947.

Donohue JF, van Noord JA, Bateman ED, et al. A 6-month, placebo-controlled study comparing lung function and health status changes in COPD patients treated with tiotropium or salmeterol. *Chest* 2002;122:47–55.

The European Respiratory Society Study on Chronic Obstructive Pulmonary Disease. Long term treatment with inhaled budesonide in persons with mild chronic obstructive pulmonary disease who continue smoking. *N Engl J Med* 1999;340: 1948–1953.

Ferguson G. Recommendations for the management of COPD. *Chest* 2000;117[2 Suppl]:S23–S28.

Global strategy for the diagnosis, management, and prevention of chronic obstructive pulmonary disease: National Heart, Lung, and Blood Institute and World Health Organization global initiative for chronic obstructive lung disease (GOLD): executive summary. *Respir Care* 2001;46(8):798–825.

Ikeda A, Nishimura K, Koyama H, Izumi T. Bronchodilating effects of combined therapy with clinical dosages of ipratropium bromide and salbutamol for stable COPD: comparison with ipratropium bromide alone. *Chest* 1995;107:401–405.

The Joint Expert Panel on Chronic Obstructive Pulmonary Disease of the American College of Chest Physicians and ACP-ASIM. Evidence base for management of acute exacerbations of chronic obstructive pulmonary disease. *Ann Intern Med* 2001;134:595–599.

Mahler DA, Donohue JF, Barbee RA, et al. Efficacy of salmeterol xinafoate in the treatment of COPD. *Chest* 1999;115:957–965.

Martin RJ, Bartelson BL, Smith P, et al. Effect of ipratropium bromide treatment on oxygen saturation and sleep quality in COPD. *Chest* 1999;115:1338–1345.

National Emphysema Treatment Trial Research Group. A randomized trial comparing lung-volume–reduction surgery with medical therapy for severe emphysema. *N Engl J Med* 2003;348:2059–2073.

Rand CS, Nides MK, Cowles RA, et al. Long-term metered-dose inhaler adherence in a clinical trial. The Lung Health Study Research Group. *Am J Respir Crit Care Med* 1995;152:580–588.

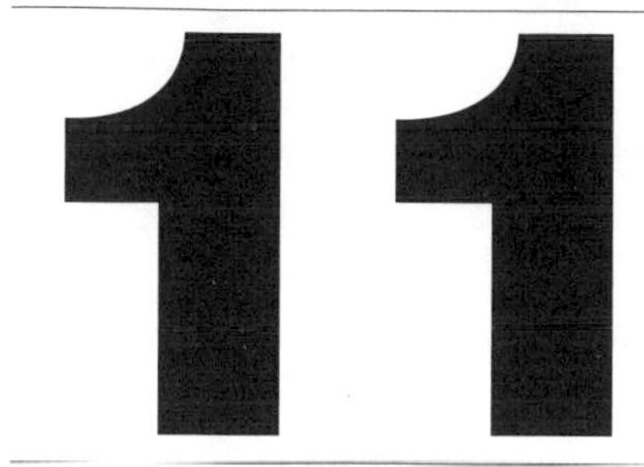

Smoking Cessation

Anne K. Nagler

INTRODUCTION

Tobacco use continues to be prevalent in society today. Although rates of tobacco use have dropped, 25% of Americans are ex-smokers, and 30% are current cigarette users. Of people who have successfully quit, most have failed 3–4 times before stopping permanently.

Nicotine activates the sympathetic nervous system, leading to elevated circulating levels of norepinephrine, epinephrine, vasopressin, growth hormone, cortisol, and endorphins. These result in increases in heart rate, BP, cardiac stroke volume, and coronary blood flow. Other effects include arousal early in the day, relaxation during stressful situations, and an increased metabolic rate with reduced hunger leading to body weight reduction.

There are multiple known carcinogens in cigarette smoke, resulting in a high risk of lung, oral, esophageal, laryngeal, and urothelial cancers. The risk of lung cancer increases in relation to the amount an individual smokes and the age at which he or she started smoking. Cigarette smoking alters immunity in the lung as well as the structure and function of the airways. Smokers have a lower forced expiratory volume over 1 sec (FEV_1) and an accelerated rate of FEV_1 decline when compared with nonsmokers, and cigarette smoking has resulted in a high prevalence of COPD. It is also an important trigger for asthma attacks.

There is evidence that smoking contributes to vascular endothelial damage, coronary vasospasm, and increased platelet aggregation. Cigarette smoking is a known risk factor for coronary artery disease, HTN, and stroke. Nicotine interacts with many medications, including warfarin (increased metabolism), heparin (increased clearance), and theophylline (decreased levels).

CESSATION FAILURE

Most smoking cessation attempts fail. Nicotine has addictive properties, and people become physiologically dependent on its effects. People who quit experience withdrawal symptoms with the peak varying from 24 hrs to 4 wks after quitting. Withdrawal symptoms include anxiety, impatience, restlessness, irritability, hostility, difficulty concentrating, nicotine cravings, awakening at night, insomnia, depression, dysphoria, and hunger. Patients with a previous history of major depression, bipolar disorder, or alcohol and drug abuse may be especially susceptible to withdrawal and relapse.

Patients should be considered **highly dependent** on nicotine if they smoke >20 cigarettes/day, smoke their first cigarette of the day within 30 mins of awakening, or if during a previous quit attempt they developed strong cravings or withdrawal symptoms. Because nicotine is an addictive substance, patients can be expected to cycle through multiple periods of relapse and remission. Physicians should support each quit attempt as they would for patients in alcohol or drug rehabilitation.

APPROACH TO SMOKING CESSATION

The following steps, initially developed by the National Cancer Institute as the "Four As" program, can be used in most outpatient settings. The Four As have been expanded to the Five As by the Clinical Practice Guidelines for Treating Tobacco Use and Dependence.

Five As

1. Ask

Ask at every visit about smoking: Do you smoke? Have you considered quitting? Are you ready to quit?

2. Advise

Advise users to quit at every visit. Personalize your advice based on both the patient's health and his or her social situation. For example, if the patient lives with children, the adverse effects of smoking on children may be a good incentive to quit.

3. Assess

Assess each individual's willingness to quit. Many smokers leave clinic visits without being asked if they smoke and without being advised to quit. Physician intervention is important, and smokers claim that a physician's advice to quit is an important motivator to attempt smoking cessation. If they are willing to try quitting, schedule a return visit to prepare a plan for smoking cessation.

Inform current smokers of the risks of smoking and the benefits of quitting. Identify roadblocks to quitting, and discuss strategies for overcoming these. Repeat all of these steps frequently, and personalize the information for each patient. In patients who have had previous failed quit attempts, the discussion should center on the reasons for the failure and developing strategies to cope with these problems. Common reasons for failure include withdrawal, cravings, stress, illness, and situational factors. Once the smoker wants to quit, a quit plan with stop date should be drawn up. Discuss counseling and candidacy for pharmacologic therapy, and arrange follow-up calls or appointments.

For previous smokers who quit in the distant past, no further intervention is needed. They should, however, be congratulated on their achievement. For smokers who quit within the past year, give reinforcement along with reeducation on the benefits of having quit. Discuss any problems that might have been encountered and their possible solutions. Again, congratulations are in order.

4. Assist

Assist with the development of a quit plan. Give consideration to drawing up a contract for the patient to sign in a similar fashion to a narcotics contract or asthma management plan. Discuss the patient's motivation for quitting and the benefits and drawbacks of quitting. A quit date needs to be established. Encourage the patient to discuss the plan with family and friends and enlist their support. Provide pharmacologic therapy after assessment of the individual's dependence and risk factors. Patients also benefit from counseling and/or scheduled follow-up. Encourage total abstinence. The smoker may also want to avoid alcohol because it is a cue for many patients to smoke. Initiating an exercise plan should be encouraged, with the goal being twofold: (a) occupying the patient's free time, leaving less time to smoke, and (b) helping avoid the weight gain associated with nicotine withdrawal. The average weight gain with smoking cessation is 2–3 kg, and it may be delayed by use of pharmacologic agents.

5. Action

Action is taken by the patient to quit smoking. A "quit visit" may help the patient by reviewing strategy, including avoiding high-risk situations and developing coping mechanisms for dealing with them should they arise. This visit could also be used to initiate medical therapy. During the action phase, follow-up needs to be arranged. The physician, a counselor, or even office staff can perform the follow-up.

Counseling

Any amount of counseling is known to be effective, even if it is simply a physician advising a smoker to quit. Studies have demonstrated that brief interventions, often no longer than 3–10 mins, can increase cessation rates. There seems to be a **dose–response relationship between intensity and effectiveness.** High-intensity counseling lasting >30 mins or at more than two visits is even more effective. Most studies of smoking cessation have a counseling component or, at the very minimum, regular appointments with medical personnel to reinforce and remind patients of their goal to quit. The components of successful smoking cessation counseling therapy are variable but may include the following.

Self-Management
The goal of self-management is to have the patient become aware of personal cues and patterns that initiate smoking.

Stimulus Control
The patient becomes aware of personal cues and attempts to avoid them. If, for example, a patient goes to happy hour after work and ends up smoking a cigarette with his or her beer, he or she should either avoid happy hour or avoid having a beer.

Aversive Conditioning
Aversive conditioning modification has fallen out of favor. A patient would be advised to take drag after drag until physically ill or increase the amount that he or she smokes to 2–3 packs/day, leading to mild intoxication. The goal is to make the patient associate smoking with offensive symptoms.

Relapse Prevention
Relapse prevention involves anticipating circumstances and cues that may cause a relapse, then trying to avoid exposure or devising strategies to cope once exposed.

Nicotine Fading
Nicotine fading involves systematized cutting back. It has not been shown to be effective.

Visualization
Visualization involves imagining the consequences of smoking and using the recollection of these images as a deterrent to cravings.

Contingency Management
Contingency management involves the establishment of a system of rewards and punishments.

Nicotine Replacement Therapy

Nicotine replacement thrapy (NRT) works via direct absorption into the circulation through the buccal mucosa, nasal mucosa, or skin. NRT should be considered for any smoker attempting cessation, but it is **contraindicated in anyone with unstable angina or within 2 wks of a coronary event.** It has not been approved for use during pregnancy, but because circulatory levels are lower than those achieved by actual cigarette smoking, NRT should in theory cause less uterine vasoconstriction and therefore be safer than smoking.

NRT may be used in a step-down method, but doing so may prolong the total duration of therapy. There is a low potential for dependence because blood nicotine levels achieved with any method of NRT are lower than levels achieved through cigarette smoking. NRT also does not produce tar and carbon monoxide, which are other substances linked to the ill effects of smoking.

Nicotine Patch
There are two types of nicotine patches available: a 24-hr release form and a 16-hr release form. They are applied to the skin and changed every day. The maximum strength of the 24-hr patch is 21 mg, whereas the maximum strength of the 16-hr patch is 15 mg. Peak action is within 2–9 hrs of application. The 21-mg patches are frequently used for 4–6 wks followed by a short taper (14 mg/day for 2–4 wks, then 7 mg/day for 2–4 wks) to wean the patient off of the patches completely. The 24-hr patch is believed to be more effective against early morning urges.

Advantages of the patch include convenience and a minimal need for instruction. Disadvantages include mild itching or erythema at the application site and possible allergy to the adhesive. Some patients also develop a generalized rash, headache, nausea, vertigo, or dyspepsia. The 24-hr patch has also been associated with a greater incidence of sleep disturbances. 6-mo quit rates with the patch range from 22% to 42%, whereas permanent cessation rates range from 5% to 28%.

Nicotine Gum

Nicotine gum was the first NRT approved for use in the United States. The gum is chewed briefly until a tingling sensation is noted, then is "parked" in the mouth for 30 mins. The location of parked gum should be rotated regularly. Because absorption of the nicotine is based on pH in the oral cavity, coffee and carbonated beverages before use may lead to poor absorption. The effects peak within 20–40 mins. Maximum dosing recommendations are 30 pieces of the 2-mg gum, or 20 pieces of the 4-mg gum, per day. It is suggested that smokers start with a fixed dose per day then progressively wean themselves.

The most obvious advantage of this method is that gum chewing is socially acceptable in most settings. The disadvantages include a higher level of instruction for proper use and difficulty of use for people with temporomandibular joint problems or dentures, or those who are edentulous. Other disadvantages include air swallowing, hiccups, indigestion, nausea, stomachache, burning sensation in the throat, and a sore jaw. The gum has also been noted to have a bad taste. The U.S. Food and Drug Administration has recently approved a new nicotine lozenge, with a delivery system similar to the gum. The lozenge should require less instruction than the gum but have similar efficacy.

Nicotine Inhaler

A nicotine inhaler consists of nicotine plugs inside hollow cigarettelike rods (a long cartridge). The nicotine levels peak in 10–15 mins after inhalation. Although it is called an inhaler, 95% of the nicotine is absorbed in the mouth and esophagus, not in the lung. The usual dosing is 6–16 nicotine cartridges/day. This form of NRT is especially good for cravings because of the quick onset of action. It also satisfies the hand-to-mouth ritual of cigarette smoking. The inhaler may cause cough and throat irritation.

Nicotine Nasal Spray

The nasal spray most closely resembles actual cigarette smoking because of the high peak blood levels obtained and the rapid onset of action in 5–7 mins. The blood levels obtained with this method, although higher than all other forms of NRT, are still lower than levels achieved with cigarette smoking. Maximum dosing is 1 spray/nostril q1–2h, not to exceed 30–40 times/day. The recommended treatment length is 12 wks including a taper. The advantage of the nasal spray is that users are able to satisfy cravings rapidly. The disadvantages include local irritation of the nose, eyes, and throat, as well as headache, burning sensation, sneezing, and watery eyes. A cold or nasal congestion negatively affects absorption.

Bupropion

The effectiveness of bupropion in smoking cessation is believed to be related to the dopaminergic and noradrenergic effects of the drug. The noradrenergic modifications may limit nicotine withdrawal symptoms, while the dopaminergic modulation may affect areas of the brain that are involved with the reinforcing properties of addictive drugs such as nicotine. Medication should commence 1 wk before quitting, at a dose of 150 mg PO qd for 3 days, and then be increased to 150 mg PO bid for 7–12 wks. Although approved at higher doses for use as an antidepressant, 300 mg/day is the maximum dose for smoking cessation.

Bupropion is pregnancy class B. It is contraindicated in patients with a seizure history, as it lowers seizure threshold, and it should not be used in patients with anorexia nervosa, bulimia nervosa, patients undergoing alcohol withdrawal, or patients who have used an MAOI in the previous 2 wks. Side effects include insomnia, dry mouth, nervousness, difficulty concentrating, rash, and constipation. A blinded, randomized,

HIV testing should be offered to all patients between the ages of 15 and 55 yrs. ***Legionella* urine antigen** is useful in cases in which *Legionella pneumophila* is suspected.

THERAPY

The premise of most guidelines for therapy of CAP is that **rapid empiric therapy,** which may be narrowed at a later time, is the most effective form of treatment. Empiric therapy must avoid excessively broad and unnecessary coverage while still providing sufficient activity to ensure eradication of all common pathogens. As such, most guidelines stratify patients into groups, identify common pathogens in each group, and devise therapeutic strategies effective for the pathogens in each group. (The ATS guidelines which have been verified clinically, are followed in slightly modified form here.)

The ATS stratifies patients based on **site of therapy** (outpatient, inpatient, or ICU) the presence or absence of **coexisting cardiopulmonary disease** (CPD) such as cardiac, lung, or renal disease; and the presence of **modifying factors** (MFs) such a patients at risk for drug-resistant organisms, gram-negative organisms, or *Pseudomonas aeruginosa*. Using the stratification system, patients may be placed into one o three site-of-therapy groups (below), which then determines the empiric treatmen used. Treatment for each group of patients is summarized in Table 12-2. Carefu attention should be paid to the route of therapy (PO or IV) and the combinations o therapy described.

Outpatients
- (a) without CPD, no MF
- (b) with CPD or MF

Inpatients
- (a) without CPD or MF
- (b) with CPD or MF

ICU patients
- (a) not at risk for *P. aeruginosa* infection
- (b) at risk for *P. aeruginosa* infection

Duration of Therapy

Scant data exist on the optimal duration of therapy for either the outpatient or inpa tient management of CAP. Traditionally, therapy has been given for 7–14 days depen ing on the severity of illness. However, the emergence of newer longer-acting dru (e.g., azithromycin) has resulted in much shorter courses of therapy, especially in th outpatient setting (the total duration of therapeutic drug levels in the serum st approaches that of traditional therapy, however). As a rule, **5–10 days** of therapy a recommended for **typical pneumonias** (even in the presence of bacteremia), and **7– days** for **atypical infections** such as *Mycoplasma pneumoniae, Chlamydia pneumoniae,* and *Legionella pneumophila.*

Switching from IV to Oral Therapy

There are also no good data on when to switch from IV to oral therapy when treati inpatient CAP. It is generally accepted that, once patients are clinically stabilized, th can be switched to oral therapy. However, the criteria for stabilization have yet to determined. Bacteremic patients generally take longer to reach a state of clinical st bility, but once stable, these patients should be switched to oral therapy in the sar fashion as nonbacteremic patients. The following criteria are recommended f switching to oral therapy:

- Improvement in symptoms
- Afebrile (<38.3°C) on two occasions >8 hrs apart
- Decreasing WBC count
- Good oral intake

placebo-controlled trial demonstrated an 18% success rate with bupropion alone and a 22% success rate with a combination of bupropion and a nicotine patch. The difference between the groups was statistically insignificant, however.

Second-Line Therapies

Nortriptyline

Nortriptyline and other antidepressants are being investigated for efficacy in smoking cessation. Bupropion remains the only antidepressant that has a smoking cessation indication.

Anxiolytics

Benzodiazepines and buspirone have been used in patients demonstrating increased anxiety during smoking cessation. Although there is no proven benefit for the use of these drugs in smoking cessation, they may be helpful in selected individuals.

Clonidine

Some physicians have tried to diminish withdrawal symptoms through clonidine use. There is little evidence to support the use of clonidine in smoking cessation.

Others

Other aids that are used but are unproven are hypnosis, acupuncture, biofeedback, and relaxation. Smoking cessation groups are often organized by hospitals or workplaces with the assistance of the American Lung Association.

CONCLUSION

Nicotine dependence warrants repeated intervention. Multiple attempts and failures should be expected before success is achieved. All patients deserve pharmacologic intervention unless medically contraindicated. Counseling is an important contributor to success. Accepted pharmacologic therapies include NRT and bupropion.

KEY POINTS TO REMEMBER

- Cigarette smoking contributes to vascular endothelial damage, coronary vasospasm, and increased platelet aggregation and is a known risk factor for coronary artery disease, HTN, and stroke.
- Nicotine has addictive properties, and people become physiologically dependent on its effects. People who quit experience withdrawal symptoms with the peak varying from 24 hrs to 4 wks after quitting.
- The "Five As" for treating tobacco use and dependence are *Ask, Advise, Assess, Assist,* and *Action.*
- All patients deserve pharmacologic intervention unless medically contraindicated.

REFERENCES AND SUGGESTED READINGS

American Lung Society (http://www.lungusa.org). Accessed September 27, 2005.

A clinical practice guideline for treating tobacco use and dependence. A U.S. Public Health Service Report. *JAMA* 2000;283:3244–3254.

Glynn TJ, Manley MW. A National Cancer Institute manual for physicians. How to help your patient stop smoking. NIH Publication No. 92-3064. Bethesda, MD: National Institutes of Health. Reprinted September 1992:1–77.

Jorenby DE, Leischow SJ, Nides MA, et al. A controlled trial of sustained-release bupropion, a nicotine patch, or both for smoking cessation. *N Engl J Med* 1999; 340(9):685–691.

National Cancer Institute (http://www.nci.nih.gov). Accessed September 27, 2005.

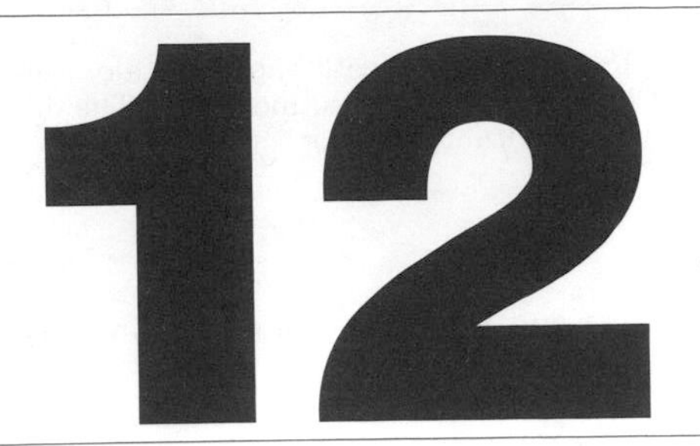

Community-Acquired Pneumonia

K. Cajal Sumino and
Adrian Shifren

INTRODUCTION

Community-acquired pneumonia (CAP) ranks sixth among all causes of death in the United States and is the number one cause of death from infection. It is also a leading cause of morbidity, resulting in >1 million hospitalizations annually. The mortality rate varies widely depending on the treatment setting (outpatient vs inpatient vs ICU), the presence or absence of associated comorbidities, and the age of the patient.

The etiology of CAP varies significantly with treatment setting too. In approximately half of all cases, an etiologic agent is never identified, making it difficult to assess infection patterns and provide empiric treatment. Although new and improved antimicrobials continue to become available, bacterial resistance is in a state of continuous flux. Recent studies have also shown that early institution of appropriate therapy for severe pneumonia has significant benefit on patient survival. Thus, **the correct management of CAP is a *high* priority** with significant patient outcome and financial implications.

The most widely recognized guidelines for the treatment of CAP include those of the American Thoracic Society (ATS), the Infectious Diseases Society of America, and the Canadian Infectious Disease Society and Canadian Thoracic Society. All take into account factors associated with a poor prognosis and provide treatment guidelines based on prognostic groups. All are excellent references, but this chapter closely follows the recommendations of the ATS, with minor modifications. It is important to note that these guidelines exclude patients with HIV.

SITE OF CARE

The initial decision to hospitalize patients or not is important. In most cases, hospitalization is an indication that patients will benefit from close observation before completing outpatient therapy. In others, however, it may indicate the need for longer-term or intensive medical care. Numerous studies have identified risk factors predicting complications (including death) associated with CAP. On inspection, most of these risk factors represent impending or existing organ failure. They are used to guide admission, because patients at risk for complications need closer observation (and therefore admission).

These risk factors are listed in Table 12-1. In general, the greater the number of risk factors, the greater the need for admission. However, the ultimate decision to admit a patient is a clinical one made by the physician and is assisted by the presence or absence of risk factors. Other information, such as outpatient support, patient level of functioning, and access to follow-up care, needs to be included in the decision.

INPATIENT TESTING

Outpatient testing for CAP should include a chest x-ray (CXR) and possibly a sputum Gram's stain (see below). Inpatient testing is usually more extensive and aids in predicting severity but is expensive. Not all testing is mandatory (and some tests are controversial). Therefore, discretion is required.

Most patients admitted through an ER already have had a routine workup performed. This evaluation usually includes a CBC and basic metabolic panel. These can

TABLE 12-1. RISK FACTORS PREDICTING COMPLICATED PNEUMONIA

History
Age >65 yrs
Coexisting illness (COPD, congestive heart failure, chronic liver disease, chronic renal failure, cerebrovascular disease, hospitalization within the last year, others)
Physical
Respiratory rate >30/min
Heart rate >125/min
Temperature >40°C or <35°C
SBP <90 mm Hg or DBP <60 mm Hg
Altered mental status
Evidence of extrapulmonary infection
Test data
WBC count $<4 \times 10^9$/L or $>30 \times 10^9$/L
Absolute neutrophil count $<1 \times 10^9$/L
Hct <30% or Hgb <9 mg/dL
Creatinine >1.2 mg/dL or BUN >20 mg/dL
Pa_{O_2} <60 mm Hg or Pa_{CO_2} >50 mm Hg breathing room air
Arterial pH <7.35
Chest x-ray
Multilobar involvement
Pleural effusion
Cavitation

Adapted from Niederman MS, Mandell LA, Anzueto A, et al. Guidelines for the management of community-acquired pneumonia: diagnosis, assessment of severity, antimicrobial therapy, and prevention. ATS Statement. *Am J Respir Crit Care Med* 2001;163:1730–1754.

be obtained on admission but are not mandatory once the decision to admit the patient has been made.

If not already performed before admission, obtaining **a good-quality posteroanterior** and **lateral CXR is mandatory.**

Sputum Gram's stain is controversial. The physician needs to get an appropriate lower respiratory tract sample, in the absence of which a Gram's stain is a useless study. Currently, no good data exist comparing sputum Gram's stains and bronchoalveolar lavage cultures (the diagnostic standard). Gram's staining is used to broaden therapeutic coverage if organisms in the specimen are not already covered. It is not used to focus therapy.

Routine sputum cultures often demonstrate the growth of pathogenic organisms, but the overall sensitivity and specificity of these cultures are poor. Positive cultures can be tested for susceptibility to various drugs and to establish isolate resistance patterns. All cultures should be obtained before antibiotic administration.

Pulse oximetry allows for the rapid evaluation of patient oxygenation only. ABG data are much more informative and should be obtained at least once in all patients with comorbid disease, especially cardiac or pulmonary disease.

Any significant **pleural effusion** (>10 mm on a lateral decubitus film) should be sampled (preferably before antibiotic therapy). This evaluation helps rule out empyema or complicated pleural effusions needing thoracostomy. Pleural fluid testing should include cell count and differential, protein, lactate dehydrogenase, pH, glucose, Gram's stain, and culture.

placebo-controlled trial demonstrated an 18% success rate with bupropion alone an 22% success rate with a combination of bupropion and a nicotine patch. The diff ence between the groups was statistically insignificant, however.

Second-Line Therapies

Nortriptyline

Nortriptyline and other antidepressants are being investigated for efficacy in smoking cessation. Bupropion remains the only antidepressant that has a smoking cessation indication.

Anxiolytics

Benzodiazepines and buspirone have been used in patients demonstrating increased anxiety during smoking cessation. Although there is no proven benefit for the use of these drugs in smoking cessation, they may be helpful in selected individuals.

Clonidine

Some physicians have tried to diminish withdrawal symptoms through clonidine use. There is little evidence to support the use of clonidine in smoking cessation.

Others

Other aids that are used but are unproven are hypnosis, acupuncture, biofeedback, and relaxation. Smoking cessation groups are often organized by hospitals or workplaces with the assistance of the American Lung Association.

CONCLUSION

Nicotine dependence warrants repeated intervention. Multiple attempts and failures should be expected before success is achieved. All patients deserve pharmacologic intervention unless medically contraindicated. Counseling is an important contributor to success. Accepted pharmacologic therapies include NRT and bupropion.

KEY POINTS TO REMEMBER

- Cigarette smoking contributes to vascular endothelial damage, coronary vasospasm, and increased platelet aggregation and is a known risk factor for coronary artery disease, HTN, and stroke.
- Nicotine has addictive properties, and people become physiologically dependent on its effects. People who quit experience withdrawal symptoms with the peak varying from 24 hrs to 4 wks after quitting.
- The "Five As" for treating tobacco use and dependence are *A*sk, *A*dvise, *A*ssess, Assist, and *A*ction.
- All patients deserve pharmacologic intervention unless medically contraindicated.

REFERENCES AND SUGGESTED READINGS

American Lung Society (http://www.lungusa.org). Accessed September 27, 2005.

A clinical practice guideline for treating tobacco use and dependence. A U.S. P Health Service Report. *JAMA* 2000;283:3244–3254.

Glynn TJ, Manley MW. A National Cancer Institute manual for physicians. help your patient stop smoking. NIH Publication No. 92-3064. Bethe National Institutes of Health. Reprinted September 1992:1–77.

Jorenby DE, Leischow SJ, Nides MA, et al. A controlled trial of susta bupropion, a nicotine patch, or both for smoking cessation. *N Engl* 340(9):685–691.

National Cancer Institute (http://www.nci.nih.gov). Accessed Septemb

12 Community-Acquired Pneumonia

K. Cajal Sumino and
Adrian Shifren

INTRODUCTION

Community-acquired pneumonia (CAP) ranks sixth among all causes of death in the United States and is the number one cause of death from infection. It is also a leading cause of morbidity, resulting in >1 million hospitalizations annually. The mortality rate varies widely depending on the treatment setting (outpatient vs inpatient vs ICU), the presence or absence of associated comorbidities, and the age of the patient.

The etiology of CAP varies significantly with treatment setting too. In approximately half of all cases, an etiologic agent is never identified, making it difficult to assess infection patterns and provide empiric treatment. Although new and improved antimicrobials continue to become available, bacterial resistance is in a state of continuous flux. Recent studies have also shown that early institution of appropriate therapy for severe pneumonia has significant benefit on patient survival. Thus, **the correct management of CAP is a *high* priority** with significant patient outcome and financial implications.

The most widely recognized guidelines for the treatment of CAP include those of the American Thoracic Society (ATS), the Infectious Diseases Society of America, and the Canadian Infectious Disease Society and Canadian Thoracic Society. All take into account factors associated with a poor prognosis and provide treatment guidelines based on prognostic groups. All are excellent references, but this chapter closely follows the recommendations of the ATS, with minor modifications. It is important to note that these guidelines exclude patients with HIV.

SITE OF CARE

The initial decision to hospitalize patients or not is important. In most cases, hospitalization is an indication that patients will benefit from close observation before completing outpatient therapy. In others, however, it may indicate the need for longer-term or intensive medical care. Numerous studies have identified risk factors predicting complications (including death) associated with CAP. On inspection, most of these risk factors represent impending or existing organ failure. They are used to guide admission, because patients at risk for complications need closer observation (and therefore admission).

These risk factors are listed in Table 12-1. In general, the greater the number of risk factors, the greater the need for admission. However, the ultimate decision to admit a patient is a clinical one made by the physician and is assisted by the presence absence of risk factors. Other information, such as outpatient support, patient level unctioning, and access to follow-up care, needs to be included in the decision.

...ENT TESTING

...t testing for CAP should include a chest x-ray (CXR) and possibly a sputum ...n (see below). Inpatient testing is usually more extensive and aids in pre...ty but is expensive. Not all testing is mandatory (and some tests are con... ...erefore, discretion is required.

... admitted through an ER already have had a routine workup per... ...uation usually includes a CBC and basic metabolic panel. These can

TABLE 12-1. RISK FACTORS PREDICTING COMPLICATED PNEUMONIA

History
- Age >65 yrs
- Coexisting illness (COPD, congestive heart failure, chronic liver disease, chronic renal failure, cerebrovascular disease, hospitalization within the last year, others)

Physical
- Respiratory rate >30/min
- Heart rate >125/min
- Temperature >40°C or <35°C
- SBP <90 mm Hg or DBP <60 mm Hg
- Altered mental status
- Evidence of extrapulmonary infection

Test data
- WBC count $<4 \times 10^9$/L or $>30 \times 10^9$/L
- Absolute neutrophil count $<1 \times 10^9$/L
- Hct <30% or Hgb <9 mg/dL
- Creatinine >1.2 mg/dL or BUN >20 mg/dL
- Pa_{O_2} <60 mm Hg or Pa_{CO_2} >50 mm Hg breathing room air
- Arterial pH <7.35

Chest x-ray
- Multilobar involvement
- Pleural effusion
- Cavitation

Adapted from Niederman MS, Mandell LA, Anzueto A, et al. Guidelines for the management of community-acquired pneumonia: diagnosis, assessment of severity, antimicrobial therapy, and prevention. ATS Statement. *Am J Respir Crit Care Med* 2001;163:1730–1754.

be obtained on admission but are not mandatory once the decision to admit the patient has been made.

If not already performed before admission, obtaining **a good-quality posteroanterior** and **lateral CXR is mandatory.**

Sputum Gram's stain is controversial. The physician needs to get an appropriate lower respiratory tract sample, in the absence of which a Gram's stain is a useless study. Currently, no good data exist comparing sputum Gram's stains and bronchoalveolar lavage cultures (the diagnostic standard). Gram's staining is used to broaden therapeutic coverage if organisms in the specimen are not already covered. It is not used to focus therapy.

Routine sputum cultures often demonstrate the growth of pathogenic organisms, but the overall sensitivity and specificity of these cultures are poor. Positive cultures can be tested for susceptibility to various drugs and to establish isolate resistance patterns. All cultures should be obtained before antibiotic administration.

Pulse oximetry allows for the rapid evaluation of patient oxygenation only. ABG data are much more informative and should be obtained at least once in all patients with comorbid disease, especially cardiac or pulmonary disease.

Any significant **pleural effusion** (>10 mm on a lateral decubitus film) should be sampled (preferably before antibiotic therapy). This evaluation helps rule out empyema or complicated pleural effusions needing thoracostomy. Pleural fluid testing should include cell count and differential, protein, lactate dehydrogenase, pH, glucose, Gram's stain, and culture.

V testing should be offered to all patients between the ages of 15 and 55 yrs.
***ionella* urine antigen** is useful in cases in which *Legionella pneumophila* is spected.

THERAPY

The premise of most guidelines for therapy of CAP is that **rapid empiric therapy,** which may be narrowed at a later time, is the most effective form of treatment. Empiric therapy must avoid excessively broad and unnecessary coverage while still providing sufficient activity to ensure eradication of all common pathogens. As such, most guidelines stratify patients into groups, identify common pathogens in each group, and devise therapeutic strategies effective for the pathogens in each group. (The ATS guidelines, which have been verified clinically, are followed in slightly modified form here.)

The ATS stratifies patients based on **site of therapy** (outpatient, inpatient, or ICU); the presence or absence of **coexisting cardiopulmonary disease** (CPD) such as cardiac, lung, or renal disease; and the presence of **modifying factors** (MFs) such as patients at risk for drug-resistant organisms, gram-negative organisms, or *Pseudomonas aeruginosa*. Using the stratification system, patients may be placed into one of three site-of-therapy groups (below), which then determines the empiric treatment used. Treatment for each group of patients is summarized in Table 12-2. Careful attention should be paid to the route of therapy (PO or IV) and the combinations of therapy described.

Outpatients
- (a) without CPD, no MF
- (b) with CPD or MF

Inpatients
- (a) without CPD or MF
- (b) with CPD or MF

ICU patients
- (a) not at risk for *P. aeruginosa* infection
- (b) at risk for *P. aeruginosa* infection

Duration of Therapy

Scant data exist on the optimal duration of therapy for either the outpatient or inpatient management of CAP. Traditionally, therapy has been given for 7–14 days depending on the severity of illness. However, the emergence of newer longer-acting drugs (e.g., azithromycin) has resulted in much shorter courses of therapy, especially in the outpatient setting (the total duration of therapeutic drug levels in the serum still approaches that of traditional therapy, however). As a rule, **5–10 days** of therapy are recommended for **typical pneumonias** (even in the presence of bacteremia), and **7–14 days** for **atypical infections** such as *Mycoplasma pneumoniae, Chlamydia pneumoniae,* and *Legionella pneumophila.*

Switching from IV to Oral Therapy

There are also no good data on when to switch from IV to oral therapy when treating inpatient CAP. It is generally accepted that, once patients are clinically stabilized, they can be switched to oral therapy. However, the criteria for stabilization have yet to be determined. Bacteremic patients generally take longer to reach a state of clinical stability, but once stable, these patients should be switched to oral therapy in the same fashion as nonbacteremic patients. The following criteria are recommended for switching to oral therapy:

- Improvement in symptoms
- Afebrile (<38.3°C) on two occasions >8 hrs apart
- Decreasing WBC count
- Good oral intake

TABLE 12-2. SITE-BASED THERAPY FOR COMMUNITY-ACQUIRED PNEUMONIA

Outpatient therapy

- Common organisms resulting in pneumonia in this group of patients include *Streptococcus pneumoniae, Mycoplasma pneumoniae, Chlamydia pneumoniae, Haemophilus influenzae, Legionella pneumophila* (less common).
- Without cardiopulmonary disease or risk factors:
  - Oral advanced generation macrolide (azithromycin, clarithromycin), or
  - Oral doxycycline
- With cardiopulmonary disease or risk factors:
  - Oral beta-lactam (cefuroxime, amoxicillin/clavulanate) and advanced generation macrolide (azithromycin, clarithromycin), or
  - Oral antipneumococcal fluoroquinolone (levofloxacin, gatifloxacin)

Inpatient therapy

- Common organisms resulting in pneumonia in this group of patients include *S. pneumoniae* (including drug-resistant strains), *M. pneumoniae, C. pneumoniae, H. influenzae, L. pneumophila* (less common), enteric gram-negatives, *Moraxella catarrhalis,* aspiration (anaerobes).
- Without cardiopulmonary disease or risk factors:
  - IV advanced generation macrolide (azithromycin), or
  - IV antipneumococcal fluoroquinolone (levofloxacin)
- With cardiopulmonary disease or risk factors:
  - IV beta-lactam (ceftriaxone, cefotaxime) and advanced generation macrolide (azithromycin, clarithromycin), or
  - IV antipneumococcal fluoroquinolone (levofloxacin, gatifloxacin)

ICU therapy

- Organisms: *S. pneumoniae* (including drug-resistant strains), *M. pneumoniae, C. pneumoniae, H. influenzae,* enteric gram-negatives, *M. catarrhalis, L. pneumophila,* aspiration (anaerobes), *Staphylococcus aureus* ± *Pseudomonas aeruginosa.*
- Without risks for *P. aeruginosa:*
  - IV beta-lactam (ceftriaxone, cefotaxime) and advanced generation macrolide (azithromycin, clarithromycin), or
  - IV antipneumococcal fluoroquinolone (levofloxacin)
- With risks for *P. aeruginosa:*
  - IV antipseudomonal beta-lactam (cefepime, imipenem, piperacillin/tazobactam) and antipseudomonal fluoroquinolone (ciprofloxacin), or
  - IV antipseudomonal beta-lactam (cefepime, imipenem, piperacillin/tazobactam) and aminoglycoside (gentamicin) and advanced generation macrolide (azithromycin, clarithromycin)

Adapted from Niederman MS, Mandell LA, Anzueto A, et al. Guidelines for the management of community-acquired pneumonia: diagnosis, assessment of severity, antimicrobial therapy, and prevention. ATS Statement. *Am J Respir Crit Care Med* 2001;163:1730–1754.

The switch to oral therapy can be made in two ways. The first is known as **sequential therapy,** which involves switching from an IV drug to the same drug in an oral formulation in which the drug levels are comparable independent of the route of administration. These drugs include the fluoroquinolones and doxycycline. The second type of switch is known as **step-down therapy,** which involves drugs in which there is an appreciable decrease in the serum levels when switching from IV to oral therapy (drug levels depend on the route of administration). These drugs include the beta-lactams and the macrolides.

When all four of the recommended criteria for switching to oral therapy are met, the likelihood of recurrence of pneumonia is very low as long as the correct oral antibiotic is selected. Most important in selection (especially when the offending pathogen is unknown) is that the spectrum of coverage is continued when the switch is made.

HOSPITAL DISCHARGE

Because the switch to oral therapy should be made when the patient is clinically stable, patients are generally fit for discharge at the time the switch to oral therapy is made. In-hospital observation of oral therapy only adds to costs and length of stay. However, not every patient who can be switched to oral therapy is eligible for discharge. Some patients may need longer stays to manage their comorbid diseases. Repeat CXR during the hospitalization is generally not recommended because radiographic resolution in response to therapy may take up to 6 wks. Rather, a **follow-up CXR** is recommended at an **outpatient visit 4–6 wks after discharge.**

KEY POINTS TO REMEMBER

- Outpatient testing for CAP should include CXR and possibly a sputum Gram's stain.
- Pleural fluid testing should include cell count and differential, protein, LDH, pH, glucose, Gram's stain, and culture.
- HIV testing should be offered to all patients between the ages of 15 and 55 years.
- In the outpatient setting, common organisms resulting in pneumonia include *S. pneumoniae, M. pneumoniae, C. pneumoniae, H. influenzae*, and *L. pneumophila* (less common).
- In the inpatient setting, common organisms resulting in pneumonia include *S. pneumoniae* (including drug-resistant strains), *M. pneumoniae, C. pneumoniae, H. influenzae, L. pneumophila* (less common), enteric gram-negatives, *M. catarrhalis, L. pneumophila*, and anaerobes (aspiration).
- Empiric therapy using multidisciplinary guidelines is currently the most effective method for treating CAP while minimizing the development of antibiotic resistance.

REFERENCES AND SUGGESTED READINGS

Arancibia F, Bauer TT, Ewig S, et al. Community-acquired pneumonia due to gram-negative bacteria and *Pseudomonas aeruginosa*: incidence, risk, and prognosis. *Arch Intern Med* 2002;162(16):1849–1858.

Arancibia F, Ewig S, Martinez JA, et al. Antimicrobial treatment failures in patients with community-acquired pneumonia. Causes and prognostic implications. *Am J Respir Crit Care Med* 2000;162:154–160.

Bartlett JG, Dowell SF, Mandell LA. Practice guidelines for the management of community-acquired pneumonia in adults. Infectious Diseases Society of America. *Clin Infect Dis* 2000;31:347–382.

Bartlett JG, Mundy LM. Current concepts: community-acquired pneumonia. *N Engl J Med* 1995;333:1618–1624.

Fine MJ, Auble TE, Yealy DM, et al. A prediction rule to identify low-risk patients with community-acquired pneumonia. *N Engl J Med* 1997;336:243–250.

Fine MJ, Smith MA, Carson CA. Prognosis and outcomes of patients with community-acquired pneumonia: a meta-analysis. *JAMA* 1996;275:134–141.

Gordon GS, Throop D, Berberian L, et al. Validation of the therapeutic recommendations of the American Thoracic Society guidelines for community-acquired pneumonia in hospitalized patients. *Chest* 1996;110:55S.

Hasley PB, Albaum MN, Li YH, et al. Do pulmonary radiographic findings at presentation predict mortality in patients with community-acquired pneumonia? *Arch Intern Med* 1996;156:2206–2212.

Lim WS, Macfarlane JT, Boswell TCJ, et al. Study of community acquired pneumonia aetiology (SCAPA) in adults admitted to hospital: implications for management guidelines. *Thorax* 2001;56(4):296–301.

Mandell LA, Marrie TJ, Grossman RF, et al. Canadian guidelines for the initial management of community-acquired pneumonia: an evidence-based update by the Canadian Infectious Diseases Society and the Canadian Thoracic Society. The Canadian Community-Acquired Pneumonia Working Group. *Clin Infect Dis* 2000;31:383–421.

Mittl RL, Schwab RJ, Duchin JS, et al. Radiographic resolution of community-acquired pneumonia. *Am J Respir Crit Care Med* 1994;149:630–635.

Niederman MS, Mandell LA, Anzueto A, et al. Guidelines for the management of community-acquired pneumonia: diagnosis, assessment of severity, antimicrobial therapy, and prevention. American Thoracic Society statement. *Am J Respir Crit Care Med* 2001;163:1730–1754.

Ramirez JA. Managing anti-infective therapy of community-acquired pneumonia in the hospital setting: focus on switch therapy. *Pharmacotherapy* 2001;21:79S.

Ruiz M, Ewig S, Marcos MA, et al. Etiology of community-acquired pneumonia: impact of age, comorbidity, and severity. *Am J Respir Crit Care Med* 1999;160: 397–405.

Skerrett SJ. Diagnostic testing for community-acquired pneumonia. *Clin Chest Med* 1999;20:531–548.

13 Hospital-Acquired Pneumonia

Shiraz A. Daud and
Marin H. Kollef

INTRODUCTION

Hospital-acquired pneumonia (HAP) can be divided into **nosocomial pneumonia (NP)** and **ventilator-acquired pneumonia (VAP).** NP is the most clinically significant hospital-acquired infection and the leading cause of death from all nosocomial infections. The rise in hospital-associated infections due to antibiotic-resistant bacteria has resulted from the increasingly recognized administration of inadequate antimicrobial regimens. Inadequate initial antibiotic treatment of NP increases the risk of hospital mortality and may also further predispose to the emergence of antibiotic-resistant bacteria. Clinicians treating patients with NP should be aware of the difficulties in establishing an accurate diagnosis of NP. **NP** is defined as **pneumonia occurring >48 hrs after admission to the hospital. VAP** occurs in 8–28% of patients requiring mechanical ventilation and is defined as **pneumonia occurring >48 hrs after intubation of the trachea and initiation of mechanical ventilation.** VAP appears to be an independent determinant of mortality in critically ill patients requiring mechanical ventilation, and mortality rates have ranged from 25% to 50% in different series. More important, emerging clinical data suggest that the application of new management strategies for the prevention and treatment of VAP could result in improved patient outcomes. It should be noted that this chapter does not include nosocomial infections involving the immunocompromised host.

ETIOLOGY AND PATHOGENESIS

Infectious organisms that commonly result in NP are generally different from those that are most commonly associated with community-acquired pneumonia. NP can be divided into early- and late-onset infections. Those that occur within the **first 4 days** of hospitalization are referred to as **early onset.** These infections are usually due to common community-acquired pathogens such as *Streptococcus pneumoniae*, methicillin-sensitive *Staphylococcus aureus*, and *Haemophilus influenzae*. Specific risk factors have been associated with certain pathogens. Aspiration has been associated with anaerobes, gram-negative enteric bacilli, and *S. aureus*. **Late-onset NP** occurs **after 4 days** of hospitalization and is associated with more virulent organisms such as methicillin-resistant *S. aureus*, *Pseudomonas aeruginosa,* and *Acinetobacter* species.

The pathogenesis of NP and VAP is linked to two separate but related processes: colonization of the aerodigestive tract with pathogenic organisms and aspiration of contaminated secretions. The **most common sources of NP pathogens** are microaspiration of oropharyngeal secretions, aspiration of esophageal/gastric contents, inhalation of infected aerosols, hematogenous spread from distant infection, exogenous penetration from the pleural space, or direct inoculation (e.g., resulting from intubation). Bacterial colonization of the oropharynx is universal, and *S. pneumoniae,* various anaerobes, and, occasionally, *H. influenzae* are found in the oropharynx of normal subjects. However, colonization with gram-negative bacilli, notably virulent organisms such as *P. aeruginosa* and *Acinetobacter* species, is rare in healthy individuals. It is known that oropharyngeal and tracheal colonization with *P. aeruginosa* and enteric gram-negative bacilli increases with length of hospital stay and with severity of illness. **Aspiration** of oropharyngeal secretions is not uncommon, even in health. Approximately 45% of healthy subjects were shown in one study to aspirate during sleep, and the rate of aspiration is higher in patients with impaired levels of consciousness and inability to protect their airway from aspiration events. Factors promoting aspiration include an overall reduced level of consciousness, a blunted gag reflex, abnormal swallowing for any reason, delayed gastric emptying, or decreased GI motility. Reflux and aspiration of nonsterile gastric contents is also a possible mechanism of pathogen entry into the lungs, although its role is generally less significant than that of oropharyngeal colonization. The stomach has been implicated, particularly in late-onset VAP, as a potential reservoir for the aspiration of contaminated secretions.

RISK FACTORS

A number of risk factors for the development of NP and VAP have been described. These risk factors generally promote either aspiration or colonization of the aerodigestive tract with pathogenic bacteria (Table 13-1).

PRESENTATION

NP or VAP is usually suspected when a patient develops a **new or progressive pulmonary infiltrate with fever, leukocytosis, and purulent tracheobronchial secretions.** However, a number of noninfectious causes of fever and pulmonary infiltrates can also occur in these patients, making clinical criteria nonspecific for the diagnosis of NP. Noninfectious causes of fever and pulmonary infiltrates that can mimic NP include chemical aspiration without infection, atelectasis, pulmonary embolism, ARDS, pulmonary hemorrhage, lung contusion, infiltrative tumor, radiation pneumonitis, and drug or hypersensitivity reactions. A number of studies have demonstrated the limitations of using clinical parameters alone for establishing the diagnosis of VAP. Autopsy results in a series of patients with acute lung injury demonstrated that clinical criteria alone led to an incorrect diagnosis of VAP in 29% of clinically suspected cases. However, the conclusion that clinical diagnosis of VAP is markedly inferior to other methods has not been universal. Clinical criteria for the diagnosis of VAP have been used to manage antibiotic therapy more effectively. One group of investigators used the **Clinical Pulmonary Infection Score** to limit the duration of antibiotic therapy for patients at low risk for VAP. The Clinical Pulmonary Infection Score is a simple scoring system evaluating temperature, blood leukocyte

TABLE 13-1. RISK FACTORS FOR HOSPITAL-ACQUIRED PNEUMONIA

Aspiration	Colonization of the aerodigestive tract
Witnessed aspiration	COPD
Supine positioning	Use of histamine type-2 antagonists
Coma	Tracheostomy
Enteral nutrition	Prior antibiotic exposure
Reintubation	Age >60 yrs
Tracheostomy	ARDS
ARDS	
Head trauma	
ICP monitoring	

count, tracheal secretions, oxygenation, and pulmonary infiltrates. Such a strategy may allow improved use of empiric antibiotics for patients with suspected VAP; however, a subsequent study failed to confirm the diagnostic accuracy of this approach.

The limitations and inaccuracies in clinical decision making have been the motivation for using other techniques to diagnose VAP. These techniques include a variety of methods for sampling material from the airways and alveoli, including bronchoscopic and nonbronchoscopic techniques. At the present time, **bronchoscopic sampling of the lower airways,** using either a protected specimen brush or bronchoalveolar lavage, is accepted as the most accurate method of diagnosing VAP, short of direct tissue examination. Quantitative or semiquantitative cultures are usually performed on the bronchoscopic specimens, with the diagnosis of VAP being made when some appropriate threshold is exceeded. From a practical standpoint, quantitative cultures between 100 and 1000 cfu/mL for protected specimen brush specimens and between 1000 and 10,000 cfu/mL for bronchoalveolar lavage specimens should probably be considered positive. It is important to note that few studies have shown that lower airway specimens obtained with bronchoscopic sampling meaningfully influence patient outcomes.

The ease with which **tracheal aspirates** can be obtained makes them an attractive alternative diagnostic technique for patients with suspected VAP. However, tracheal aspirates are nonspecific for establishing the diagnosis of VAP, because tracheobronchial bacterial colonization is common in critically ill patients as a consequence of biofilm formation on the surface of ETTs. As a result, tracheal aspirates have been of limited utility because of the increased accuracy of specimens obtained by bronchoscopy. Nevertheless, tracheal aspirate specimens have good overall sensitivity for the identification of pathogens associated with VAP.

MANAGEMENT

There are two overriding principles that make up the strategy of antibiotic treatment of HAP. The first is to **provide an adequate initial antimicrobial regimen** that is likely to be active against the pathogen(s) causing infection. The second principle is to **limit the unnecessary use of antibiotics.** The strategy of deescalation attempts to unify these two principles into a single strategy that optimizes patient outcomes while minimizing the emergence of antibiotic resistance. The first principle of antibiotic deescalation requires the administration of an adequate empiric regimen to patients with suspected HAP. Decisions regarding antibiotic selection often occur in the absence of identified pathogens. It is imperative that clinicians be aware of the microorganisms likely to be associated with infection and inadequate antimicrobial treatment in their patient population. The most common pathogens associated with the administration of inadequate antimicrobial treatment in patients with HAP include potentially antibiotic-resistant gram-negative bacteria (*P. aeruginosa, Acinetobacter* species, *Klebsiella pneumoniae,* and *Enterobacter* species) and *S. aureus,* especially the strains with methicillin resistance. However, it is important to recognize that the **predominant pathogens** associated with hospital-associated infections **may vary between hospitals** as well as **between specialized units within individual hospitals.** Therefore, clinicians should be aware of the prevailing bacterial pathogens in their hospitals and their associated antimicrobial susceptibilities. This awareness should help in the selection of empiric antibiotic regimens that are less likely to provide inadequate treatment for hospital-associated infections. The second goal of antibiotic deescalation is to avoid the unnecessary administration of antibiotics. Physicians practicing in the hospital setting are frequently faced with the dilemma of caring for acutely ill patients with suspected nosocomial infection owing to the presence of nonspecific clinical findings (fever, leukocytosis, hemodynamic instability). Failure to provide treatment with an adequate initial antimicrobial regimen may result in greater morbidity, whereas unnecessary antibiotic treatment can lead to colonization or

TABLE 13-2. THERAPY FOR VENTILATOR-ACQUIRED PNEUMONIA (VAP)

Early-onset VAP, no specific risk factors

Organisms: Enteric gram-negatives, including *Enterobacter* spp., *Escherichia coli, Klebsiella* spp., *Proteus* spp., *Serratia marcescens.* Also *Streptococcus pneumoniae, Haemophilus influenzae,* and methicillin-sensitive *Staphylococcus aureus.*

Therapy: Nonpseudomonal third-generation cephalosporin (ceftriaxone) or beta-lactam–beta-lactamase inhibitor combination (ampicillin/sulbactam). For penicillin-allergic patients, fluoroquinolone or clindamycin plus aztreonam.

Late-onset VAP

Organisms: Any of the above organisms plus *Pseudomonas aeruginosa, Acinetobacter baumanii,* methicillin-resistant *S. aureus.*

Therapy: Aminoglycoside or antipseudomonal fluoroquinolone (ciprofloxacin) plus antipseudomonal penicillin (imipenem) ± vancomycin.

infection with antibiotic-resistant pathogens. Recommended therapies are summarized in Table 13-2.

Duration of Therapy

Despite the thoroughness of many guidelines, durations of therapy remain an imprecise science. Treatment for 7–10 days has been advocated for treatment of *S. aureus* or *H. influenzae* infection, whereas a long course of antibiotics has been proposed for gram-negative necrotizing pneumonias or with isolation of *Pseudomonas* spp. Recently, the results of a large randomized trial comparing 8 days of adequate antibiotic therapy for VAP to 15 days of treatment showed similar efficacy. However, the longer course of antibiotic therapy was associated with statistically greater emergence of multiply resistant bacteria.

There have been promising data that show that scheduled alterations in antibiotic prescription patterns, or **antibiotic rotation,** are associated with declining antibiotic resistance patterns.

PREVENTION STRATEGIES

A number of pharmacologic and nonpharmacologic maneuvers have been studied as modalities to minimize NP and VAP. The strategies with best clinical evidence include those in Table 13-3.

TABLE 13-3. EFFECTIVE PREVENTION STRATEGIES FOR HOSPITAL-ACQUIRED PNEUMONIA

Effective hand washing by hospital personnel

Protective gowns and gloves

Avoiding large gastric volumes

Oral (nonnasal) intubation

Stress ulcer prophylaxis using non–pH-lowering agents in intubated patients

Avoiding unnecessary antibiotics

Adequate initial empiric antibiotic therapy

Antibiotic class rotation

KEY POINTS TO REMEMBER

- NP is defined as pneumonia occurring >48 hrs after admission to the hospital. VAP is defined as pneumonia occurring >48 hrs after intubation of the trachea and initiation of mechanical ventilation.
- Bronchoscopic sampling of the lower airways, using either a protected specimen brush or bronchoalveolar lavage, is accepted as the most accurate method of diagnosing VAP, short of direct tissue examination.
- Clinicians should be aware of the prevailing bacterial pathogens in their hospitals and their associated antimicrobial susceptibilities. This should help in the selection of empiric antibiotic regimens that are less likely to provide inadequate treatment for hospital-associated infections.
- There are promising data that scheduled alterations in antibiotic prescription patterns, or antibiotic rotation, are associated with declining antibiotic resistance patterns.

REFERENCES AND SUGGESTED READINGS

Adair CG, Gorman SP, Feron BM, et al. Implications of endotracheal tube biofilm for ventilator-associated pneumonia. *Intensive Care Med* 1999;25:1072–1076.

Andrews CP, Coalson JJ, Smith JD, Johanson WG Jr. Diagnosis of nosocomial bacterial pneumonia in acute, diffuse lung injury. *Chest* 1981;80:254–258.

Atherton ST, White DJ. Stomach as a source of bacteria colonizing respiratory tract artificial ventilation. *Lancet* 1978;2:968–969.

Bergmans DC, Bonten MJ, van Tiel FH, et al. Cross-colonization with *Pseudomonas aeruginosa* of patients in an intensive care unit. *Thorax* 1998;53:1053–1058.

Chastre J, Fagon JY. Ventilator-associated pneumonia. *Am J Respir Crit Care Med* 2002;165:867–903.

Chastre J, Wolff M, Fagon JY, Chevret S. Comparison of two durations of antibiotic therapy to treat ventilator-associated pneumonia (VAP). *Am J Respir Crit Care Med* 2003;167:A21.

Cook DJ, Kollef MH. Risk factors for ICU-acquired pneumonia. *JAMA* 1998;279:1605–1606.

Cross JT, Campbell GD. Therapy of nosocomial pneumonia. *Med Clin North Am* 2001;85:1583–1594.

du Moulin GC, Paterson DG, Hedley-Whyte J, Lisbon A. Aspiration of gastric bacteria in antacid-treated patients: a frequent cause of postoperative colonization of the airway. *Lancet* 1982;1:242–245.

Fabregas N, Ewig S, Torres A, et al. Clinical diagnosis of ventilator associated pneumonia revisited: comparative validation using immediate post-mortem lung biopsies. *Thorax* 1999;54:867–873.

Fagon JY, Chastre J, Hance AJ, et al. Detection of nosocomial lung infection in ventilated patients: use of a protected specimen brush and quantitative culture techniques in 147 patients. *Am Rev Respir Dis* 1988;138:110–116.

Fagon JY, Chastre J, Hance AJ, et al. Evaluation of clinical judgment in the identification and treatment of nosocomial pneumonia in ventilated patients. *Chest* 1993;103:547–553.

Fagon JY, Chastre J, Wolff M, et al. Invasive and noninvasive strategies for management of suspected ventilator-associated pneumonia. A randomized trial. *Ann Intern Med* 2000;132:621–630.

Fartoukh M, Maitre B, Honore S, et al. Diagnosing pneumonia during mechanical ventilation: the clinical pulmonary infection score revisited. *Am J Respir Crit Care Med* 2003;168:173–179.

Heyland DK, Cook DJ, Marshall J, et al. The clinical utility of invasive diagnostic techniques in the setting of ventilator-associated pneumonia. *Chest* 1999;115:1076–1084.

Kirtland SH, Corley DE, Winterbauer RH, et al. The diagnosis of ventilator pneumonia: a comparison of histologic, microbiologic, and clinical criteria. *Chest* 1997;112:445–457.

Kollef MH. Epidemiology and risk factors for nosocomial pneumonia. *Clin Chest Med* 1999;20:653–670.

Kollef MH, Sherman G, Ward S, Fraser VJ. Inadequate antimicrobial treatment of infections. A risk factor for hospital mortality among critically ill patients. *Chest* 1999;115:462–474.

Lynch JP. Hospital-acquired pneumonia: risk factors, microbiology, and treatment. *Chest* 2001;119[Suppl 2]:373S–384S.

Meduri GU. Diagnosis and differential diagnosis of ventilator-associated pneumonia. *Clin Chest Med* 1995;16:61–93.

Niederman MS, Torres A, Summer W. Invasive diagnostic testing is not needed routinely to manage suspected ventilator-associated pneumonia. *Am J Respir Crit Care Med* 1994;150:565–569.

Prod'hom G, Leuenberger P, Koerfer J, et al. Nosocomial pneumonia in mechanically ventilated patients receiving antacid, ranitidine, or sucralfate as prophylaxis for stress ulcer. A randomized controlled trial. *Ann Intern Med* 1994;120:653–662.

Singh N, Rogers P, Atwood CW, et al. Short-course empiric antibiotic therapy for patients with pulmonary infiltrates in the intensive care unit. A proposed solution for indiscriminate antibiotic prescription. *Am J Respir Crit Care Med* 2000;162:505–511.

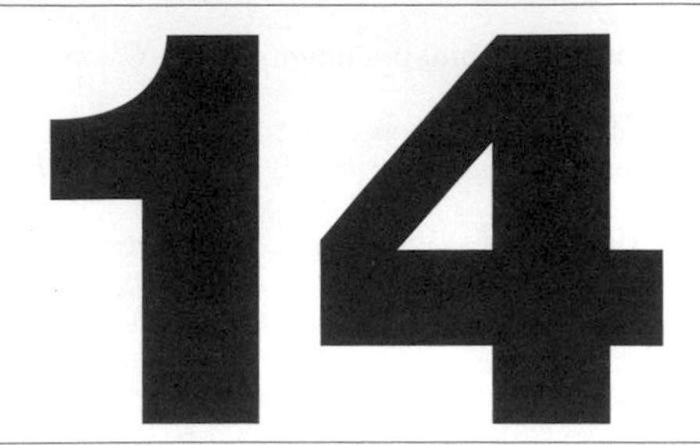

Tuberculosis

Ramsey R. Hachem

INTRODUCTION

TB has affected humans since the beginning of recorded history. Approximately 30% of the world's population is infected, and 2 million people die yearly because of TB worldwide. In the United States, TB rates declined steadily through the 1970s and early 1980s. In the mid-1980s and early 1990s, however, there was a resurgence of TB largely because of the HIV epidemic and increased emigration rates from countries with high rates of TB infection. This increase in TB was concentrated among young, urban, racial and ethnic minorities. Since its peak in 1992, the case rate for TB has decreased steadily. In 2000, 16,377 cases were reported to the CDC. This decrease in incidence is attributed to improved awareness and public health efforts aimed at controlling the spread of TB. However, reactivation of latent TB infection (LTBI) remains a constant source of new disease. Furthermore, in contrast to the current TB situation in the United States, TB remains a significant worldwide public health problem.

CLINICAL PRESENTATION

Mycobacterium tuberculosis is transmitted by airborne particles that are 1–5 μ in diameter. Infection results when a few bacteria are deposited in an alveolus. **Primary infection** is often a self-limited respiratory illness that generally goes undiagnosed. At this stage, chest radiographs often show infiltrates in the middle or lower lobes. Remnants of healed parenchymal lesions appear radiographically as calcified nodules (Ghon's lesions) and are often associated with ipsilateral hilar lymphadenopathy (Ranke's complex). In a small group of patients, rupture of a subpleural caseous focus results in pleuritis. The pleural reaction represents a delayed hypersensitivity reaction to tuberculous proteins. Mycobacterial cultures of pleural fluid in this situation are often negative. The natural history of an untreated, isolated tuberculous effusion is spontaneous resolution, only to recur as active parenchymal disease at a later date.

After primary infection, a precarious balance exists between the host and the bacteria. In approximately 5%, the infection progresses to active disease within 2 yrs of the initial infection. Factors causing this progression are poorly understood. Certain conditions that predispose to reactivation are HIV infection, malnutrition, chronic renal failure, diabetes mellitus, medical immunosuppression, and alcoholism.

Reactivation appears clinically as a subacute illness with classic systemic symptoms including fever, night sweats, and weight loss. Productive cough, hemoptysis, and pleuritic chest pain are common respiratory symptoms. Radiographically, reactivation TB typically presents as fibronodular infiltrates, often with cavitation, in the upper lobes. However, in patients with an impaired cellular immune system, such as those with advanced AIDS, mediastinal lymphadenopathy in the absence of parenchymal infiltrates is more common. In the past, it had been generally accepted that the radiographic findings differ in primary and reactivation TB. Midlobe and lower-lobe infiltrates, mediastinal adenopathy, and pleural effusions were believed to represent primary TB from recent infection, whereas upper-lobe cavitary infiltrates were attributed to reactivation TB from remote infection. Recent evidence suggests that this dichotomy in radiographic findings is not truly present and that those with recent and remote infections often have similar radiographic findings.

DIAGNOSIS

The diagnosis of TB rests on isolation of the organism from infected specimen material. In cases of pulmonary parenchymal TB, **sputum analysis** by **acid-fast stain for AFB** and **mycobacterial cultures** are paramount. Cultures are necessary to determine drug susceptibility and because smears alone miss up to 50% of samples with positive cultures. In the past, 6–8 wks were necessary for culture results. Newer lab techniques using rapid radiometric culture assays have shortened the required time to as little as 1–2 wks. In the right clinical setting, when sputum analysis is nondiagnostic, **fiber-optic bronchoscopy** with bronchoalveolar lavage, transbronchial lung biopsies, and brushings may be diagnostic either of TB or of an alternative diagnosis. All specimens should be evaluated with acid-fast stains and cultures. The histopathologic finding of **caseating granulomatous inflammation** is strongly supportive of the diagnosis of TB while cultures are pending.

Nucleic acid amplification (NAA) tests may facilitate the rapid detection of microorganisms. Commercial kits for the detection of *M. tuberculosis* have been approved by the U.S. Food and Drug Administration. However, specificity is poor when applied to AFB smear–negative specimens, and sensitivity is inadequate when applied to smear-positive specimens. These tests appear to be most helpful by indicating a high likelihood of TB when AFB smears are positive and cultures are pending. Conversely, a negative NAA test does not exclude TB. Therefore, the decision to use NAA tests should be individualized.

Tuberculin Skin Testing

The tuberculin skin test is a valuable tool in the investigation of TB infection. The CDC recommends targeted testing: testing persons at high risk for TB exposure or infection and those at high risk for developing TB disease once infected. Groups that are not at high risk for TB should not be tested routinely because positive skin tests in low-risk persons may not represent TB infection. In general, **persons at high risk for TB exposure or infection** include close contacts of persons who have active TB, foreign-born persons from areas where TB is endemic, residents of high-risk congregate settings (such as correctional facilities and homeless shelters), health care workers caring for high-risk patients, and illicit drug abusers. **Persons at high risk for TB disease** once infected include those with HIV infection, persons recently infected with TB, and those who have chronic medical illnesses (such as diabetes mellitus and renal failure).

The **tuberculin skin test** is performed by injecting a standardized dose of 5 tuberculin units of purified protein derivative intradermally. This injection usually produces a 5- to 10-mm wheal at the time of injection. The reaction should be read **48–72 hrs** after the injection. The area of induration, not erythema, should be measured and recorded. The **interpretation of the skin test** is based on an individual's risk factors for TB infection (Table 14-1). Therefore, a tuberculin reaction ≥**5 mm** is classified as positive in persons infected with HIV, close contacts of someone with active TB, persons with radiographic findings of TB, and others who are immunosuppressed. A tuberculin reaction ≥**10 mm** is classified as positive in foreign-born persons from areas where TB is highly prevalent, injection drug users, persons with underlying medical conditions such as chronic renal failure or diabetes mellitus, and residents of long-term facilities. Finally, a ≥**15-mm** tuberculin reaction is classified as positive in all other persons tested. **Conversion** is defined as an increase in induration of 10 mm in those aged <35 yrs and 15 mm in those aged >35 yrs within a 2-yr period. In all patients, a positive skin test, as defined above, indicates infection with TB.

The skin test is imperfect. Infection with nontuberculous mycobacteria and vaccination with bacille Calmette-Guérin can lead to **false-positive results.** Conversely, immunosuppression may result in anergy and a false-negative result. Other causes of

TABLE 14-1. POSITIVE TUBERCULIN SKIN TESTS

Tuberculin reaction (mm)	Risk factors for TB infection
≥ 5	HIV infection, close contacts of someone with active TB, x-ray findings of TB
≥ 10	Foreign-born persons from areas where TB is endemic, injection drug users, chronic medical illness (renal failure, diabetes)
≥ 15	All others tested

false-negative reactions include recent infection with TB, very young age (<6 mos), and overwhelming TB infection. Finally, up to 25% of patients with documented active TB may have a negative tuberculin skin test.

TREATMENT

Treatment of TB requires the dedicated efforts of clinicians and public health workers. TB infection should be **reported to the public health department** to ensure adequate therapy of the individual, to evaluate close contacts, and to identify potential outbreaks. There are several fundamental principles of TB therapy. Treatment is significantly **longer** than for other infectious diseases because *M. tuberculosis* is a slow-growing organism. However, the shortest adequate course of therapy is necessary to ensure **compliance.** It should consist of **multiple antimycobacterial agents** to which the organism is susceptible to avoid the emergence of drug resistance. Finally, **directly observed therapy** promotes adherence to treatment plans and should be considered for all patients. However, when therapy is self-administered, fixed-dose combination tablets enhance adherence.

First-line antituberculous drugs are listed in Table 14-2. These agents are proven to be effective and are relatively well tolerated. Other, second-line agents, listed in Table 14-3, have been shown to be less effective or more toxic, or have not been studied as extensively as first-line agents. The primary goals of therapy are the eradication of *M. tuberculosis* organisms within the host and the prevention of the emergence of drug resistance.

Within the host, **tuberculous organisms exist in various environments,** and different antituberculous drugs target organisms in different environments. Extracellular organisms growing rapidly along cavity walls and in a liquid necrotic medium are killed best by isoniazid. Slower-growing extracellular organisms found in caseous material that exhibit spurts of growth are killed most effectively by rifampin, which has an onset of action fast enough to kill the organisms during a growth spurt. Slowly growing organisms found within macrophages are targeted most effectively by pyrazinamide, which works best in the intracellular acid pH of macrophages. Finally, there are dormant organisms that cannot be killed until they begin to grow. These mechanisms explain the philosophy of using a multidrug regimen in treating active TB. Other reasons include a rapid decrease in the burden of organisms and a decreased chance for the emergence of drug resistance. The low burden of organisms in the setting of TB infection without active disease (LTBI) allows for the possible use of a single agent, isoniazid, for adequate therapy.

The **duration of therapy** depends on the drugs used, the organism's susceptibility results, and the patient's response to therapy. Table 14-4 shows multiple regimens that may be used. Most patients can be treated with short-course regimens. All regimens of ≤ 9 mos must contain isoniazid and rifampin; 6-mo regimens must contain isoniazid, rifampin, and initially pyrazinamide. The addition of pyridoxine (vitamin B_6), 25–50 mg PO qd, (to prevent neuropathy) should be considered in those patients taking isoniazid. Adults with smear- or culture-positive pulmonary TB can be treated with a 6-mo course consisting of an 8-wk induction phase with isoniazid, rifampin, and pyrazinamide. In areas where primary isoniazid resistance is ≥ 4%, ethambutol or

TABLE 14-2. FIRST-LINE AGENTS

Drug	Daily oral dose (max dose)	Twice weekly (max dose)	Thrice weekly (max dose)	Adverse reactions	Monitoring
Isoniazid	5 mg/kg (300 mg)	15 mg/kg (900 mg)	15 mg/kg (900 mg)	Rash, hepatitis, neuropathy, drug interactions	LFTs
Rifampin	10 mg/kg (600 mg)	10 mg/kg (600 mg)	10 mg/kg (600 mg)	Rash, hepatitis, drug interactions	CBC, LFTs
Rifabutin	5 mg/kg (300 mg)	5 mg/kg (300 mg)	Unknown	Rash, hepatitis, thrombocytopenia, uveitis	CBC, LFTs
Pyrazinamide	15–30 mg/kg (2 g)	50–70 mg/kg (4 g)	50–70 mg/kg (3 g)	Rash, hepatitis, hyperuricemia	Uric acid, LFTs
Ethambutol	15–25 mg/kg	50 mg/kg	25–30 mg/kg	Optic neuritis, rash	Visual acuity, color vision
Streptomycin	15 mg/kg (1 g)	25–30 mg/kg (1.5 g)	25–30 mg/kg (1.5 g)	Ototoxicity, renal dysfunction	Renal function, hearing tests

LFTs, liver function tests.
From Centers for Disease Control and Prevention. Treatment of tuberculosis. American Thoracic Society, CDC, and Infectious Diseases Society of America. *MMWR* 2003;52(RR-11):4–5, with permission.

streptomycin should be included in the induction phase until the organism is proven to be susceptible to both isoniazid and rifampin. The remainder of the 6-mo course consists of isoniazid and rifampin (maintenance phase). Because of the organisms' slow replication times, intermittent dosing (twice or thrice weekly) is effective in the setting of directly observed therapy. When isoniazid, pyrazinamide, and ethambutol are given twice or thrice weekly, their dose must be increased (see Table 14-2); however, the dose of rifampin is the same when given daily or intermittently.

HIV-infected patients do not have a higher incidence of treatment failure or relapse. Therefore, the duration of therapy is similar to that for non–HIV-infected patients as long as there is an appropriate clinical and microbiological response. However, the treatment of TB in the setting of HIV infection is complex because of drug interactions. Protease inhibitors and nonnucleoside reverse transcriptase inhibitors interact with rifampin, resulting in subtherapeutic blood levels of the antiretroviral agents and toxic levels of rifampin. Rifabutin is another rifamycin that is active against *M. tuberculosis* and has fewer interactions with protease inhibitors and nonnucleoside reverse transcriptase inhibitors. This drug can be substituted for rifampin when HIV-infected patients are receiving these antiretrovirals.

Multidrug-Resistant Tuberculosis

Drug-resistant TB is determined on the basis of susceptibility testing of culture data. In the setting of isoniazid resistance, patients should receive rifampin, pyrazinamide,

TABLE 14-3. SECOND-LINE AGENTS

Drug	Oral dose (max dose)	Adverse reactions	Monitoring	Comments
Capreomycin	15–30 mg/kg (1 g)	Ototoxicity, renal	Hearing tests, renal	Dose reduction after response
Kanamycin	15–30 mg/kg (1 g)	Ototoxicity, renal	Hearing tests, renal	Dose reduction after response
Amikacin	15–30 mg/kg (1 g)	Ototoxicity, renal, dizziness	Hearing tests, renal	Dose reduction after response
Ethionamide	15–20 mg/kg (1 g)	Hepatotoxicity, GI upset, metallic taste	LFTs	May cause hypothyroidism, titrate dose
Para-aminosalicylic acid	150 mg/kg	Hepatotoxicity, GI upset, hypersensitivity	LFTs	May cause hypothyroidism, titrate dose
Cycloserine	15–20 mg/kg (1 g)	Rash, depression, psychosis, seizures, headaches	Mental status	Titrate dose, pyridoxine may reduce CNS effects
Ciprofloxacin	1500 mg/day	GI upset, hypersensitivity	Drug interactions	Not FDA approved for TB therapy
Ofloxacin	800 mg/day	GI upset, hypersensitivity	Drug interactions	Not FDA approved for TB therapy
Levofloxacin	500 mg/day	GI upset, hypersensitivity	Drug interactions	Not FDA approved for TB therapy
Clofazimine	300 mg/day	GI upset, skin discoloration, crystal deposition	Drug interactions	Not FDA approved for TB therapy, unproven efficacy

FDA, U.S. Food and Drug Administration; LFTs, liver function tests.
From Centers for Disease Control and Prevention. Treatment of tuberculosis. American Thoracic Society, CDC, and Infectious Diseases Society of America. *MMWR* 2003;52(RR-11):4–5, with permission.

and ethambutol for 6 mos. Rifampin-resistant isolates should be treated with isoniazid and ethambutol for 18 mos or isoniazid, pyrazinamide, and streptomycin for 9 mos. **Isolates resistant to isoniazid and rifampin are defined as multidrug resistant.** The necessary therapy is complex and must be individualized based on the patient's medication history and susceptibility testing. Adequate data are unavailable on the effectiveness of various regimens for the treatment of multidrug-resistant TB. Furthermore, multidrug-resistant isolates are often resistant to first-line agents other than isoniazid and rifampin. In this setting, at least three drugs to which the organism is susceptible should be given. This regimen should be continued until sputum cultures are negative, followed by at least 12 mos of two-drug therapy. Surgical resection, when feasible, can offer significantly improved cure rates; however, drug therapy is still necessary to sterilize remaining disease.

During therapy, patients should be monitored for adverse effects **monthly.** A **chest radiograph** should be obtained at the initiation and completion of therapy to serve as a baseline for future reference. The rapidity of symptom resolution is highly variable.

TABLE 14-4. REGIMENS FOR TREATMENT OF ACTIVE TB

	Indication	Duration (wks)	Induction drugs	Interval and duration	Maintenance drugs	Interval and duration
1	Active TB	24	INH, RIF, PZA, EMB or SM	Daily for 8 wks	INH, RIF	Daily, twice, or thrice per week for 16 wks
2	Active TB	24	INH, RIF, PZA, EMB or SM	Daily for 2 wks, then twice/wk for 6 wks	INH, RIF	Twice/wk for 16 wks
3	Active TB	24	INH, RIF, PZA, EMB or SM	Thrice/wk for 24 wks	—	—
4	Smear and culture negative	16	INH, RIF, PZA, EMB or SM	Regimen 1, 2, or 3 for 8 wks	INH, RIF, PZA, EMB or SM	Daily, twice, or thrice per week for 8 wks
5	Active TB without PZA	36	INH, RIF, EMB or SM	Daily for 4–8 wks	INH, RIF	Daily or twice/wk for 28–32 wks

EMB, ethambutol; INH, isoniazid; PZA, pyrazinamide; RIF, rifampin; SM, streptomycin.
From Centers for Disease Control and Prevention. Treatment of tuberculosis. American Thoracic Society, CDC, and Infectious Diseases Society of America. *MMWR* 2003;52(RR 11):3, with permission.

Therefore, in patients with **positive sputum cultures**, specimens should be obtained monthly until conversion is documented to objectively assess the response to therapy. Finally, a **sputum culture** should be obtained at the **completion of therapy** to document a cure.

Latent Tuberculosis Infection

When targeted tuberculin skin testing is performed, all persons with positive tests, as defined above, should be treated. Before initiating therapy for LTBI, **careful evaluation to rule out active TB disease is necessary.** Table 14-5 shows multiple accepted treatment regimens. During therapy, patients should be monitored for adherence to the regimen, for signs and symptoms of active TB disease, and for signs of hepatitis. Up to 20% of persons taking isoniazid have mild, asymptomatic elevation of liver enzymes. These elevations tend to resolve even when isoniazid is continued. However, if liver enzymes are elevated >3–5× the upper limit of normal, isoniazid should be stopped.

CONCLUSION

In the coming years, public health efforts to control and prevent the spread of TB need to be maintained. According to the CDC, these efforts should include three strategies: identifying and treating all persons with active TB disease, identifying and evaluating all close contacts of TB patients, and testing and appropriately treating all persons at high risk for TB infection. The role of the clinician will be to remain vigi-

TABLE 14-5. REGIMENS FOR THE TREATMENT OF LATENT TUBERCULOUS INFECTION

Regimen	Duration (mos)	Daily oral dose (max dose)	Twice/wk dose (max dose)	Comments
INH	9	5 mg/kg (300 mg)	15 mg/kg (900 mg)	Preferred regimen in adults.
INH	6	5 mg/kg (300 mg)	15 mg/kg (900 mg)	Adequate for HIV-negative adults; not for HIV-positive or children.
RIF and PZA	2	10 mg/kg (600 mg) and 15–20 mg/kg (2 g)	10 mg/kg (600 mg) and 50 mg/kg (3.5 g)	Appropriate for HIV-positive adults; rifabutin should be substituted for RIF if taking protease inhibitors or nonnucleoside reverse transcriptase inhibitors.
RIF	4	10 mg/kg (600 mg)	—	For persons intolerant of PZA.

INH, isoniazid; PZA, pyrazinamide; RIF, rifampin.
From Centers for Disease Control and Prevention. Targeted tuberculin testing and treatment of latent tuberculosis infection. *MMWR* 2000;49(RR-6):2, with permission.

lant in identifying cases of active TB disease and persons with LTBI who are candidates for treatment. In contrast to the dedicated public health and governmental efforts in the United States to make the control and eradication of TB a real possibility in the future, the limited resources in third-world countries where TB is endemic keep the disease a persistent global public health problem.

KEY POINTS TO REMEMBER

- *M. tuberculosis* is transmitted by airborne particles (1–5 μ in diameter). Infection results when even a few bacteria are deposited in an alveolus.
- The diagnosis of TB rests on isolation of the organism from infected specimen material. In cases of pulmonary parenchymal TB, sputum analysis by acid-fast stain for AFB and mycobacterial cultures are paramount. The histopathologic finding of caseating granulomatous inflammation is strongly supportive of the diagnosis of TB while cultures are pending.
- The tuberculin skin test is a valuable tool, and the interpretation is based on the individual's risk factors for TB infection.
- Treatment for TB is significantly longer than for other infectious diseases, since *M. tuberculosis* is a slow-growing organism. However, the shortest adequate course of therapy is necessary to ensure compliance.
- During therapy for LTBI, patients should be monitored for adherence to the regimen, for signs and symptoms of active TB disease, and for signs of hepatitis.

REFERENCES AND SUGGESTED READINGS

Bass JB Jr, Farer LS, Hopewell PC, et al. Treatment of tuberculosis and tuberculosis infection in adults and children. American Thoracic Society and Centers for Disease Control and Prevention. *Am J Respir Crit Care Med* 1994;149:1359–1368.

Centers for Disease Control and Prevention. Targeted tuberculin testing and treatment of latent tuberculosis infection. *MMWR* 2000;49(RR-6).

Centers for Disease Control and Prevention. Treatment of tuberculosis. American Thoracic Society, CDC, and Infectious Diseases Society of America. *MMWR* 2003;52(RR-11).

Christie JD, Callihan DR. The laboratory diagnosis of mycobacterial diseases. *Clin Lab Med* 1995;15:279–288.

Cohen RA, Muzaffar S, Schwartz D, et al. Diagnosis of pulmonary tuberculosis using PCR assays on sputum collected within 24 hours of hospital admission. *Am J Respir Crit Care Med* 1998;157:156–161.

Friedman LN. Tuberculosis: current concepts and treatment, 2nd ed. Boca Raton, FL: CRC Press, 2001.

Halvir DV, Barnes PF. Tuberculosis in patients with human immunodeficiency virus infection. *N Engl J Med* 1999;340(5):367–373.

Jones BE, Ryu R, Yang Z, et al. Chest radiographic findings in patients with tuberculosis with recent or remote infection. *Am J Respir Crit Care Med* 1997;156:1270–1273.

McAdams HP, Erasmus JE, Winter JA. Radiologic manifestations of pulmonary tuberculosis. *Radiol Clin North Am* 1995;33:655–659.

McCray E, Weinbaum CM, Braden CR, Onorato IM. The epidemiology of tuberculosis in the United States. *Clin Chest Med* 1997;18(1):99–113.

McKenna MT, McCray E, Onorato I. The epidemiology of tuberculosis among foreign-born persons in the United States, 1986 to 1993. *N Engl J Med* 1995;332(16):1071–1076.

Small PM, Fujiwara PI. Management of tuberculosis in the United States. *N Engl J Med* 2001;345(3):189–200.

15 Fungal Pulmonary Infections

Nitin J. Anand

INTRODUCTION

Infections of the lung with both opportunistic and endemic fungi are increasingly common, a result of the increasing population of immunocompromised hosts resulting from AIDS, chemotherapy, organ transplantation, and chronic steroid use. Both neutropenia and lymphocytic deficiencies predispose to mycotic infection, with pulmonary involvement being the most common form of invasive fungal disease observed in immunocompromised hosts. This chapter examines the clinical presentation, diagnostic approach, and treatment of specific fungal infections of the lung. Fungi that infect the lung include those that appear as budding forms (yeasts), hyphae (molds), or both (dimorphic fungi). The yeasts include *Candida* and *Cryptococcus;* the molds, *Aspergillus* and mucormycosis; and the dimorphic fungi, *Histoplasma, Blastomyces,* and *Coccidioides. Pneumocystis jiroveci* (formerly known as *Pneumocystis carinii*) is commonly classified as a fungus based on its microsomal and ribosomal features and is also discussed.

ASPERGILLUS

The *Aspergillus* species cause a spectrum of **clinical syndromes** in the lung. These include (a) aspergillomas or fungal balls, (b) invasive pulmonary aspergillosis, (c) chronic necrotizing aspergillosis, and (d) allergic bronchopulmonary aspergillosis (ABPA). *Aspergillus fumigatus* is the most commonly implicated organism, but any of the *Aspergillus* species including *A. flavus* and *A. niger* can cause disease. *Aspergillus* is a ubiquitous soil-dwelling organism found in debris, dust, compost, foods, spices, and rotted plants. It has a worldwide distribution. Inhalation of the spores is common, but disease is rare. Neutropenia and prolonged steroid use are the most common predisposing factors to *Aspergillus* infection, but aspergillus has increasingly been identified as a lung pathogen in patients with AIDS and patients receiving chemotherapy for malignancies or immunosuppression for transplantation.

Aspergilloma

An aspergilloma, or fungus ball, is the **most common form of pulmonary aspergillosis** and usually occurs in patients with preexisting cavitary lung disease, such as TB, sarcoidosis, neoplasm, cystic fibrosis, or severe emphysema. Rare cases of *de novo* aspergilloma in patients without preexisting cavitary lung disease have been reported.

Fungal balls cause **few clinical symptoms.** Hemoptysis, reported in up to 75% of patients, is usually mild but may on occasion be severe. It is believed to be due to bleeding from bronchial blood vessels lining the lung cavity. Other symptoms include chest pain, dyspnea, malaise, and fever. Aspergillomas are often noticed as **incidental** findings on chest radiograph (CXR) or in the initial workup for hemoptysis. They classically appear as upper lobe intracavitary masses surrounded by a radiolucent crescent (crescent sign).

Repeated sputum cultures for aspergillus should be obtained. However, these may be negative in up to 50% of patients given the limited communication between cavities and the bronchial tree. A positive sputum culture in the correct clinical setting is highly suggestive of an aspergilloma.

An aspergilloma that is clinically quiescent or causing only minimal symptoms can be observed. The mainstay of therapy in patients with severe hemoptysis is surgical resection, but resection is often limited by the extent of the underlying lung disease. In patients who are actively bleeding, bronchial artery embolization can be a useful temporizing measure. Systemic, inhaled, and intracavitary antifungal agents have all failed to show benefit in the clinical course, morbidity, or mortality of aspergillomas, although reduction in size of fungus balls with prolonged itraconazole therapy has been reported.

Invasive Aspergillosis

Invasive pulmonary aspergillosis (IA) occurs most commonly in the immunocompromised host. Unlike aspergilloma and chronic necrotizing aspergillosis, there is **direct vascular invasion** by the fungus, often with **dissemination to other organs.**

IA should be suspected in the **immunocompromised host with high fevers** that persist despite empiric treatment with broad-spectrum antibiotics. Pleuritic chest pain (due to microinfarctions), hemoptysis, and dyspnea may also be present. The CXR is nonspecific and may reveal patchy infiltrates or nodular opacities. The chest CT scan typically shows multiple nodules and may demonstrate the *halo sign*—an area of infiltrate surrounded by a rim of air (representing pulmonary necrosis).

The **diagnosis of IA** requires histologic demonstration of vascular invasion by typical septate, acute-angle–branching hyphae. Thus, **lung tissue,** often from **thoracoscopic** or **open-lung biopsy,** is the gold standard for diagnosis of IA. The presence of aspergillus in the sputum is commonly due to the colonization of the airways, but in immunosuppressed patients at risk for invasive disease, it has a positive predictive value of 80–90%. Bronchoalveolar lavage (BAL) fluid has high specificity for aspergillus, but a sensitivity of only 35–50%, and is often useful in patients with diffuse lung involvement. There are no useful serologic tests for the diagnosis of IA.

Given the difficulty of making a definitive diagnosis of IA (with the lack of sensitivity of diagnostic testing), empiric presumptive antifungal therapy among high-risk patients is mandatory. Given the lethal nature of the disease, **IV amphotericin B** at a dose of 1–1.5 mg/kg/day should be initiated as soon as the diagnosis is suspected and should be continued despite modest increases in creatinine. In patients who cannot tolerate amphotericin B owing to renal dysfunction, the less toxic lipid formulations may be tried. The optimal duration of therapy is unknown, but patients may be switched to oral itraconazole for prolonged therapy only after immunosuppression has ended and there has been a definite clinical response. **Voriconazole** (6 mg/kg IV bid on day one, then 4 mg/kg IV × 7 days, then 200 mg PO qd) has also been approved for the treatment of IA and may be used as an alternative initial regimen. Caspofungin (70 mg load followed by 50 mg IV qd) is used as salvage therapy for IA. Surgical resection of infected tissue should be considered when there is massive hemoptysis or a localized focus of infection, especially if further immunosuppression is planned in the future.

Chronic Necrotizing Aspergillosis

Chronic necrotizing aspergillosis (CNA) is distinct from both an aspergilloma and IA and is a more indolent form of invasive infection characterized by **local invasion of lung tissue.** It usually occurs in association with an aspergilloma at the interface of the fungus ball and the normal lung, although a preexisting cavity is not needed for CNA to occur.

CNA is usually encountered in **elderly patients with underlying chronic lung disease,** especially COPD. Other predisposing lesions include inactive TB, previous lung resection, and scarring from prior radiation therapy. It can also occur in patients with cystic fibrosis. The patient typically presents with cough, low-grade fever, mild hemoptysis, and weight loss of 1–6 mos' duration. The CXR or chest CT scan shows a slowly progressive lesion, usually with an infiltrate in the upper lobes or the superior segments of the lower lobes. One-half of lesions are associated with a fungus ball.

As with the diagnosis of IA, the **definitive diagnosis of CNA is histologic.** Given the relatively indolent nature of the infection and the morbidity of the underlying lung disease, the **diagnosis** is usually made **clinically,** and a lung biopsy is often not pursued.

Amphotericin B may be considered, but oral **itraconazole** (400 mg/day) has increasingly been used for therapy of CNA. Treatment is usually prolonged (3–9 mos), and the optimal duration and criteria for discontinuing therapy are currently uncertain. In those patients with isolated disease and adequate pulmonary reserve, surgical resection may be considered.

Allergic Bronchopulmonary Aspergillosis

Allergic bronchopulmonary aspergillosis (ABPA) is a **hypersensitivity reaction** (and not a true infection) occurring in patients colonized by aspergillus. It most commonly occurs in patients with asthma or cystic fibrosis. ABPA is typically suspected when patients present with severe asthma—wheezing, occasional productive cough, fever, chest pain, and peripheral blood eosinophilia—responsive only to systemic corticosteroid therapy. Occasionally, patients complain of expectoration of thick brown plugs, which are due to aspergillus-laden mucoid bronchial casts. The CXR may be clear or show transient migratory infiltrates that occur during acute exacerbations, usually in the upper lobes. In the later stages of ABPA, the chest CT scan may show mucoid impaction, bronchial thickening, or frank bronchiectasis, usually in a central upper-lobe distribution.

The evaluation of patients suspected of having ABPA should be performed in a particular order. The evaluation begins with an aspergillus skin prick test, followed by assays for aspergillus serum precipitins and total serum IgE, and then assays for specific IgE and IgG directed against *A. fumigatus.* A negative skin prick test is followed by an intradermal skin test. Negative reactivity to both the skin prick and intradermal tests virtually excludes the diagnosis of ABPA and generally allows termination of the evaluation. The **diagnosis of ABPA** is usually confirmed by the following clinical, radiologic, and immunologic criteria: (a) a history of asthma, (b) immediate skin reactivity to aspergillus (using the skin prick test), (c) serum precipitins to *A. fumigatus,* (d) total serum IgE >1000 ng/mL, (e) increased serum levels of IgE and/or IgG directed against *A. fumigatus,* (f) current or previous pulmonary infiltrates, (g) central bronchiectasis, and (h) peripheral eosinophilia (>1000 cells/μL). Patients meeting criteria b, c, and d are labeled ABPA-S (ABPA seropositive).

ABPA should be treated with **oral corticosteroids** at a dose of 0.5/mg/kg/day for 2 wks, followed by a slow taper over 3–6 mos. Clinical response should be monitored using monthly total serum IgE levels and symptoms. **Oral itraconazole** has also been reported to be useful in the treatment of ABPA.

CRYPTOCOCCUS

Cryptococcosis is caused by *Cryptococcus neoformans,* a yeast in both its natural habitat as well as in humans and animals. Cryptococcus is found in soil around the world, particularly in areas frequented by birds such as pigeons. The vast majority of infections in normal hosts are **asymptomatic,** although it can **occasionally cause severe pneumonias.** It is usually encountered as an opportunistic pathogen in immunocompromised hosts, especially those with AIDS or lymphoma or in those on chronic corticosteroid therapy.

In the **normal host,** infections are **frequently asymptomatic** but can present as pneumonia characterized by cough with scant sputum production. In the **immunocompromised host,** cryptococcal infection is often **disseminated** at the time of diagnosis, and patients most commonly present with **CNS findings,** especially meningoencephalitis, in addition to fever and cough. The CXR may range from diffuse well-defined nodular infiltrates (more common in normal hosts) to diffuse alveolar infiltrates (more common in the immunosuppressed host). Masses mimicking lung carcinoma may also be seen. Pleural effusions and cavitation are uncommon.

Definitive diagnosis requires culture of the organism. Sputum cultures may grow *Cryptococcus* in up to 50% of patients. Cultures of BAL fluid increase the yield to close to 90%, and examination of **BAL smears** with **India ink** may allow for a rapid diagnosis. Nodular lesions can be biopsied by fine-needle aspiration or transbronchial biopsy if accessible. Cryptococcal capsular antigen should be obtained in serum and CSF but is only positive if disease has disseminated beyond the lung.

In the healthy host, cryptococcosis isolated to the lung should be treated with **oral fluconazole** (200–400 mg/day) for 3 mos. In the immunocompromised host, **IV amphotericin B** at a dose of 0.5–1.0 mg/kg/day should be initiated and should be continued despite modest increases in creatinine. In patients who cannot tolerate amphotericin B secondary to renal dysfunction, the less toxic lipid formulations may be used. After 10 wks of induction therapy, patients with continued immunocompromise should be continued on **lifelong maintenance therapy** with oral fluconazole (200 mg/day).

CANDIDIASIS

Candida is a dimorphic fungus. It is a common human saprophyte, found normally in the GI tract and other mucocutaneous regions. Although *Candida albicans* is the most important pathogen, other *Candida* organisms may also lead to infection. Increased colonization of the organism, especially in the oropharynx, skin, and vagina, is the **major risk factor** for development of systemic candidiasis. Diabetes mellitus, indwelling urinary and venous catheters, and prolonged use of antibiotics, total parenteral nutrition, and corticosteroids all predispose to increased colonization. Even in immunocompromised patients, pulmonary candidiasis is rare and is more commonly manifest as part of a systemic hematogenous infection from a primary extrapulmonary site—usually the GI tract. When primary pulmonary candidiasis occurs, it is usually the result of aspiration of organisms from the oropharynx.

Pulmonary candidiasis, when part of a disseminated disease, is often a terminal event in debilitated, immunocompromised patients receiving antibiotics, steroids, or immunosuppressive therapy. The pulmonary symptoms are nonspecific and include cough, purulent sputum, and hemoptysis. Extrapulmonary manifestations including skin lesions, endophthalmitis, and multiple organ failure may be seen at the time of diagnosis of candida fungemia. The CXR may show a focal or diffuse patchy infiltrate with primary disease. A miliary nodular pattern is more common in disseminated disease.

The definitive **diagnosis** of pulmonary candidiasis requires documentation of candida **invasion of the bronchi or lungs.** The isolation of candida from sputum does not establish the diagnosis because it is often a contaminant from the oropharynx. Bronchial washings and BAL fluid are more representative of lung pathology but may also be contaminated by oropharyngeal secretions. Thus, a diagnosis of candidiasis can be made using these methods in the appropriate clinical setting, especially if samples show repeated heavy growth of the organism, but a definitive diagnosis requires tissue obtained either by bronchoscopic or open-lung biopsy. Blood cultures are often positive for candida in disseminated disease.

IV amphotericin B in doses of 0.5–1.5 mg/kg/day for 2–4 wks is the mainstay for treatment of pulmonary candidiasis. The lipid preparations of amphotericin have not been studied for this indication but should be considered if the patient is unable to tolerate amphotericin B. Fluconazole has been studied in patients with candidemia with good results; however, its efficacy in pulmonary candidiasis has not been well established. When using fluconazole for the treatment of candidiasis, it is important to know both the species of candida and the sensitivity of the organism to the drug as resistance has been reported. This resistance may be innate (e.g., *C. krusei* and *C. glabrata*) or acquired (e.g., *C. albicans*).

MUCORMYCOSIS

Rhizopus, Rhizomucor, and *Cunninghamella* are the most common causes of mucormycosis. The fungi are commonly found on decaying organic material such as fruit or bread and have a worldwide distribution. This opportunistic infection almost always occurs in patients with underlying chronic disease, especially diabetes, chronic renal failure, lymphoma, and leukemia.

Rhinocerebral mucormycosis, most commonly seen in diabetics, is a fatal disease that involves the nose and sinuses and frequently spreads to the orbits and brain. It presents with high fevers, purulent nasal discharge, and sinus pain. It may extend to the lungs through aspiration. Patients with **primary pulmonary mucormycosis,** a less common entity, present with high fevers, chest pain, and hemoptysis. Massive hemoptysis may occur as a result of invasion of the pulmonary artery. CXR findings are nonspecific, and mucormycosis may manifest as a diffuse infiltrate or a mass.

The diagnosis of pulmonary mucormycosis usually requires histopathologic evidence of invasion of lung tissue, usually obtained using transbronchial, percutaneous needle, or open-lung biopsy. Silver or hematoxylin and eosin stains of infected tissues show the classic **broad, nonseptate hyphae** occurring at **right angles.** Blood, sputum, and nasal swabs are usually of little diagnostic utility because the species are extremely difficult to isolate and culture.

The prognosis of pulmonary (and rhinocerebral) mucormycosis is grave, with mortality >65%. Therapy involves regulation of blood sugars in diabetics, rapid reduction of immunosuppression, and institution of maximum (at least 1.0 mg/kg/day) tolerated doses of amphotericin B. Aggressive debridement of necrotic tissue can be attempted in localized disease.

HISTOPLASMOSIS

Histoplasmosis is caused by *Histoplasma capsulatum,* a dimorphic fungus that grows as mold in the soil and as a budding yeast in culture. It is endemic in the southeastern, mid-Atlantic, and central states. It is found in greater quantity in soil with large amounts of bird and bat excrement.

>95% of histoplasma infections are either **asymptomatic** or so **mild** that medical attention is not sought. **Acute pulmonary histoplasmosis** infection is characterized by flulike symptoms, cough, fever, malaise, earache, and retrosternal discomfort. It is occasionally associated with erythema nodosum. A heavy inoculum of *H. capsulatum* can cause acute pulmonary histoplasmosis even in the immunocompetent host. Disseminated histoplasmosis is rare and usually only occurs in patients who are immunosuppressed or at extremes of age. The CXR of a patient with severe symptomatic acute histoplasmosis reveals one or more areas of patchy air space consolidation. Hilar adenopathy is often present. In disseminated disease, a miliary pattern with bilateral discrete nodular shadows up to 3–4 mm in diameter may be seen.

A definitive diagnosis of acute histoplasmosis requires culture of the organism or histologic exam of infected tissue. A diagnosis of histoplasmosis may be presumed with detection of the **histoplasma polysaccharide antigen** in the serum, urine, or BAL fluid. The urine antigen test has a high sensitivity (75–90%) and specificity (98%). Fungal stains of tissue, especially bone marrow or pulmonary biopsy specimens, may reveal the organism. Cultures of blood, bone marrow, or mucosal lesions provide the strongest proof for histoplasmosis but are limited by low sensitivity (10–15%) as well as extremely slow growth of the organism. Histoplasmin skin tests are not useful diagnostically given the high rates of background skin positivity in endemic areas.

Patients with **life-threatening pulmonary or disseminated histoplasmosis** manifest as respiratory failure should be started on **IV amphotericin B** (1 mg/kg/day) as soon as infection is suspected. Those with non–life-threatening histoplasmosis restricted to the lung may be treated with **itraconazole** (200 mg IV tid for 3 days followed by 200–400 mg/day PO). Fluconazole has no efficacy in the treatment of histoplasmosis.

Chronic cavitary histoplasmosis occurs in patients with chronic lung disease and is characterized by gradual onset (over weeks or months) of increasing cough, weight loss, and occasionally night sweats. The disease has a predilection for males aged >40 yrs but may also occur in females. The CXR reveals fibronodular apical infiltrates that may cavitate. Culture of respiratory specimens is usually positive for the organism, whereas antigen tests are almost always negative. Treatment consists of induction with IV itraconazole or amphotericin B followed by a prolonged course of oral itraconazole (at least 6 mos) until sputum cultures are negative and radiographic findings have resolved.

BLASTOMYCOSIS

Blastomycosis is caused by inhalation of the spores of *Blastomyces dermatitidis*. The spores are found in the soil and are endemic in the Ohio and Tennessee River valleys. Blastomycosis is rare, and the disease is much less common than histoplasmosis or coccidioidomycosis.

Blastomycosis can range from **asymptomatic** to **acute pulmonary disease** characterized by the abrupt onset of fevers, chills, productive cough, and pleuritic chest pain. It is occasionally associated with erythema nodosum, arthralgia, and myalgias.

Even 50% of immunocompetent hosts present with disseminated disease characterized by skin lesions (due to epidermal hyperplasia) that appear as **painless erythematous nodules.** Other common sites of dissemination include the CNS, joints, bone, and genitourinary tract. In the immunocompromised host, the disease is usually more severe and almost always disseminated at the time of presentation. CNS involvement, especially, is far more common than in the normal host.

Culture of organisms from bronchoscopy specimens, CSF, brain, skin, or blood is the gold standard. Cultures from one of these sites exhibit growth in >95% of patients with disseminated disease. In addition, direct microscopic exam of sputum and secretions using fungal stains may provide a more rapid diagnosis by allowing visualization of the broad-based budding yeast forms. The organism can also be identified with **DNA probes.** There are no useful serologic or antigen detection tests for blastomycosis.

The initial treatment for severe pulmonary blastomycosis causing respiratory failure or disseminated disease is **IV amphotericin B** (1–1.5 mg/kg/day), especially in the immunosuppressed host. Milder forms may be treated with **itraconazole** (200 mg/day PO). The duration of therapy is unclear but in general should be continued until clinical and lab findings have normalized. Maintenance therapy should be considered in immunosuppressed patients.

COCCIDIOIDOMYCOSIS

Coccidioides immitis is a dimorphic fungus that is endemic to the southwestern United States. Its natural habitat is the desert soil. Only 20% of patients infected with coccidioidomycosis have clinical manifestations of the disease—almost all live in or have recently traveled to an endemic region. Patients with AIDS or organ transplants are especially susceptible to the disease.

Symptomatic coccidioidomycosis or **valley fever** presents as a **nonspecific flulike illness** accompanied by **fever, nonproductive cough, and headache** approximately 1–3 wks after exposure. Occasionally, arthralgias or a generalized erythematous rash is present. The CXR initially shows patchy infiltrates, occasionally with mediastinal adenopathy. Most CXRs resolve as symptoms improve, but 5% of cases progress to form nodular coin lesions (coccidioidomas), which are commonly located in the middle and upper lung zones. Some patients with resolved disease may also develop residual thin-walled cavities. Despite the appearance of their CXRs, these patients are usually asymptomatic, although the nodules or cavities may serve as foci for reactivation of disease.

It is estimated that 1% of patients with **primary pulmonary coccidioidomycosis** develop disseminated disease. Specific risk factors include HIV or AIDS, solid organ transplantation, chronic steroid use, hematologic malignancies, diabetes, chemotherapy, and the third trimester of pregnancy. Sites most commonly infected include the skin, meninges, bone, and joints, but dissemination may occur to almost any organ. CXRs in patients with disseminated coccidioidomycosis usually show diffuse reticulonodular infiltrates, although miliary infiltrates, nodules, and cavities may also be seen.

The visualization of organisms from **sputum** using **fungal stains** allows for rapid diagnosis. If the sputum examination is negative, **BAL fluid** may improve the diagnostic yield. Tissue cultures are usually positive and show growth within 3–5 days. Organisms may also be rapidly identified from culture using **DNA probe** testing. Blood cultures are rarely positive. Coccidioidomycosis serology is also useful: An **IgM antibody** to **coccidioidin** can be measured using several methods, and IgG complement fixing antibody can be quantified. The IgG is present in low titer in early disease but is higher in patients with disseminated disease and can be used to monitor disease activity. A titer of ≥ 1:16 should prompt an evaluation for disseminated disease. Antibody titers should also be quantified in the CSF if meningitis is suspected. Delayed type hypersensitivity skin testing for coccidioidomycosis may be useful as a diagnostic screening test.

Immunocompetent hosts with mild symptoms or those with nodules or cavities on CXR after resolution of symptoms **do not require antifungal therapy,** and the vast majority recover over a few weeks to months. IV amphotericin B is the cornerstone of therapy for severe pulmonary involvement resulting in hypoxia or disseminated disease or in those patients who are immunosuppressed. IV fluconazole has been used as an alternative to amphotericin B for coccidioidomycosis meningitis given its lower toxicity and excellent penetration into the CSF. **Lifelong oral maintenance therapy** is indicated for **HIV-infected patients** and patients with continued immunosuppression. Itraconazole (200 mg PO bid) or fluconazole (200–400 mg PO qd) should be used. Surgical resection should be considered as an adjunct to medical therapy in patients with adequate lung reserve and isolated chronic foci of pulmonary infection.

PNEUMOCYSTIS

P. jiroveci (previously *P. carinii*) is an opportunistic pathogen of the lung that has a worldwide distribution. The natural reservoir of the organism remains unknown, but it has been found in the lungs of many animals. The initial infection, which occurs in childhood, is extremely common. Clinically significant *P. jiroveci* pneumonia (PJP) is believed to represent **reactivation of latent disease** in susceptible hosts such as those with HIV, underlying malignancy, and recent or current prolonged glucocorticoid therapy, and in children with primary immunodeficiency syndromes.

Patients with PJP present with **severe dyspnea, nonproductive cough, and fever out of proportion to their clinical and radiographic findings.** Physical exam findings include fever, tachypnea, tachycardia, and occasionally crackles (50% of patients have a normal chest exam). Elevated serum levels of lactate dehydrogenase are common. In HIV-infected patients, PJP generally occurs when the CD4 count is <200. In patients on prolonged steroid therapy, symptoms often begin as the dose is being tapered.

There is no radiographic pattern that is pathognomonic for PJP. The CXR may be normal or have bilateral diffuse interstitial infiltrates beginning in the perihilar regions. Nodular lesions and cavities may also be seen.

A definitive diagnosis should be sought because PJP can have atypical presentations and appear similar to other lung pathogens and because therapy may have significant toxicity. The diagnosis requires visualization of the organism in a respiratory specimen with appropriate **histologic staining (Wright-Giemsa, methenamine silver,** or **direct immunofluorescence).** Routine sputum specimens are often inadequate, and sputum samples should be obtained by induction with hypertonic saline. The yield of an induced specimen ranges from 30% to 75%, with higher yields in HIV patients. If organisms are not seen on induced sputum, a BAL should be obtained. The yield is >50% in all patients with PCP and >95% in patients with AIDS. In rare cases, a transbronchial or open-lung biopsy may be necessary to make the diagnosis.

Because PJP is often fatal, **empiric treatment** should be initiated as soon as the diagnosis is considered. Short courses of treatment (<48 hrs) should not impair the ability for definitive diagnosis. The treatment of choice is **TMP-SMX** (15–20 mg/kg/day of the TMP component) given PO or IV in three to four divided doses for 14 days in non–HIV-infected patients and 21 days in HIV-infected patients. The therapy should be continued despite development of mild side effects including neutropenia, rash, and transaminase elevation. In patients unable to tolerate TMP-SMX as a result of severe side effects such as nephrotoxicity, Stevens-Johnson syndrome, or bone marrow suppression, **IV pentamidine** (4 mg/kg/day) or dapsone may be used. The use of adjunctive steroid therapy (**prednisone,** 60 mg PO or IV tid–qid) is recommended in AIDS patients with marked hypoxemia (Pa_{O_2} <70 mm Hg). Its use in non–HIV-infected patients has not been established but can be considered.

TMP-SMX is highly effective as **primary prophylaxis** against *P. jiroveci* and should be used in immunocompromised hosts at risk for the development of PJP, including AIDS patients, organ transplant recipients, patients on chemotherapeutic regimens, and patients on prolonged (>2 wks) steroid regimens. Oral prophylactic therapy consists of one double-strength tablet (160 mg of TMP plus 800 mg of SMX) daily or 3 times/wk.

KEY POINTS TO REMEMBER

- Fungi that infect the lung include those that exist as budding forms (yeasts), hyphae (molds), or both (dimorphic fungi).
- With the increase in organ transplantation, immunosuppressive therapies for medical diseases, and HIV, fungal diseases are becoming increasingly prevalent.
- Pulmonary fungal infections are often asymptomatic or minimally symptomatic in immunocompetent hosts.
- An aspergilloma, or fungus ball, is the most common form of pulmonary aspergillosis and usually occurs in patients with preexisting cavitary lung disease, such as TB, sarcoidosis, neoplasm, cystic fibrosis, or severe emphysema.
- Given the difficulty of making a definitive diagnosis of IA, empiric presumptive antifungal therapy among high-risk patients with hematologic malignancies and neutropenia is mandatory.

REFERENCES AND SUGGESTED READINGS

Bradsher RW. Histoplasmosis and blastomycosis. *Clin Infect Dis* 1996;22[Suppl 2]:S102–S111.

Catanzaro A. Fungal pneumonias. *Curr Opin Pulm Med* 1997;3(2):146–150.

Fishman AP, ed. *Fishman's pulmonary diseases and disorders*, 3rd ed. New York: McGraw-Hill, 1998.

Fishman JA. Common pulmonary infections in immunocompromised patients. In: *UpToDate*, Rose BD, ed. Waltham, MA: UpToDate, 2004.

Fraser RS, Colman NC, Paré PD, et al., eds. *Diagnosis of diseases of the chest*, 4th ed. Philadelphia: WB Saunders, 1999.

Goldman M, Johnson PC, Sarosi GA. Fungal pneumonias. The endemic mycoses. *Clin Chest Med* 1999;20(3):507–519.

Klein NC, Cunha BA. New antifungal drugs for pulmonary mycoses. *Chest* 1996;110(2):525–532.

Lee FY, Mossad SB, Adal KA, et al. Pulmonary mucormycosis: the last 30 years. *Arch Intern Med* 1999;159(12):1301–1309.

Meyer KC, McManus EJ, Maki DG. Overwhelming pulmonary blastomycosis associated with the adult respiratory distress syndrome. *N Engl J Med* 1993;329(17):1231–1236.

Pound MW, Drew RH, Perfect RJ. Recent advances in the epidemiology, prevention, diagnosis, and treatment of fungal pneumonia. *Curr Opin Infect Dis* 2002;15(2):183–194.

Saubolle MA. Fungal pneumonias. *Semin Respir Infect* 2000;15(2):162–177.

Soubani AO, Chandrasekar PH. The clinical spectrum of pulmonary aspergillosis. *Chest* 2002;121:1988–1999.

Tasci S, Ewig S, Burghard A, et al. *Pneumocystis carinii* pneumonia. *Lancet* 2003;362(9378):124.

Wheat LJ, Goldman M, Sarosi G. State-of-the-art review of pulmonary fungal infections. *Semin Respir Infect* 2002;17(2):158–181.

16 Viral Pulmonary Infections

Sabu Thomas

INTRODUCTION

Viral respiratory infections are exceedingly common, with an estimated incidence of 3 cases/person/yr, and account for nearly 50% of all acute respiratory diseases. Economically, these diseases represent a significant burden to society in terms of lost time and productivity. In fact, an estimated 30–50% of time lost from work can be attributed to the effects of viral respiratory infections, with the common cold alone costing the U.S. economy an estimated $3.5 billion/year.

There are approximately **200 antigenically distinct viruses** that result in multiple clinical syndromes. These include the common cold, influenza, pharyngitis, croup (laryngotracheobronchitis), tracheitis, bronchitis, bronchiolitis, and pneumonia. Given that significant clinical overlap exists between different viruses and clinical syndromes, lab methods must often be used to establish a specific diagnosis. However, the often benign and self-limited nature of many viral illnesses usually makes specific diagnoses unnecessary.

Immunosuppression resulting from diseases such as AIDS, chemotherapeutic treatment in cancer patients, and immunosuppressive regimens in transplant patients has forced the modern clinician to be familiar with the various opportunistic viral infections seen in these populations. Severe acute respiratory syndrome (SARS), a respiratory viral infection linked to a common cold virus, has recently received significant media attention after affecting thousands of patients in Asia, North America, and Europe. The purpose of this chapter is to introduce the major respiratory viruses in clinical practice and address the recent SARS epidemic and the clinical implications that this disease imposes.

RHINOVIRUS

Rhinoviruses are members of the Picornaviridae family. They are nonenveloped, single-stranded RNA-containing agents with a diameter up to 30 nm. They grow preferentially at 34°C, the temperature encountered in the nasal passages. There are 100 different serotypes and 1 subtype.

Rhinoviruses are responsible for **up to 40% of common colds.** Infection rates are highest among young children and infants, with an average of approximately 6 infections/year in this group. Generally, infection rates steadily decrease with advancing age except in the twenties, during which another peak is seen. Infections are introduced into families by children aged <6 yrs, explaining the slight increase in infection rates among 20- to 29-year-old subjects who often are the primary care givers for these young children. Attack rates increase with increasing family size, especially in families with children who attend elementary schools or preschools.

Rhinovirus infections occur throughout the year but have notable seasonal peaks in early autumn and spring in North America and Europe. They are more active during the rainy season in tropical regions of the world. Rhinovirus activity is generally lower in the winter months when coronaviruses and other agents are responsible for causing common colds. Rhinoviruses are usually **spread via direct contact with infected secretions.** Subsequent self-inoculation of the nasal or conjunctival mucosa leads to infection. **Aerosolized virus** from sneezing or coughing is another important mode of transmission. Rhinoviruses can survive for hours on contaminated surfaces, resulting in fomite-mediated spread.

Despite anecdotal evidence and popular beliefs, cold temperature exposure, fatigue, and sleep deprivation have not been associated with increased rates of transmission.

Clinically, rhinoviruses cause the **typical symptoms** recognized as the common cold. Typically, there is a 1- to 2-day incubation period before the onset of symptoms. Viral shedding occurs with the onset of symptoms and can last up to 3 wks. The nasal mucosa becomes edematous and hyperemic and produces a mucoid discharge. The nasal turbinates often become engorged, which can lead to sinus cavity obstruction and subsequent bacterial superinfection. Symptoms typically last 4–9 days and then resolve spontaneously. They include rhinorrhea and sneezing in 50–70% and sore throat in 50% of cases. Some patients report sore throat as their initial complaint. Occasionally, patients complain of malaise and mild headaches. Fever, chills, and myalgias are unusual and should prompt the clinician to search for other potential causes, such as influenza. Hoarseness and cough are less common but can be associated with complications of the cold such as sinusitis and bronchitis. Rhinovirus infections are associated with COPD and asthma exacerbations in susceptible patients. Other complications include ostial meatal swelling leading to eustachian tube occlusion and otitis media.

Rhinovirus infection is usually **recognized on clinical grounds alone.** However, clinical characteristics do not allow the clinician to differentiate between rhinovirus and other etiologies of the common cold. Specific diagnosis can be obtained via nasal secretion or nasal washing culture. Given the many different serotypes of rhinovirus, serum antibody tests remain impractical.

Aggressive treatment of rhinovirus infection is usually unnecessary given the **benign and self-limited nature** of the illness. Treatment is supportive and symptom based. Despite advances in the understanding of this disease, there is no cure for the common cold. The host immune system clears the infection but also contributes to the bothersome symptoms with which we are all familiar.

Symptom alleviators include analgesics, decongestants, antihistamines, steroids, mast cell stabilizers, and localized hyperthermia. Antihistamines such as brompheniramine (4 mg PO q4–6h) and clemastine (1–2 mg PO q8–12h) have been shown to reduce sneezing rates and rhinorrhea. These benefits must be balanced against the side effects of sedation and confusion caused by the drugs. Nonsedating antihistamines such as loratadine also produce symptom control, but comparison with first-generation antihistamines is lacking.

Decongestant agents such as pseudoephedrine (30–60 mg PO q4–6h) and oxymetolazone (2–3 sprays per nostril bid) also decrease rhinorrhea and congestive symptoms. These agents are often found in combination preparations with antihistamines. Side effects of this class of drugs include insomnia and dry mouth. Nasal decongestants should also not be used for >3 days because of the risk of rhinitis medicamentosa (rebound nasal congestion) resulting from prolonged use.

Analgesic agents such as NSAIDs and acetaminophen can be used to relieve the symptoms of headache and sore throat. Steroids may reduce symptoms over the first few days of infection but do not affect symptoms thereafter and are not recommended for uncomplicated rhinovirus infections. Several small studies looking at the effect of mast cell stabilizers such as cromolyn show reduction in symptoms. They have minimal side effects but, similar to steroids, do not affect the duration of illness or viral shedding.

Some studies have suggested a mild improvement in symptoms with respiratory hyperthermia produced by warm steam inhalation. Recent studies looking at various zinc preparations have been equivocal, as have clinical trials of *Echinacea,* a common herbal remedy. Vitamin C supplementation did not have any effect on reducing the incidence of colds, although some have argued that it results in symptom improvement.

CORONAVIRUS

Coronaviruses are another important cause of the common cold. More recently, they have been implicated as the causative agent in the recent SARS epidemic. They contain a crownlike envelope and a single-stranded RNA, and have a diameter of 80–160 nm. There are three antigenically distinct subgroups that are important in human disease. They are fastidious organisms that are difficult to culture *in vitro*. In fact, some strains do not even grow well in standard tissue culture and require human tracheal organ culture to grow.

These viruses are responsible for **10–20% of cases of the common cold.** In temperate climates, they appear to cause disease in late fall, winter, and early spring and are associated with outbreaks every 2–4 yrs. Respiratory coronavirus infections are spread in a manner similar to that of rhinoviruses—i.e., via direct contact with infected secretions or via large aerosol droplets. Compared with rhinoviruses, however, their incubation period is slightly longer at 3 days. Fortunately, the illness duration is shorter: approximately 6–7 days.

Clinically, in adults, these viruses produce acute upper respiratory infections (URIs) that are very similar to rhinovirus infections. They are also implicated as important causes of **acute otitis media** in children and **triggers of asthma exacerbations** as well. Normally, these viruses are not associated with lower respiratory infections but can cause **pneumonia** in infants and immunocompromised adults. Similar to rhinovirus, coronavirus does not seem to damage respiratory epithelial cells, and therefore the host immune system may be responsible for the pathogenesis of lower respiratory tract disease.

Diagnosis of coronavirus infection is usually clinical. Again, **clinical diagnosis** cannot rule out other causes for URI, and lab methods are needed for a specific diagnosis. Until recently, there were no practical methods for detecting this virus. PCR techniques and indirect immunofluorescence have solved this problem and are equally able to detect the virus.

These infections are usually managed with **supportive therapy** similar to that for rhinovirus infections. **Preventative measures** include frequent hand washing and appropriate disposal of infected secretions. Interestingly, several antiseptic solutions such as chloroxylenol, benzalkonium, and chlorhexidine (which are effective against rhinoviruses) are ineffective against coronavirus.

SEVERE ACUTE RESPIRATORY SYNDROME

In 2002, a variant of the coronavirus causing a severe acute respiratory syndrome known as SARS was identified. Initial cases were seen in China, Singapore, Vietnam, Hong Kong, and Canada. The **current case definition** for suspected SARS is an individual presenting with

- Fever >38°C, plus
- Cough or difficulty breathing, plus
- Sick contact with someone diagnosed with SARS and/or travel to an area with recent local transmission of SARS within 10 days of onset of symptoms

A **probable** case is defined as

- A suspected case with chest radiograph findings consistent with findings of pneumonia or ARDS, or
- A suspected case of SARS based on lab assays, or
- A suspected case with an unexplained respiratory illness resulting in death and an autopsy demonstrating the pathology of ARDS without an identifiable cause

The first cases of this disease were noted in China. Health care workers and their contacts seemed to be involved first. The index case was a physician from mainland China who traveled to Hong Kong. Cases in Singapore, Vietnam, Thailand, and Canada arose in travelers coming from mainland China or Hong Kong. Most cases have occurred in adults. In younger children, SARS seems to be a milder illness.

RESPIRATORY SYNCYTIAL VIRUS

Respiratory syncytial viruses (RSVs) are the foremost causes of **lower respiratory viral infection** in **infants and young children.** RSV can also infect certain adult populations. They are members of the Paramyxoviridae family. RSVs are enveloped, single-stranded RNA viruses with a diameter of 150–300 nm. They replicate by causing fusion of neighboring cells into large multinucleated syncytia. They are divided into two distinct groups (RSV-A and RSV-B), both of which are present during outbreaks.

RSVs are mainly a respiratory pathogen of young children. The highest rates of illness are seen in infants aged 1–6 mos, with peak rates occurring at 3 mos. Up to 80,000 pediatric hospitalizations and approximately 500 deaths each year are attributed to RSV. RSV are also an unrecognized cause of lower respiratory tract infection in the elderly and immunocompromised populations. One study found that RSV was identified as commonly as influenza A in hospitalized patients with flulike illness. Annual epidemics occur in late fall through early spring.

Primarily, **RSV transmission** is by self-inoculation of mucous membranes of the eyes, nose, and mouth by infected secretions. Transmission from fomites may also occur. RSV can survive outside the body for several hours, making good hand washing and contact isolation precautions critical in disease prevention.

Previous infection with RSV does not confer complete protection against reinfection. Humoral immunity, however, may reduce the severity of subsequent RSV infections. Antibodies acquired transplacentally do not protect infants against infection but, again, may reduce the severity of disease. Elderly patients who have lower antibody titers are more likely to develop symptomatic disease.

Clinical characteristics of **URIs** include cough, coryza, rhinorrhea, conjunctivitis, and otitis media. Apneic episodes may be seen in approximately 25% of infants admitted with RSV infections, but the exact mechanism remains unclear. These RSV-induced apneic episodes may also be responsible for up to one-third of cases of sudden infant death syndrome.

RSV infection of the **lower respiratory tract** can result in bronchospasm, bronchiolitis, pneumonia, and in severe cases, respiratory failure. Patients at risk for lower respiratory tract disease include infants (<6 mos of age), children with underlying structural lung and heart disease, patients of any age group with significant asthma or COPD, institutionalized elderly patients, and immunocompromised patients.

RSV infection is a **self-limited process** with no apparent long-term pulmonary sequelae in most individuals. However, there may be a correlation between RSV infection in infancy and the later development of reactive airways disease. One study found that approximately 25% of infants with RSV infection requiring hospitalization subsequently develop bronchospastic disease later in childhood. How this correlation translates to the development of reactive airway disease in adults remains unknown.

Acquiring secretions for **culture** using nasal or throat swabs allows the diagnosis of RSV to be made definitively. In patients who are intubated, tracheal aspirates, bronchial washings, and even bronchoalveolar lavage (BAL) samples can be obtained for culture. Syncytium formation with positive immunofluorescent staining of the viral cultures confirms the diagnosis. However, this test takes days to weeks. Antigen capture techniques allow for rapid diagnosis in <30 mins with sensitivities and specificities >90%. Diagnostic serology is unhelpful because individuals may have high levels of antibodies in circulation from previous RSV infections.

Treatment for RSV infection consists primarily of **supportive management** with **bronchodilators and oxygen supplementation.** One in two infants with bronchospasm responds to bronchodilator therapy, but to date no reliable method exists to determine which will respond. Inhaled epinephrine may improve airway obstruction in RSV bronchiolitis but should be stopped if no effect is demonstrated within 6–12 hrs of use. Mechanical ventilation may be required when oxygenation becomes significantly impaired. This impairment occurs in 5% of hospitalized infants, 10% of hospitalized elderly patients, and 50% of infected leukemic patients who are neutropenic secondary to chemotherapy. The use of steroids, antiviral agents, and immunoglobulins for treatment is controversial.

The American Academy of Pediatrics consensus statement indicates that **ribavirin** may be considered in infants with structural heart or lung disease, infants who are immunosuppressed, or those whose disease has progressed to require mechanical ventilation. In bone marrow and stem cell transplantation recipients, the early use of ribavirin (30–45 mg/kg/day) has been shown to reduce morbidity and mortality compared to historic controls. Ribavirin is contraindicated in pregnancy.

The use of **steroids** is not supported by compelling clinical evidence. Nebulized corticosteroids have shown no significant effects on symptom duration, hospitalization rates, or other treatment endpoints when compared to placebo.

RSV IV immunoglobulin (1.5 g/kg IV) may reduce viral shedding and improve oxygenation. There is, however, no evidence to support any change in the length of hospitalization. **Palivizumab,** an RSV-specific humanized monoclonal antibody, may also reduce viral shedding and improve oxygenation but also without an effect on length of hospitalization. Combination therapy with ribavirin and RSV IV immunoglobulin in adult bone marrow transplant patients was found to reduce mortality by 22% in one study. Therefore, combination therapy may be considered in certain immunocompromised patients. Efforts to develop an RSV vaccine have been unsuccessful to date.

PARAINFLUENZA VIRUS

Parainfluenza viruses (PIVs) are members of the Paramyxoviridae family. They are single-stranded RNA viruses with a pleomorphic shape. They range in diameter from 150 to 200 nm. There are four major serotypes that include PIV-1, 2, 3, and 4. PIV-3 is the most prevalent serotype, with 90–100% of children being seropositive by age 5; this serotype is associated with **pneumonia** and **bronchiolitis.** Adult infections are almost universally due to PIV-4, which usually causes **mild URIs.** PIV-1 and PIV-2 are associated with **croup** in children.

PIV primarily infects nasal and oropharyngeal epithelial cells, with subsequent distal spread to the large and small airways. Viral replication occurs 24 hrs after infection in the nasal and pulmonary passageways, peaking after 2–5 days. PIV-1 and 2 infect the larynx and trachea, whereas PIV-3 infects the distal airways. Very little direct damage is caused by the virus, and host immune response is probably a major contributor to clinical disease.

Approximately 18% of acute respiratory tract infections in hospitalized children can be attributed to human PIV. Spread of the virus occurs through large droplet inhalation, and the virus is **easily spread by person-to-person contact.** PIV-1 and 2 occur in epidemics every 2 yrs during the fall. PIV-3 occurs in annual spring epidemics. Seasonal patterns of PIV-4 infection are unclear. Non-Caucasian males are most likely to develop bronchiolitis from PIV.

PIV can cause **upper and lower respiratory infections** in both adults and children. In adults, this virus usually causes mild URIs. Lower respiratory disease in adults is usually seen in immunocompromised hosts. In infants and young children, PIV ranks as the second most common cause of lower respiratory tract infections.

There are many different **clinical presentations of PIV** depending on the viral serotype and host infected. PIV-1 is the main agent responsible for croup in children. PIV-2 also causes croup, but symptoms are milder. These patients present with fever, rhinitis, and pharyngitis that eventually develops into the characteristic barking cough. The symptoms usually last up to 4 days. The presentation can be complicated by stridor, dyspnea, and respiratory distress. Hypoxemia is rare but can be seen with lung parenchymal involvement. PIV-3 is associated with bronchiolitis and pneumonia and is often mistaken for RSV infection. Increased airways reactivity has been associated with PIV-3 infection, similar to that connected with RSV bronchiolitis. PIV-4 usually causes mild upper respiratory tract symptoms in both adults and children.

Immunocompromised hosts are susceptible to serious PIV infections. Here, mild upper respiratory tract symptoms can progress to pneumonias or even disseminated infections. Bone marrow and stem cell transplantation patients have infection rates ranging from 2% to 7% with mortality rates among infected patients as high as 30%.

The virus has also been associated with COPD and asthma exacerbations. Secondary bacterial pneumonias may occur in institutionalized elderly patients. Other complications from PIV infection include sinusitis, otitis media, meningitis, pericarditis, myocarditis, and Guillain-Barré syndrome. The last three complications are very rare.

The diagnosis of PIV infection is often made clinically (i.e., not by identifying the causative organism). The gold standard is **culture of PIV** from nasopharyngeal or lower respiratory secretions. Rapid antigen detection is available with 75–90% sensitivity. Serologic testing is impractical even though it is possible. PCR for PIVs is available, with sensitivities and specificities being >95%.

Treatment is largely **supportive.** There are no antiviral agents with activity against PIV infections in immunocompetent hosts. Ribavirin has been used to treat bone marrow transplant recipients, but few data exist on its efficacy in this setting. Combination therapy with ribavirin and immunoglobulin did not alter the duration of illness or mortality in clinical studies. Cold mist inhalation has been used to treat croup, but very little evidence exists for its efficacy. Bronchodilators can be useful, but data from prospective randomized trials are lacking. Steroids have had variable success in anecdotal reports, but prospective trials have not been completed. Currently, no effective vaccine for PIV has emerged, although active research is ongoing.

ADENOVIRUS

Adenoviruses are double-stranded DNA viruses. There are 52 different serotypes with 6 subgroups, A–F. Viruses readily infect human epithelial and fibroblast cell lines, leading to cytolysis. This cytopathic effect is used to isolate the viruses from clinical specimens.

Adenoviruses have a worldwide distribution, and infections occur year round. They cause **5–10% of all febrile illnesses in children.** They are so prevalent that by age 10 most individuals have serologic evidence of infection. URI is most common, usually resulting from infection with viruses of subgroup C. This virus is commonly encountered in households and daycare centers where young children are found. Transmission may occur via fomites, aerosolized particles, and the fecal-oral route. Adenoviruses can cause persistent infections, and the virus may be shed in the feces for months. Adenoviral infections have been transmitted to kidney and liver transplant recipients, suggesting that reactivation of latent virus (possibly in the transplanted organ) may be another important mode of transmission. Vertical transmission has been reported in infants who were exposed to infected cervical secretions.

The **presentation** of infection depends primarily on the **age** and **immune status** of the infected host. In children, adenoviruses are the most common cause of febrile respiratory illness. Adenoviruses cause **upper respiratory tract illnesses** such as coryza, pharyngitis, croup, and bronchitis but can also cause lower respiratory tract disease—i.e., pneumonia. Bacterial superinfection can also occur, which can increase the duration and severity of the illness. Adenovirus is the most common cause of tonsillitis in infants. Exudative tonsillitis and palpable cervical adenopathy may be seen, making differentiation from strep throat in older children difficult. Pneumonia is most common in infants and rare in immunocompetent adults. **Complications** include bronchiectasis in children and acute respiratory disease (ARD) in young adults. ARD is especially common in close-quarter dwellings. Patients with ARD develop fever, pharyngitis, cough, hoarseness, and conjunctivitis.

Bone marrow transplant patients may develop a wide range of respiratory clinical syndromes, including **pneumonia.** Solid organ transplant recipients may develop asymptomatic shedding, all manner of respiratory syndromes, and even fatal disseminated disease. Adenoviral pneumonia is a well-known early complication of lung transplantation.

The **diagnosis** of adenoviral infection is difficult to make on clinical grounds alone as the virus can cause a multitude of syndromes. There are multiple diagnostic methods for determining whether adenovirus infection is present.

Viral culture is the most sensitive and specific test. All adenoviruses except serotypes 40 and 41 cause a characteristic cytopathic effect in culture. Samples for culture can be obtained from nasopharyngeal swabs or aspirates, throat washings or swabs, rectal swabs, urine, and CSF or tissue biopsies. Because prolonged shedding may be seen in immunocompromised patients without overt disease, culture positivity should be interpreted with respect to the clinical situation.

Viral antigen assay is a direct detection method for detecting adenovirus antigens. Usually, an ELISA or a simple immunofluorescence assay is used. It is not as sensitive as viral culture but much more rapid.

Restriction endonuclease assay can be used to differentiate clinical isolates of the same serotype.

PCR is a highly sensitive and specific assay that can be used to detect adenovirus in multiple different samples.

Histopathology provides definitive diagnosis of adenovirus in tissue biopsies.

Serologies are less commonly used. A fourfold increase in antibodies to adenovirus can indicate active infection. Anything less than fourfold is likely to be secondary to prior exposures.

Treatment for adenoviral infection in the immunocompetent host is usually **supportive,** as most disease is **self-limited.** No compelling role for antiviral agents has been documented. Ganciclovir has limited activity against adenoviruses *in vitro* as do ribavirin and vidarabine. There is some debate about the utility of cidofovir, which is currently approved only for the treatment of CMV infections.

Vaccines have been used in certain circumstances. **Oral vaccine** consisting of enteric-coated viruses (type 4 and 7) has been used to prevent disease in military recruits, although recently the manufacturer has stopped producing this vaccine.

INFLUENZA VIRUS

Influenza is an acute respiratory illness caused by **type A or type B influenza virus** infection. It usually occurs as epidemics in the winter months. Systemic and respiratory symptoms are usually present. Usually, this illness is benign in that its course is self-limited with supportive therapy, although in high-risk populations, there can be significant morbidity and mortality.

Symptoms in the immunocompetent host usually begin with the abrupt onset of fever, myalgias, and headache, often associated with respiratory symptoms such as cough and sore throat. The spectrum of presentations varies, with some patients having symptoms resembling a simple cold without systemic symptoms and others having systemic symptoms without respiratory complaints. Patients usually appear hot and flushed with oropharyngeal hyperemia. Mild cervical lymphadenopathy may be present in younger patients. Lung exam is usually clear to auscultation. **Postinfluenza asthenia** refers to weakness and fatigue after an influenza attack that may last several weeks.

In complicated cases of influenza, pneumonia may develop. **Pneumonia** is especially common in patients with underlying lung or cardiovascular disease, diabetes, renal disease, immunosuppression (of any etiology), or hemoglobinopathies; who are in nursing homes; and who are of advanced age (>65 yrs). Pneumonias can be either primary viral or secondary bacterial infections. Patients with primary influenza pneumonia usually have persistent or worsening symptoms. They have very high fevers and dyspnea with or without cyanosis. Bacterial pneumonias develop owing to injury of tracheobronchial epithelium predisposing to infection by *Streptococcus pneumoniae*, *Staphylococcus aureus,* and *Haemophilus influenza.* These patients usually show some improvement in their influenza-related symptoms before developing worsening fever and respiratory complaints.

Diagnosis of influenza is usually made on **clinical grounds** alone, especially in the midst of influenza epidemics. More definitive diagnosis can be made through a variety of lab methods.

Viral culture samples are obtained from throat or nasal swabs, sputum, or BAL fluid and grown in tissue culture. Isolation of virus from culture can take 48–72 hrs.

Rapid testing is increasingly used. There are a variety of different techniques for making a rapid diagnosis of influenza infection. They include immunofluorescence assays, enzyme immunoassays, and PCR.

Serology may occasionally be used. Antibody titer increases in excess of fourfold (diagnostic of infection) can be established in acute illness primarily by the hemagglutination inhibition reaction.

Treatment consists mainly of **supportive measures,** although a number of targeted treatment strategies are becoming more commonplace. General supportive measures for influenza infection include treatment of headaches, myalgias, and fever with acetaminophen. Salicylates should be avoided in patients aged <18 yrs owing to the possibility of the development of Reye's syndrome. Antitussives may also be used, and adequate hydration is essential. Antibiotics are reserved for bacterial superinfections, including pneumonia, otitis media, and sinusitis.

A number of antiviral agents are used in both the prevention and treatment of influenza. **Amantadine** (100 mg PO bid ×5 days) and **rimantadine** (100 mg PO bid ×5 days) are two currently approved drugs for the prevention of influenza. They are only active against influenza A and have been reported to be 70–100% effective. Both these medications should be administered daily throughout the influenza season. They are used primarily in patients not immunized against influenza and to prevent outbreaks in institutions. Both agents can be used to treat influenza as well. When administered within 2 days of the onset of symptoms, the duration of illness can be reduced by 50% in most cases.

Neuraminidase inhibitors, such as inhaled zanamivir and oral oseltamivir, have activity against both type A and type B influenza viruses. **Zanamivir** (10 mg bid inhaled ×5 days) can be used to treat influenza in patients aged >7 yrs but has no approved indication for prophylaxis. It can cause bronchospasm and should be avoided in patients with chronic pulmonary disease. **Oseltamivir** can be used to treat patients >18 yrs old (treatment dose: 75 mg PO bid) and can be used as prophylaxis in patients aged >13 yrs (preventive dose: 75 mg PO qd). It can cause nausea and vomiting. Both of these agents can reduce the severity and duration of illness by 1 day.

Immunization is the major measure for prevention of influenza. Current vaccines are available as whole virus or *split products* (inactivated subcomponents of the virion). Whole virus vaccine is not readily available in the United States. The efficacy of the vaccine is determined by how closely related the current strains are to those from the previous year, as vaccines are manufactured based on the most common strains found the year before. Current vaccines are well tolerated, although **reactions** can be seen in up to 5% of cases. These include low-grade fever and mild systemic symptoms. Patients who have serious documented allergies to eggs or egg components should not receive this vaccine because it is prepared in egg cultures. In the mid-1970s, there was an increase of Guillain-Barré syndrome noted in patients who received the swine vaccine, but this reaction has not been seen in those immunized with egg-cultured vaccines.

Current **recommendations** for annual influenza vaccination include

- Persons aged ≥ 50 yrs
- Nursing home or long-term-care facility residents
- Patients with chronic pulmonary or cardiovascular disease
- Patients requiring medical care or hospitalization for diabetes, renal disease, hemoglobinopathy, or immunosuppression
- Adolescents or children on long-term ASA who may be at risk for Reye's syndrome
- Women in the second or third trimester of pregnancy during the influenza season
- Health care workers

AVIAN INFLUENZA (BIRD FLU)

Avian influenza is caused by certain strains of influenza virus. These strains occur naturally among wild birds but may on occasion infect domesticated birds, including chickens, ducks, and turkeys. Domesticated birds may become infected through direct contact with infected waterfowl or through contact with surfaces (e.g., cages) or materials (e.g., feed) that have been contaminated with the virus through the secretions and excretions of infected birds. Infection in domesticated birds results in two forms of disease. The *low pathogenic* form usually causes only mild disease (e.g., decreased egg production), whereas the *highly pathogenic* form spreads more rapidly, resulting in multisystem disease with a mortality rate reaching 90–100%, often within 48 hrs.

Influenza A (H5N1) virus—also called **H5N1 virus**—is an influenza A virus occurring mainly in birds. Outbreaks of avian H5N1 influenza in domesticated birds occurred in eight countries in Asia (Cambodia, China, Indonesia, Japan, Laos, South Korea, Thailand, and Vietnam) during late 2003. By March 2004, the outbreak was reported to be under control, but since June 2004, new outbreaks have been reported by several countries (Cambodia, China, Indonesia, Kazakhstan, Malaysia, Mongolia, Russia, Thailand, and Vietnam). It is believed that these outbreaks are ongoing.

Although H5N1 virus does not usually infect humans, more than 130 human cases have been reported by the WHO since January 2004 in Cambodia, China, Indonesia, Thailand, and Vietnam. Most cases occurred as a result of direct or close contact with infected poultry or contaminated surfaces; however, a few cases of human-to-human spread of H5N1 have been documented. In the current outbreak, the mortality has exceeded 50%. However, it is probable that only the most severe cases were reported, and that the full range of illness caused by the H5N1 virus has yet to be defined. Spread of H5N1 virus from person to person has been rare and has not been documented to continue beyond single cases of transmission. Nonetheless, concern that the H5N1 virus may mutate into a form both infectious to and transmissible between humans is both real and concerning, because there is little or no innate immunity in the human population. If this were to occur, the result could be an influenza pandemic.

The H5N1 virus currently infecting humans in Asia is resistant to both amantadine and rimantadine. However, both oseltamivir and zanamivir have shown promise in early studies and are believed to be effective in treating H5N1 disease. There currently is no available vaccine, although vaccine development is occurring at a furious pace. The first studies testing vaccine against H5N1 virus began in April 2005, and a series of clinical vaccine trials is under way.

CYTOMEGALOVIRUS

CMV is a member of the Herpesviridae family. CMV usually produces asymptomatic infection in immunocompetent hosts with the virus remaining latent. Although the cells of latency are unknown, CMV can be recovered from the salivary glands and the uterine cervix. Seroprevalence increases with age and number of sexual partners. CMV itself is immunosuppressive and can worsen *Pneumocystis jiroveci* pneumonia.

Severe disease tends to occur in **immunocompromised patients.** Solid organ and bone marrow transplantation patients are at highest risk of infection during the first 100 days after transplantation. The main pulmonary manifestation is CMV pneumonitis, which may occur in up to 15% of transplant populations. The disease is usually severe, with a high incidence of **respiratory failure** and a mortality rate exceeding 80%. Patients may present with focal infiltrates, bilateral patchy infiltrates, or diffuse interstitial infiltrates. Pulmonary manifestations are also seen in HIV patients but are becoming less prevalent with the advent of highly active antiretroviral therapy. In immunocompetent patients, infection is mostly asymptomatic, but pharyngitis is usually the main respiratory symptom if any occur.

Diagnosis of infection is by viral isolation from **culture** of sputum, bronchial washings, and BAL fluid. To confirm the diagnosis of CMV pneumonitis, transbronchial (or rarely surgical lung) **biopsies** demonstrating giant CMV-infected pneumocytes are required. Serologies for IgM in immunocompetent patients may be of some utility. Quantitative antigen detection in blood, urine, or CSF using PCR can be helpful in making the diagnosis.

There are **no vaccines** available to date. The antiviral agents that are effective against CMV include ganciclovir, foscarnet, or cidofovir. **Ganciclovir** (5 mg/kg q12h IV ×14–21 days for induction therapy of CMV retinitis, then 6 mg/kg IV for 5 days every week or 5 mg/kg IV qd; oral dose is 1000 mg PO tid with food) is the first-line therapeutic agent, with the other agents being used as salvage therapy owing to their significant incidence of adverse effects. In transplant patients with life-threatening CMV infection, **CMV immune globulin** (150 mg/kg 2×/wk) has been used in addition to the antiviral agents mentioned. See Chap. 32, Lung Transplantation, for more information on diagnosis and treatment of CMV infection.

OTHER VIRAL INFECTIONS

Epstein-Barr virus infection has been implicated in the development of posttransplant lymphoproliferative disease (see Chap. 32, Lung Transplantation).

VZV manifests with chickenpox on primary exposure and as zoster with reactivation. Primary pneumonias are rare but can have a high mortality rate. Immunocompromised patients are at greatest risk of VZV pulmonary infection. Infections are treated with IV acyclovir. Preventative measures in immunocompromised patients may include vaccination of seronegative patients before transplantation, administration of varicella zoster immune globulin to exposed patients or the use of prophylactic acyclovir.

KEY POINTS TO REMEMBER

- Rhinoviruses are responsible for up to 40% of common colds. They are usually spread via direct contact with infected secretions; cold temperature exposure, fatigue, and sleep deprivation have not been associated with increasing rates of transmission.

- Coronaviruses are an important cause of the common cold, and more recently, they have been implicated as the causative agent in the recent SARS epidemic.
- RSV is the foremost cause of lower respiratory viral infection in infants and young children.
- Adenoviruses may be responsible for "acute respiratory disease" in young adults.
- Influenza is generally a benign and self-limited disease, although in high-risk populations, significant morbidity and mortality can occur.
- Current influenza vaccines are well tolerated, although reactions can be seen in up to 5% of cases. Patients who have serious documented allergies to eggs or egg components should not receive this vaccine.
- CMV infection generally occurs in patients who have undergone organ transplantation and are immunosuppressed.

REFERENCES AND SUGGESTED READINGS

Atmar RL, Guy E, Guntupalli KK, et al. Respiratory tract viral infections in inner-city asthmatic adults. *Arch Intern Med* 1998;158:2453.

Centers for Disease Control and Prevention. Key facts about avian influenza (bird flu) and avian influenza A (H5N1) virus. Available at http://www.cdc.gov/flu/avian/gen-info/facts.htm. Accessed December 12, 2005.

Cohen JI, Corey GR. Cytomegalovirus infection in the normal host. *Medicine (Baltimore)* 1985;64:100.

Denny FW Jr. The clinical impact of human respiratory virus infections. *Am J Respir Crit Care Med* 1995;152:S4.

Dolin R. Influenza: current concepts. *Am Fam Physician* 1976;14:72.

Engel JP. Viral upper respiratory infections. *Semin Respir Infect* 1995;10:3.

Evans AS. Infectious mononucleosis and related syndromes. *Am J Med Sci* 1978;276: 325.

Gwaltney J, Hendley J, Simon G, et al. Rhinovirus infections in an industrial population. *N Engl J Med* 1966;275:1261.

Hall CB. Respiratory syncytial virus and parainfluenza virus. *N Engl J Med* 2001;344: 191.

Ho M. Epidemiology of cytomegalovirus infections. *Rev Infect Dis* 1990;12[Suppl 7]:S701.

Horwitz CA, Henle W, Henle G, et al. Clinical and laboratory evaluation of cytomegalovirus-induced mononucleosis in previously healthy individuals. Report of 82 cases. *Medicine (Baltimore)* 1986;65:124.

Kilbourne ED, Loge JP. Influenza A prime: a clinical study of an epidemic caused by a new strain of virus. *Ann Intern Med* 1950;33:371.

Klemola E, Kaarianinen L. Cytomegalovirus as a possible cause of a disease resembling infectious mononucleosis. *BMJ* 1965;2:1099.

Lai MM, Cavanagh D. The molecular biology of coronaviruses. *Adv Virus Res* 1997;48:1.

Makela M, Puhakka T, Ruuskanen O, et al. Viruses and bacteria in the etiology of the common cold. *J Clin Microbiol* 1998;36:539.

Monto A, Ullman B. Acute respiratory illness in an American community: the Tecumseh study. *JAMA* 1974;227:164.

Ottolini MG, Hemming VG. Prevention and treatment recommendations for respiratory syncytial virus infection—background and clinical experience 40 years after discovery. *Drugs* 1997;54:867.

Preliminary clinical description of severe acute respiratory syndrome. *MMWR Morb Mortal Wkly Rep* 2003;52:255.

Respiratory syncytial virus activity—United States, 1999–2000 season. *MMWR Morb Mortal Wkly Rep* 2000;49(48):1091.

Shay DK, Holman RC, Newman RD, et al. Bronchiolitis-associated hospitalizations among US children, 1980–1996. *JAMA* 1999;282:1440.

Shay DK, Holman RC, Roosevelt GE, et al. Bronchiolitis-associated mortality and estimates of respiratory syncytial virus–associated deaths among US children, 1979–1997. *J Infect Dis* 2001;183:16.

Siddell S, Wege H, Ter MV. The biology of coronaviruses. *J Gen Virol* 1983;64(4):761.

Stuart-Harris CH. Twenty years of influenza epidemics. *Am Rev Respir Dis* 1961;83:54.
Tsang KW, Ho PL, Ooi GC, et al. A cluster of cases of severe acute respiratory syndrome in Hong Kong. *N Engl J Med* 2003;348:1977.
Turner R. Epidemiology, pathogenesis and treatment of the common cold. *Ann Allergy Asthma Immunol* 1997;78:531.
Update: Influenza activity—United States, 2002–03 season. *MMWR Morb Mortal Wkly Rep* 2003;52:224.
Update: Influenza activity—United States and worldwide, 2002–03 season, and composition of the 2003–04 influenza vaccine. *MMWR Morb Mortal Wkly Rep* 2003;52:516.
Wald TG, Miller BA, Shult P, et al. Can respiratory syncytial virus and influenza A be distinguished clinically in institutionalized older persons? *J Am Geriatr Soc* 1995;43:170.
Walsh EE, Falsey AR, Hennessey PA. Respiratory syncytial and other virus infections in persons with chronic cardiopulmonary disease. *Am J Respir Crit Care Med* 1999;160:791.
Wendt CH, Hertz MI. Respiratory syncytial virus and parainfluenza virus infections in the immunocompromised host. *Semin Respir Infect* 1995;10:224.
Winther B, Gwaltney JM Jr, Mygind N, Hendley JO. Viral-induced rhinitis. *Am J Rhinol* 1998;12:17.
Wood A, Payne D. The action of three antiseptics/disinfectants against enveloped and non-enveloped viruses. *J Hosp Infect* 1998;38:283.
World Health Organization. Avian influenza frequently asked questions. Available at http://www.who.int/csr/disease/avian_influenza/avian_faqs/en/index.html. Accessed December 12, 2005.
Zhao H, De BP, Das T, Banerjee AK. Inhibition of human parainfluenza virus-3 replication by interferon and human MxA. *Virology* 1996;220:330.

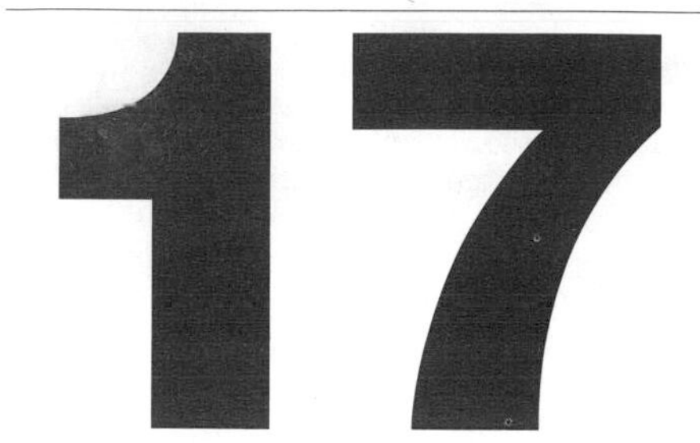

Cystic Fibrosis

Stephen Ryan

INTRODUCTION

Cystic fibrosis (CF) is the most common lethal inherited disease affecting the white population. The incidence is approximately 1 in 3300 white births, but all races are affected to some degree. Pediatricians traditionally provided most of the care for CF patients, but with the significant increase in life expectancy over the past five decades, internists increasingly participate in the management of this condition. The median age of survival in the United States is approximately 32 yrs.

A genetic mutation leading to an abnormal protein is the basic molecular defect responsible for CF. The protein is called the **CF transmembrane conductance regulator (CFTR).** The CFTR is an ion channel on the apical surface of epithelial cells that primarily plays a role in chloride transport. In CF, this protein is missing or malfunctioning, leading to a mishandling of chloride transport. The CFTR also plays a role in the regulation of other ion channels that may be important in the pathogenesis of CF. Many of the specific mechanisms by which the molecular defect of CF leads to clinical disease remain unclear and are the subject of current investigations.

CLINICAL MANIFESTATIONS

The clinical presentation of CF in the adult patient can be separated by organ system.

Pulmonary

Pulmonary consequences of CF are the source of considerable morbidity and mortality. Nearly all patients have **chronic sinusitis** on radiographic studies. More important are the **chronic lower airway infections** that are characteristic of this disease. Chronic infection causes inflammation, increased mucus secretion and obstruction, and direct destruction of pulmonary parenchyma. Classically, infectious colonization is described as happening in a stepwise fashion. *Haemophilus influenzae* and *Staphylococcus aureus* are early colonizers of the lung. Later, *Pseudomonas aeruginosa* becomes the dominant lung pathogen in a majority of CF patients. Progressive inflammation and lung damage are most closely correlated with this organism. Other organisms such as *Burkholderia cepacia* can lead to a fulminant course with a high mortality rate. Colonization with *Aspergillus fumigatus* is common, but invasive disease from this organism is relatively rare.

Acute exacerbation of CF is a common presentation of pulmonary disease. The specific factors important in the genesis of exacerbations are unclear, but viral infections have been implicated in some studies. The typical exacerbation presents with some combination of symptoms, including increased cough, changing sputum, increased shortness of breath, decreased exercise tolerance, and weight loss. Low-grade fever is common but not universal. Occasionally, a reduction in pulmonary function on spirometry may be the only abnormality. Chest radiographs are often unchanged during exacerbations but are useful to exclude other pulmonary complications of CF.

A number of less common pulmonary complications can lead to hospitalization. **Pneumothorax** is a relatively common pulmonary condition that presents in CF. The incidence of pneumothorax rises with increasing age secondary to worsening lung disease. Patients typically present with chest pain and dyspnea (but may present atypically) because of decreased compliance in the CF lung. A second pulmonary complication is minor **hemoptysis,** which is extremely common and often occurs with acute exacerbations of this disease. More significant hemoptysis ranging from moderate to massive has an incidence from 5% to 61% depending on the series studied. Hypertrophic bronchial arteries from chronic inflammation are the typical source of bleeding. Respiratory failure is the most concerning pulmonary presentation of CF. Unless reversible etiologies are responsible, this complication often indicates end-stage lung disease and carries a poor prognosis for recovery.

Gastrointestinal

GI manifestations are common in CF. Approximately 90% of CF patients exhibit pancreatic insufficiency. Patients with pancreatic insufficiency have significantly lower life expectancies than those with pancreatic sufficiency. Pancreatic sufficiency is more common in patients who present later in life. Pancreatic exocrine insufficiency can lead to steatorrhea, chronic malnutrition, edema secondary to hypoalbuminemia, and various vitamin deficiencies. Vitamin deficiencies are slightly more common in adolescents and adults. Vitamin A deficiency can lead to poor bone mineralization. Vitamin E deficiency can lead to ataxia and absent deep tendon reflexes.

Other GI complications involve nearly all segments of the GI tract. **Gastroesophageal reflux disease** is more common than in non-CF patients and is possibly linked to worsening lung disease. Another presentation of GI disease is the **distal intestinal obstruction syndrome,** which can be considered an adult equivalent of meconium ileus. Colicky abdominal pain with a palpable mass is a typical presentation. Radiographic patterns consistent with partial or complete obstruction can be seen on obstructive series. Caution must be exercised, however, because these signs and symptoms are present in other abdominal conditions that present in CF patients. CF can be associated with an asymptomatic increase in bilirubin and a mild transaminitis in up to one-third of patients, whereas biliary cirrhosis is much less common. However, a small percentage of patients do have significant disease with 3–5% of deaths in CF patients attributed to **liver disease.**

Endocrine

Endocrine and reproductive physiology can be affected in both sexes in CF. Men are usually infertile secondary to obstructive azoospermia. Women have reduced fertility because of thick cervical mucus as well as other, less understood factors. Puberty is often late in onset owing to malnutrition.

Diabetes mellitus is common in CF, affecting 12–15% of adults. Diabetes in CF is primarily due to deficient insulin production, although insulin resistance may play a role as well. CF patients may be dependent on insulin for glucose control, but diabetic ketoacidosis is rare.

DIAGNOSIS

The diagnosis of CF is based on **clinical presentation** coupled with confirmatory testing. **Pilocarpine iontophoresis,** or **sweat testing,** is the most common confirmatory test. A quantitative test with a chloride value of >60 mmol/L is consistent with CF. Other conditions produce abnormal sweat tests but can usually be differentiated from CF based on their clinical presentation. Nasal potential difference can be used as confirmatory testing in the rare instance in which CF is suspected clinically but sweat testing is inconclusive. This testing is only available at specialized centers. Genetic testing for CF is available but usually is not used as the initial diagnostic test. There are >600 known mutations and a number of unknown mutations that can lead to CF disease. The **most common mutation, ΔF508,** is responsible for between 70% and 80% of cases, making genetic testing a viable alternative. However, if a patient has known CF-causing mutation, genetic testing can be used to diagnose the disease and its carrier state in family members, irrespective of the frequency of its occurrence.

Other diagnostic evaluation can support the presence of CF but is generally neither specific nor sensitive for the diagnosis. Pulmonary function tests show an obstructive pattern early in the disease and tend to change to a mixed obstructive and restrictive pattern later when more fibrosis is present. Early in the disease, radiology tends to show hyperinflated lungs. Bronchiectasis with cyst formation is a later finding.

TREATMENT

Management of the acute pulmonary exacerbation is probably the most common reason for the **hospital admission** of CF patients. **Immunizations** should be kept up to date in an attempt to prevent exacerbations. **Antibiotics** are the main treatment for acute exacerbations. Antibiotic use in CF patients differs from that in other patients. First, higher doses of antibiotics are needed because of increased clearance and volumes of distribution. Second, longer courses of antibiotics are required. Fourteen- to twenty-one-day courses are typical of effective regimens. Sputum culture and sensitivity results should guide antibiotic choice. Oral antibiotics are appropriate for mild exacerbations. The main barrier to using oral antibiotics is the limited number of agents active against ***Pseudomonas***. **Ciprofloxacin** (400 mg IV bid or 750 mg PO bid) is one choice. Use of this drug should be limited to 3-wk courses given the rapid rise of resistant organisms when longer courses are used. For moderate to severe exacerbations or failed oral treatment courses, IV regimens are the standard of care. A typical two-drug regimen consists of an **aminoglycoside** (gentamycin/tobramycin, 3 mg/kg IV q8h or 10 mg/kg q24h following peak and trough levels) plus an **extended-spectrum penicillin** (piperacillin/tazobactam, 4.5 g IV q6h) or **cephalosporin** (cefepime, 2g IV q8h). Traditional dosing of aminoglycosides with measurement of peaks and troughs should be used. Occasionally, methicillin-resistant *S. aureus* is isolated from the sputum and requires **IV vancomycin** (15 mg/kg adjusted to maintain a trough of approximately 1s) for adequate coverage. One recent innovation in antibiotics for CF has involved a mode of delivery rather than a new agent. Inhaled tobramycin in 520 patients used in 28-day cycles was shown to improve pulmonary function and decrease the rate of hospitalization.

The issue of using **home IV antibiotics** arises frequently. There is some evidence that home IV treatment can be as effective as hospital treatment. However, the decision of inpatient vs outpatient treatment must be made on an individual basis. Resources available in the hospital such as intensive monitoring and extensive chest physical therapy are generally unavailable at home.

In the United States, IV antibiotics are generally reserved for the treatment of acute exacerbations owing to the concern of creating pathogen resistance with overuse of antibiotics. However, trials in other countries have shown scheduled IV antibiotics to be effective in CF. The Danish CF center sponsored a trial of intensive treatment of pseudomonal colonization against a historical control of patients treated with usual therapy. Patients treated with scheduled courses of antipseudomonal antibiotics were less likely to develop chronic pseudomonal infection. In addition, they were significantly less likely to have a reduction in pulmonary function compared to the control group.

Antibiotics are only one part of the treatment of pulmonary exacerbations in CF. **Respiratory therapy,** including chest percussion and postural drainage, has long been known to be efficacious in exacerbations. Recently, new techniques of physiotherapy have been used. For example, one trial looked at a mask using positive expiratory pressure **(PEP)** compared with conventional postural drainage and percussion. They found that PEP outperformed conventional therapy as shown by greater improvements in forced vital capacity and forced expiratory volume over 1 sec (FEV_1). Other techniques including percussors, pneumatic compression vests, and flutter valves are available to assist in **airway clearance.** Inflammation in CF is an additional target for CF therapeutics. One trial compared **prednisone** therapy with 1 mg/kg vs 2 mg/kg vs placebo on alternate days. The prednisone group had a higher percentage of predicted forced vital capacity. However, complications of steroid therapy, such as growth retardation and glycemic control, have limited the use of this therapy. **High-dose ibupro-**

fen has been used with some success but is again limited by side effects including renal failure and ulcer disease. Although traditional mucolytics have been disappointing in the treatment of CF, an **inhaled recombinant DNAse** that reduces the viscosity of CF sputum has been shown to be effective in reducing sputum viscosity and improving pulmonary function.

Complications including pneumothorax and hemoptysis are relatively common in CF. **Pneumothorax** is an indication for hospital admission. If small (<20% of the hemithorax volume), pneumothoraces can be managed conservatively with serial chest radiographs. If the pneumothorax enlarges or is symptomatic, a chest tube should be placed. Obliterative procedures should be considered for persistent and recurrent pneumothoraces. Chemical pleurodesis and surgical correction are the two primary options. Surgical correction is probably preferred if lung transplantation is a consideration. **Hemoptysis** is usually minor and responds to conservative treatment with IV antibiotics. Moderate to massive hemoptysis usually requires a more interventional approach. Basic treatment involves correction of coagulation parameters, withholding chest physiotherapy, and stopping inhaled antibiotics. Bronchial artery embolization plays an important role in massive or recurrent hemoptysis. A small study showed decreased bleeding and pulmonary exacerbations as well as increased quality of life when early bronchial artery embolization was used. Surgery is the last option if bronchial artery embolization fails to control the bleeding.

Treatment for respiratory failure is usually unsatisfactory. Noninvasive ventilation or even intubation has been used as a bridge to lung transplantation. **Bilateral lung transplantation** is the treatment of choice. The challenges of lung transplantation for this population are formidable given the incidence of preexisting infections and poor nutrition. However, success rates compare favorably to other indications for transplantation. Many cases are complicated by bronchiolitis obliterans.

Achieving **adequate nutrition** in CF patients affects both pulmonary status and overall mortality. **Replacement of pancreatic enzymes** as supplements is important for this goal. The usual starting dose is 500 lipase units/kg PO, which can be increased to maximum dose of 2500 units/kg. A typical regimen is to take one-third of the supplement at the start of the meal, one-third in the middle, and the last third at the end of the meal. Acid suppression may be necessary in some patients. Adequate proportions of fat and protein calories need to be ingested, which usually requires increased caloric intake. CF patients need to ingest 110–120% of the calories of their age-controlled peers to meet their metabolic needs. Fat-soluble vitamins should be provided in supplements.

The preferred treatments for **other GI complications** are less clear. Ursodeoxycholic acid probably has a role to play in the management of CF-induced cholestasis. Management of end-stage liver disease and the resulting complications of portal HTN is the same as in other etiologies of end-stage liver disease. Some literature available on the treatment of distal intestinal obstruction syndrome is available. A balanced intestinal lavage fluid has proven to be effective in mild cases. With the presence of partial or complete obstruction, diatrizoate meglumine and diatrizoate sodium (Hypaque) enemas can be used as both a diagnostic and a therapeutic maneuver. Surgery is rarely required.

Glucose intolerance as well as diabetes mellitus are more common in CF patients. Screening with blood glucose should probably be done yearly. Management of CF-related diabetes mellitus generally relies on insulin therapy.

Most males are **infertile** secondary to obstructive azoospermia. Microsurgical epididymal sperm aspiration with intracytoplasmic sperm injection into the ova shows promise for overcoming male infertility. Likewise, intrauterine insemination has overcome many of the factors that decrease fertility rates for female CF patients.

SPECIAL CONSIDERATIONS

Corresponding with the increasing life expectancy are increasing rates of pregnancy in CF patients. **Pregnancy** is more complicated but not insurmountable for CF patients. Women with mild lung disease and reasonable nutrition status generally do

QMUL Library
Whitechapel Library

Check loans & holds, pay fines
and much more online at:

www.library.ac.uk/self_service

Renewed Items 19/04/2013 09:28
XXXXXX6342

Item Title	Due Date
* The Washington manual pi	26/04/2013
* Self-assessment colour rev	17/05/2013

Thank you for using
QMUL Medical Libraries.

well. FEV_1 is probably the best predictor of problems in pregnancy. For example, in a UK study by Edinburgh, women with FEV_1 <60% delivered more preterm infants and had a greater decrease in lung function during the pregnancy compared to those with milder disease. Women should be encouraged to reach 90% of their ideal weight before their pregnancy. Nocturnal NG feeds can be used in those patients having difficulty gaining weight. Exacerbations should be treated aggressively. Cephalosporins and synthetic penicillins are generally safe. Aminoglycosides potentially cause fetal ototoxicity but may be necessary. Families should be counseled on the genetic risk of CF. All children of a parent with CF carry a single CF mutation; their chances of having CF disease depend on the genetics of the father.

EMERGING THERAPIES

Aggressive treatment of pulmonary infections and inflammation as well as attention to the **nutritional issues** involved in CF have largely been responsible for the significant improvement in mortality over the past five decades. New understanding of the genetic and molecular basis of CF holds the promise for similar advances in the decades ahead. New therapies can be divided into those that attempt to improve the function of the mutant CFTR protein and those that attempt to treat the genetic defect directly. Two drugs that are able to alter chloride transport independent of CFTR function are amiloride and uridine triphosphate. Amiloride showed promise in early trials but has not been shown to be clinically effective in larger trials. Uridine triphosphate has a half-life too short to be clinically useful, but longer-acting agents with similar action are in development.

Since the isolation of the CF gene in 1989, there has been interest in applying the principles of **gene therapy** to CF. The theoretical promise of this approach is still great, but there are many technical difficulties to overcome before this becomes a common approach to CF therapy.

CONCLUSION

Most diagnoses of CF are made by age 5 yrs. However, advances over the last three to five decades, with a corresponding increase in longevity, have led to an increasing role for internists in the management of this disease. Some medical issues are shared by both pediatric and adult CF patients, whereas other issues such as reproductive issues and treatment of end-stage disease tend to affect adults predominately. New research on the molecular basis of this disease coupled with therapeutics based on this new understanding will contribute to the improved management of CF in the coming years.

KEY POINTS TO REMEMBER

- CF is the most common lethal inherited disease affecting the white population.
- The median age of survival in the United States is around 32 years.
- CF is caused by a genetic mutation leading to a missing or malfunctioning protein, CFTR. CFTR is an ion channel in the apical surface of epithelial cells that plays a role in chloride transport.
- The typical CF exacerbation presents with some combination of symptoms including increased cough, changing sputum, increased shortness of breath, decreased exercise tolerance, and weight loss.
- Pneumothorax is a relatively common pulmonary complication occurring in CF.
- Approximately 90% of CF patients exhibit pancreatic insufficiency.
- Pilocarpine iontophoresis, or sweat testing, is the most common confirmatory diagnostic test. A quantitative test with a chloride value of >60 mmol/L is consistent with CF.

REFERENCES AND SUGGESTED READINGS

Antonelli M, Midulla F, Tancredi G, et al. Bronchial artery embolization for the management of nonmassive hemoptysis in cystic fibrosis. *Chest* 2002;121:796–801.

Cleghorn GJ, Forstner GG, Stringer DA, Durie PR. Treatment of distal intestinal obstruction syndrome with a balanced intestinal lavage solution. *Lancet* 1986;1(8471):8–11.

Collinson J, Nicholson KG, Cancio E, et al. Effects of upper respiratory tract infections in patients with cystic fibrosis. *Thorax* 1996:51:1115–1122.

Cystic Fibrosis Foundation. Cystic Fibrosis Foundation patient registry annual data report 1998. Bethesda, MD: Cystic Fibrosis Foundation, 1999.

Cystic Fibrosis Foundation. Cystic Fibrosis Foundation patient registry annual data report 2000. Bethesda, MD: Cystic Fibrosis Foundation, 2001.

Eigen H, Rosenstein B, Fitzsimmons S, et al. A multicenter study of alternate-day prednisone therapy in patients with cystic fibrosis. *J Pediatr* 1995;126:515–523.

Frederiksen B, Koch C, Hoiby N. Antibiotic treatment of initial colonization with *Pseudomonas aeruginosa* postpones chronic infection and prevents deterioration of pulmonary function in cystic fibrosis. *Pediatr Pulmonol* 1997;23:330–335.

Fuchs HJ, Borowitz DS, Christiansen DH, et al. Effect of aerosolized recombinant human DNAse on exacerbations of respiratory symptoms and on pulmonary function in patients with cystic fibrosis. *N Engl J Med* 1994;331:637–642.

Hilman B, Aitken M, Constantinescu M. Pregnancy in patients with cystic fibrosis. *Clin Obstet Gynecol* 1996;39:70–86.

Konstan MW, Byard PJ, Hoppel CL, et al. Effect of high-dose ibuprofen in patients with cystic fibrosis. *N Engl J Med* 1995;332:848–854.

LeGrys V. Sweat testing for the diagnosis of cystic fibrosis: practical considerations. *J Pediatr* 1996;129:892–897.

McIlwaine M, Wong L, Peacock D, Davidson G. Long-term comparative trial of conventional postural drainage and percussion versus positive expiratory pressure physiotherapy in the treatment of cystic fibrosis. *J Pediatr* 1997;131:570–574.

Mendeloff E, Huddleston C, Mallory G, et al. Pediatric and adult lung transplantation for cystic fibrosis. *J Thorac Cardiovasc Surg* 1998;115:404–413.

Orenstein D, Winnie G, Altman H. Cystic fibrosis: a 2002 update. *J Pediatr* 2002;2: 156–164.

Pond MN, Newport M, Joanes D, Conway SP. Home versus hospital intravenous antibiotic therapy in the treatment of young adults with cystic fibrosis. *Eur Respir J* 1994;7:1640–1644.

Ramsey B, Pepe MS, Quan JM, et al. Intermittent administration of inhaled tobramycin in patients with cystic fibrosis. *N Engl J Med* 1999;340:23–30.

Rubin B. Emerging therapies for cystic fibrosis lung disease. *Chest* 1999;115:1120–1126.

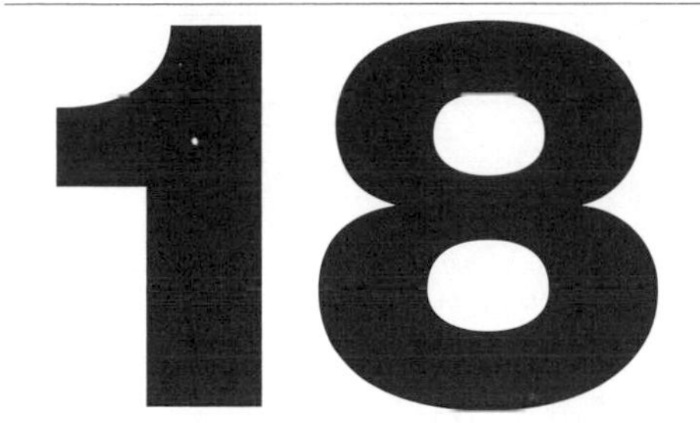

Hemoptysis

Tonya D. Russell

INTRODUCTION

Hemoptysis refers to the expectoration of blood originating from the lower airway or lung. **Massive hemoptysis** is the form that requires urgent attention; however, the definition of massive hemoptysis is variable in the literature and has ranged from 100 mL/24 hrs to 1000 mL/24 hrs. The most commonly accepted definition of massive hemoptysis is ≥ 600 mL/24 hrs. Massive hemoptysis accounts for 1.5–5% of all patients presenting with hemoptysis.

ETIOLOGY

In determining the cause of hemoptysis, other processes that could be confused with hemoptysis, such as hematemesis or bleeding from the upper airway, must first be eliminated. Table 18-1 outlines many of the possible causes of hemoptysis.

In a retrospective study of Veterans Administration patients, Santiago et al. noted that the four most commonly found causes for hemoptysis in their patient population were **cancer** (29%), **chronic bronchitis** (23%), **no identifiable cause** (22%), and **TB** (6%). Other identified causes included a variety of infections, sarcoidosis, pulmonary fibrosis, and bronchiectasis. In contrast, Hirshberg et al. performed a retrospective analysis of an Israeli patient population. The most commonly identified causes of hemoptysis were **bronchiectasis** (20%), cancer (19%), bronchitis (18%), and **pneumonia** (16%). Compared to the Santiago et al. study, unknown cause was listed only for 8% of patients and TB for 1.4% of patients. Given that both of these studies are retrospective and involve very different patient populations, it is difficult to compare them directly. However, they do give an idea of the more common causes of hemoptysis.

The circulation of the lung consists of two components—pulmonary and bronchial. In normal patients, the pulmonary artery system is a low-pressure system with systolic pressures of 15–20 mm Hg and diastolic pressures of 5–10 mm Hg. The bronchial artery arises from the aorta and thus represents systemic pressures. Therefore, in patients with normal pulmonary artery pressures, bleeding from the pulmonary artery only accounts for approximately 5% of massive hemoptysis cases.

DIAGNOSIS

The three traditional methods of evaluating the etiology of hemoptysis include chest x-ray (CXR), CT scan, and bronchoscopy. Although **CXR** is traditionally the first step in evaluating hemoptysis, it is normal in 20–30% of patients. For certain diagnoses such as bronchiectasis, **CT scan (high resolution)** has a much higher yield than CXR (sensitivity of 82–97% vs 37%).

Bronchoscopy has an overall diagnostic yield of 26%. In patients with abnormal, but nonlocalizing CXRs, the diagnostic yield is 34–55%. In patients with localizing CXRs, the yield of bronchoscopy has been as high as 82%. In patients with moderate to severe hemoptysis, Hirshberg et al. found that bronchoscopy was able to localize the site of bleeding in 64–67% of patients. CT scan has been touted as a mode complementary to bronchoscopy in determining the etiology of hemoptysis. Hirshberg et al. noted that

TABLE 18-1. CAUSES OF HEMOPTYSIS

- Infectious
  - Pneumonia
  - Lung abscess
  - Bronchitis
  - Bronchiectasis
  - Mycetoma
- Malignancy
  - Primary bronchogenic carcinoma
  - Extrapulmonary cancer with metastases to the lung
- Trauma/foreign body
  - Foreign body
  - Broncholith
  - Direct trauma
  - Tracheovascular fistula
- Cardiac/pulmonary vascular
  - Mitral stenosis
  - Pulmonary embolism/infarction
  - Pulmonary artery rupture
  - Arteriovenous malformation
- Alveolar hemorrhage
  - Goodpasture's syndrome
  - Wegener's granulomatosis
  - Henoch-Schönlein purpura
  - Scleroderma
  - Systemic lupus erythematosus
  - Rheumatoid arthritis
  - Behçet's syndrome

Adapted from Stoller JK. Diagnosis and management of massive hemoptysis: a review. *Respir Care* 1992;37:564–581; and Dwiek RA, Arroliga AC, Cash JM. Alveolar hemorrhage in patients with rheumatic disease. *Rheum Dis Clin North Am* 1997;23:395–410.

when used alone, CT scan had the higher yield (abnormal finding leading to final diagnosis) when compared to bronchoscopy alone: 67% vs 42%. In their study, 54% of patients with an abnormal CT scan had a positive bronchoscopy, and 38% of patients with a normal CT scan had a positive bronchoscopy. When **CT scan and bronchoscopy** were used together, the diagnostic yield was 93%.

There is still controversy over whether to use flexible bronchoscopy or rigid bronchoscopy in the setting of massive hemoptysis. There are no clear data favoring one method over the other. Flexible bronchoscopy has the advantage of better visualization of airways and the ability to navigate into small subsegments. In addition, it can be performed at the bedside of a patient in the ICU. However, the ability to suction blood with flexible bronchoscopy is inferior compared to that with rigid bronchoscopy. Rigid bronchoscopy is performed in the OR. It allows only visualization of larger airways, but as mentioned above, the ability to clear blood from the airway is better. In addition, more therapeutic interventions can be performed through the rigid bronchoscope.

MANAGEMENT

In patients with **nonmassive hemoptysis,** the therapy essentially involves treating the underlying cause (i.e., antibiotics for an infection, radiation therapy or laser therapy for an endobronchial tumor). The more urgent need for treatment arises in patients with **massive hemoptysis.**

The first priorities are **airway protection** and **stabilization of the patient.** The patient with massive hemoptysis usually requires intubation. If it is known which lung contains the site of bleeding, the patient can be selectively intubated. **Selective intubation** can be performed in several manners. One method requires the use of a double-lumen ETT, which allows for the lumen of the bleeding side to be clamped and for selective ventilation of the nonbleeding side. The placement of the double-lumen ETT requires the help of a physician skilled in this procedure. If the right lung is the bleeding site, a regular ETT can be inserted into the left mainstem bronchus to allow for selective ventilation of the left lung. Right mainstem intubation is not recommended when the left side is bleeding because it is easy to occlude the orifice to the right upper-lobe bronchus with the ETT and cause collapse of the right upper lobe. Instead, if the left lung is the bleeding site, an ETT can be placed in the trachea, and a Fogarty catheter can be inserted via a bronchoscope into the left mainstem bronchus.

Other strategies to help minimize the risk of aspirating blood into the nonbleeding side include positioning the patient with the bleeding side down and the use of strong cough suppressants (i.e., codeine). Large-bore IV access and fluid resuscitation should be started. Any coagulopathy should be corrected. A patient with massive hemoptysis should be observed in the ICU, even if not intubated.

Once **bronchoscopy** has been performed to localize the site of bleeding, **therapeutic options** can be performed through the bronchoscope, including iced saline lavage, topical epinephrine, endobronchial tamponade, and laser photocoagulation.

Bronchial artery embolization is frequently used to try to stop massive hemoptysis or recurrent hemoptysis (from sources such as mycetomas). The short-term success rate of bronchial artery embolization has been reported as between 64% and 100%. The recurrence rate of hemoptysis after bronchial artery embolization has been noted to be between 16% and 23%. Bronchial artery embolization may not be able to be performed if the anterior spinal artery arises from the bronchial artery owing to the possibility of spinal cord ischemia. The overall risk of spinal cord ischemic injury is <1%.

Surgery is another potential therapeutic option. To be considered a surgical candidate, a patient must be able to tolerate a lobectomy or possibly a pneumonectomy. Surgical mortality rates that have been reported vary between 1% and 50%.

CONCLUSION

The management of massive hemoptysis requires hemodynamic stabilization of the patient with protection of the airway in the nonbleeding lung. A multidisciplinary approach with input from both a pulmonologist and a thoracic surgeon is usually best.

KEY POINTS TO REMEMBER

- Hemoptysis refers to the expectoration of blood originating from the lower airways or lung parenchyma. Massive hemoptysis, the form that requires urgent attention, accounts for 1.5–5% of all patients presenting with hemoptysis.
- The three traditional methods of evaluating the etiology of hemoptysis include CXR, CT scan, and bronchoscopy.
- The patient with massive hemoptysis usually requires intubation. If it is known which lung is bleeding, the patient can be selectively intubated to protect the opposite lung from filling with blood.
- If the right lung is the bleeding site, insert a regular ETT into the left mainstem bronchus. Right mainstem intubation is not recommended when the left side is bleeding; instead, insert an ETT in the trachea and insert a Fogarty catheter via a bronchoscope into the left mainstem bronchus.

REFERENCES AND SUGGESTED READINGS

Dweik RA, Arroliga AC, Cash JM. Alveolar hemorrhage in patients with rheumatic disease. *Rheum Dis Clin North Am* 1997;23:395–410.

Dweik RA, Stoller JK. Role of bronchoscopy in massive hemoptysis. *Clin Chest Med* 1999;20:89–105.

Hirshberg B, Beran I, Glazer M, Kramer MR. Hemoptysis: etiology, evaluation and outcomes in a tertiary hospital. *Chest* 1997;112:440–444.

Jean-Baptiste E. Clinical assessment and management of massive hemoptysis. *Crit Care Med* 2000;28:1642–1647.

O'Neil KM, Lazarus AA. Hemoptysis: indications for bronchoscopy. *Arch Intern Med* 1991;151:171–174.

Santiago S, Tobias J, Williams AJ. A reappraisal of the causes of hemoptysis. *Arch Intern Med* 1991;151:2449–2451.

Stoller JK. Diagnosis and management of massive hemoptysis: a review. *Respir Care* 1992;37:564–578.

Tasker AD, Flower CDR. Imaging the airway: hemoptysis, bronchiectasis, and small airways disease. *Clin Chest Med* 1999;20:761–773.

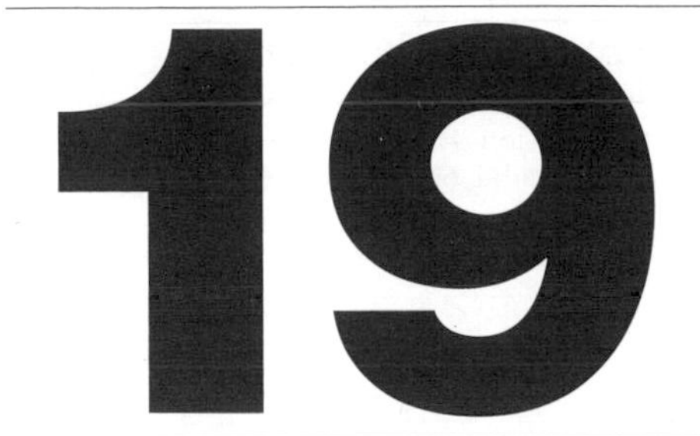

Diffuse Alveolar Hemorrhage

Steven L. Leh

INTRODUCTION

Diffuse alveolar hemorrhage (DAH) encompasses a heterogeneous group of pulmonary and nonpulmonary disorders characterized by widespread intraalveolar bleeding. The exact incidence and prevalence of DAH are unknown owing to the variety of underlying etiologies. Clinically, DAH should be suspected whenever a patient presents with **hemoptysis, dyspnea, and a predisposing condition,** such as an underlying connective tissue disorder, systemic vasculitis, or certain drug or occupational exposures. Hemoptysis, a presumed cardinal symptom of DAH, may be absent in up to one-third of cases despite pronounced and life-threatening alveolar hemorrhage. Differentiation from localized etiologies (Table 19-1) of pulmonary hemorrhage is difficult to ascertain on history and physical exam alone; diagnostic procedures such as chest radiography (CXR) and fiber-optic bronchoscopy are often needed. **Rapid diagnosis of DAH is mandatory** given the potential for excessive morbidity (renal failure, restrictive and obstructive lung disease) and mortality rates approaching 70–80% in untreated subsets of patients.

DIAGNOSIS

Appropriate diagnosis of DAH requires high clinical suspicion and a thorough history and physical exam. DAH is infrequently the initial presentation of an underlying systemic disorder (Table 19-2). 20% of patients with SLE and 5–10% of patients with Goodpasture's syndrome present with DAH as the initial or sole manifestation. Therefore, emphasis should be placed on the rheumatologic, renal, pulmonary, and cardiac review of systems.

A **detailed history of past and present medications** (prescribed, over-the-counter, and recreational) and **occupational exposures** should be obtained. Amiodarone, retinoic acid, sirolimus, penicillamine, and crack cocaine have all been implicated as causative agents of DAH. Inhalation of trimellitic anhydride, a chemical found in paints, varnishes, and plastics, has also been reported as a cause of DAH.

Physical exam findings are nonspecific and may include fever, hypoxemia, tachypnea, and diffuse rales. Identification of signs suggesting an underlying systemic disorder should be sought. These signs may include sinusitis, iritis, oral ulcers, arthritis, synovitis, palpable purpura, neuropathy, and cardiac murmurs. The definitive diagnosis of DAH, however, is based on radiologic, lab, bronchoscopic, and pathologic findings.

Standard posteroanterior and lateral **CXR** in DAH is nonspecific for any of the underlying etiologies and often reveals bilateral alveolar infiltrates during the acute episode. High-resolution chest CT is generally not indicated in DAH, as it adds little information to the CXR. It may, however, point to alternative diagnoses for hemoptysis or better localize parenchymal findings such as cavitary lung disease or malignancy. With recurrent episodes of DAH, pulmonary fibrosis or severe obstructive lung disease may develop. Accordingly, persistent interstitial infiltrates or hyperinflation may be evident on successive CXRs.

Lab evaluation is crucial for the diagnosis of DAH. A CBC, coagulation parameters, basic metabolic profile, urinalysis, and drug screen should be obtained on all patients. Anemia is commonly found, and repeated bouts of DAH may lead to an iron deficiency. Thrombocytopenia or elevated coagulation parameters should raise the possibility of hemorrhage secondary to an acquired coagulopathy or antiphospholipid antibody syndrome. If an abnormal creatinine is present, urine microscopy should be assessed for dysmorphic RBCs or RBC casts. Most urine drug screens are adequate to assess for cocaine use.

TABLE 19-1. CAUSES OF LOCALIZED PULMONARY HEMORRHAGE

Upper airway or GI bleeding with resultant aspiration—i.e., epistaxis or hematemesis (may be difficult to distinguish from diffuse alveolar hemorrhage)
Neoplasm (primary bronchogenic, Kaposi's)
Cavitary lung disease (secondary to TB, aspergillus)
Pulmonary infarction
Bronchitis
Bronchiectasis
Broncholithiasis
Necrotizing bronchopneumonia
Arteriovenous malformations

Serologic markers should also be obtained and their selection guided by the differential diagnosis. Patients suspected of developing a **pulmonary-renal syndrome** should be tested for serum ANCA and antiglomerular basement membrane antibodies (anti-GBM). ANCA are commonly found in patients with Wegener's granulomatosis, microscopic polyangiitis, Churg-Strauss syndrome, and isolated pauciimmune capillaritis.

Cytoplasmic ANCA (c-ANCA) is associated with **Wegener's granulomatosis** and is specifically directed against serine proteinase-3, a 29-kDa proteinase in neutrophil pri-

TABLE 19-2. CAUSES OF DIFFUSE ALVEOLAR HEMORRHAGE

Rheumatologic
SLE
Rheumatoid arthritis
Mixed connective tissue disorder
Systemic sclerosis
Behçet's disease
Juvenile rheumatoid arthritis
Polymyositis
Vasculitis
Wegener's granulomatosis
Microscopic polyangiitis
Henoch-Schönlein purpura
Pulmonary
Isolated pulmonary capillaritis
Idiopathic pulmonary hemosiderosis
Acute lung transplant rejection
Pulmonary venoocclusive disease
Pulmonary capillary hemangiomatosis
Renal
IgA nephropathy
Idiopathic glomerulonephritis
Poststreptococcal glomerulonephritis

(*continued*)

TABLE 19-2. (*continued*)

Hematologic
Autologous or allogeneic stem cell transplant
Thrombotic thrombocytopenic purpura
Idiopathic thrombocytopenic purpura
DIC
Cryoglobulinemia
Antiphospholipid antibody syndrome
Multiple myeloma
Cardiac
Mitral stenosis
Bacterial endocarditis
Gastrointestinal
Ulcerative colitis
Medication
Penicillamine
Propylthiouracil
Phenytoin
Retinoic acid
Nitrofurantoin
Amiodarone
Warfarin
Abciximab
Tirofiban
Crack cocaine
Occupational exposures
Trimellitic anhydride
Radiation exposure
Asbestosis
Welder's pneumoconiosis

mary granules. The level of c-ANCA has been used to follow disease activity, and its sensitivity is greater in active or generalized disease. In a literature review by Rao et al., the sensitivity of c-ANCA in active Wegener's granulomatosis was 91% vs 63% in inactive disease. The specificity was equivalent in both situations and approached 99%.

Perinuclear ANCA (p-ANCA), antibodies directed against **myeloperoxidase,** is less specific and may be associated with many clinical syndromes. p-ANCA is found in 80% of patients with microscopic polyangiitis. p-ANCA has also been identified in 15–20% of patients with Wegener's granulomatosis and up to 20–30% of patients with Goodpasture's syndrome.

Goodpasture's syndrome, characterized by antibodies (predominantly IgG) directed against the noncollagenous domain of (α3) type IV collagen, is diagnosed by the presence of anti-GBM. The sensitivity and specificity of anti-GBM approach 98%. 2–3% of patients with renal biopsy–proven Goodpasture's syndrome may have negative serum anti-GBM, making renal (and not lung) biopsy the gold standard for diagnosis.

Other markers of rheumatologic disease including ANA, anti-double-stranded DNA, complement levels, rheumatoid factor, extractable nuclear antigens, and anti-scleroderma antibody should be obtained to assess for etiologies such as SLE, rheumatoid arthritis, mixed connective tissue disorder, and progressive systemic sclerosis.

Fiber-optic bronchoscopy has a vital role in identifying the clinical syndrome of DAH. **Bronchoscopy with bronchoalveolar lavage (BAL)** rules out infectious etiologies and confirms the presence of DAH. Accepted bronchoscopic criteria for DAH include progressively bloodier returns from sequential BAL performed in three separate subsegmental bronchi or >20% hemosiderin-laden macrophages. False-positive results can occur in smokers ("smokers' macrophages"—the most common cause of hemosiderin-laden macrophages) and with distal bronchiolar sources of hemorrhage. A false-negative may occur if bronchoscopy is performed too early or too late. On average, 48–72 hrs are necessary for hemosiderin-laden macrophages to be seen in alveoli and interstitial spaces. After 2–4 wks, hemosiderin-laden macrophages generally clear.

Once BAL confirms the presence of DAH, the role of bronchoscopic biopsies in determining the underlying etiology of DAH is less significant. Only 17.6% of directed endobronchial biopsies were diagnostic of Wegener's granulomatosis in the setting of observed ulcerating tracheobronchitis. Typical **light microscopic findings** of DAH—including pulmonary capillaritis, diffuse alveolar damage, and bland pulmonary hemorrhage—can be found on transbronchial biopsy. The yield, however, is diminished owing to the small sample size and sampling error. If the diagnosis is not clearly made by history, physical exam, and serologic markers, video-assisted thoracoscopy or open-lung biopsy is the procedure of choice.

Lung biopsy specimens (from video-assisted thoracoscopy or open-lung biopsy) typically reveal one of three light microscopic patterns: pulmonary capillaritis, diffuse alveolar damage, or bland pulmonary hemorrhage. The most common histologic finding in DAH is pulmonary capillaritis (fibrin thrombi occluding capillaries, fibrinoid necrosis of capillary walls, neutrophils and nuclear dust in the interstitium and surrounding alveoli, and interstitial RBCs and hemosiderin). In one series of 34 patients with biopsy-proven DAH, 88% of patients displayed pulmonary capillaritis. Diffuse alveolar damage, a stereotypic response to lung injury, is characterized by interstitial edema, intraalveolar hyaline membranes, and type 2 alveolar cell hyperplasia in the acute phase. Bland pulmonary hemorrhage, conversely, reveals nonspecific alveolar septal thickening without any evidence of vasculitis, necrosis, or inflammation. None of these patterns is pathognomonic for any specific disease. In fact, multiple histologic findings can be associated with the same disease process. Pulmonary capillaritis, diffuse alveolar damage, and bland pulmonary hemorrhage have all been associated with DAH secondary to SLE.

TREATMENT

Treatment of DAH **depends primarily on the underlying disorder,** and the details are beyond the scope of this chapter. Therapies ranging from watchful waiting in idiopathic pulmonary hemosiderosis to high-dose corticosteroids and cytotoxic therapy in ANCA-associated vasculitides have significantly decreased the morbidity and mortality associated with these disorders. Typical regimens for life-threatening alveolar hemorrhage include cyclophosphamide, 3–5 mg/kg/day initially, with methylprednisolone, 1 g/day IV for 3 days, followed by prednisone (1 mg/kg/day for 3 mos followed by a 3-mo taper until discontinued) and subsequent prolonged maintenance therapy with cyclophosphamide (dosed to keep absolute neutrophil count ~1500). In certain immunologically mediated diseases such as Goodpasture's syndrome, therapeutic plasmapheresis is also indicated.

CONCLUSION

In summary, DAH encompasses a group of heterogeneous disorders characterized by widespread intraalveolar bleeding. If not readily diagnosed and treated, morbidity and mortality are exceedingly high. A high index of suspicion, thorough clinical history, appropriate serologic markers, and tissue biopsy remain the mainstays of diagnosis.

KEY POINTS TO REMEMBER

- DAH should be suspected whenever a patient presents with hemoptysis, dyspnea, and a predisposing condition such as an underlying connective tissue disorder, systemic vasculitis, or certain drug or occupational exposures.
- Hemoptysis, however, may be absent in up to one-third of cases.

- A CBC, coagulation parameters, basic metabolic profile, urinalysis, and drug screen should be obtained in all patients.
- Serological markers should be obtained and their selection guided by the differential diagnosis.

REFERENCES AND SUGGESTED READINGS

Afessa B, Tefferi A, Litzow MR, et al. Diffuse alveolar hemorrhage in hematopoietic stem cell transplant recipients. *Am J Respir Crit Care Med* 2002;166:641–645.

Ali A, Patil S, Grady KJ, Schreiber TL. Diffuse alveolar hemorrhage following administration of tirofiban or abciximab: a nemesis of platelet glycoprotein IIb/IIIa inhibitors. *Cathet Cardiovasc Intervent* 2000;49:181–184.

Barnett VT, Bergmann F, Humphrey H, Chediak J. Diffuse alveolar hemorrhage secondary to superwarfarin ingestion. *Chest* 1992;102:1301–1302.

Colby TV, Fukuoka J, Ewaskow SP, et al. Pathologic approach to pulmonary hemorrhage. *Ann Diagn Pathol* 2001;5:309–319.

Crausman RS, Achenbach GA, Pluss WT, et al. Pulmonary capillaritis and alveolar hemorrhage associated with the antiphospholipid antibody syndrome. *J Rheumatol* 1995;22:554–556.

Daum TE, Specks U, Colby TV, et al. Tracheobronchial involvement in Wegener's granulomatosis. *Am J Respir Crit Care Med* 1995;151:522–526.

Fontenot AP, Schwarz MI. Diffuse alveolar hemorrhage. In: Schwarz MI, King TE, eds. *Interstitial lung disease,* 4th ed. Philadelphia: BC Decker, 2003.

Gal AA, Velasquez A. Antineutrophil cytoplasmic autoantibody in the absence of Wegener's granulomatosis or microscopic polyangiitis: implications for the surgical pathologist. *Mod Pathol* 2002;15(3):197–204.

Green RJ, Ruoss SJ, Kraft SA, et al. Pulmonary capillaritis and alveolar hemorrhage. Update on diagnosis and management. *Chest* 1996;110:1305–1316.

Haim DY, Lippmann ML, Goldberg SK, Walkenstein MD. The pulmonary complications of crack cocaine. A comprehensive review. *Chest* 1995;107:233–240.

Hudson BG, Tryggvason K, Sundaramoorthy M, Neilson EG. Alport's syndrome, Goodpasture's syndrome, and type IV collagen. *N Engl J Med* 2003;348:2543–2556.

Jantz MA, Sahn SA. Corticosteroids in acute respiratory failure. *Am J Respir Crit Care Med* 1999;160:1079–1100.

Kalluri R, Meyers K, Mogyorosi A, et al. Goodpasture's syndrome involving overlap with Wegener's granulomatosis and anti-glomerular basement membrane disease. *J Am Soc Nephrol* 1997;8:1795–1800.

Katzenstein AA. *Katzenstein and Askin's surgical pathology of non-neoplastic lung disease,* 3rd ed. Philadelphia: WB Saunders, 1997.

Mark EJ, Matsubara O, Tan-Liu NS, Fienberg R. The pulmonary biopsy in the early diagnosis of Wegener's (pathergic) granulomatosis: a study based on 35 open lung biopsies. *Hum Pathol* 1988;19:1065–1071.

Mark EJ, Ramirez JF. Pulmonary capillaritis and hemorrhage in patients with systemic vasculitis. *Arch Pathol Lab Med* 1985;109:413–418.

Martinex AJ, Maltby JD, Hurst DJ. Thrombotic thrombocytopenic purpura seen as pulmonary hemorrhage. *Arch Intern Med* 1983;143:1818–1820.

Metcalf JP, Rennard SI, Reed EC, et al. Corticosteroids as adjunctive therapy for diffuse alveolar hemorrhage associated with bone marrow transplantation. *Am J Med* 1994;96(4):327–334.

Nicolls MR, Terada LS, Tuder RM, et al. Diffuse alveolar hemorrhage with underlying pulmonary capillaritis in the retinoic acid syndrome. *Am J Respir Crit Care Med* 1998;158:1302–1305.

Rao JK, Weinberger M, Oddone EZ, et al. The role of antineutrophil cytoplasmic antibody testing in the diagnosis of Wegener's granulomatosis. A literature review and meta-analysis. *Ann Intern Med* 1995;123:925–932.

Salama AD, Dougan T, Levy JB, et al. Goodpasture's disease in the absence of circulating anti-glomerular basement membrane antibodies as detected by standard techniques. *Am J Kidney Dis* 2002;39:1162–1167.

Schwarz MI, Zamora MR, Hodges TN, et al. Isolated pulmonary capillaritis and diffuse alveolar hemorrhage in rheumatoid arthritis and mixed connective tissue disease. *Chest* 1998;113:1609–1615.

Travis WD, Colby TV, Lombard C, Carpenter HA. A clinicopathologic study of 34 cases of diffuse pulmonary hemorrhage with lung biopsy confirmation. *Am J Surg Pathol* 1990;14(12):1112–1125.

Vizioli LD, Cho S. Amiodarone-associated hemoptysis. *Chest* 1994;105:305–306.

Vlahakis NE, Rickman OB, Margenthaler T. Sirolimus-associated DAH. *Mayo Clin Proc* 2004;79(4):541–545.

Winters JL, Pineda AA, McLeod BC, Grima KM. Therapeutic apheresis in renal and metabolic diseases. *J Clin Apheresis* 2000;15:53–73.

Zamora MR, Warner ML, Tuder R, Schwarz MI. Diffuse alveolar hemorrhage and systemic lupus erythematosus: clinical presentation, histology, survival, and outcome. *Medicine* 1997;76(3):192–202.

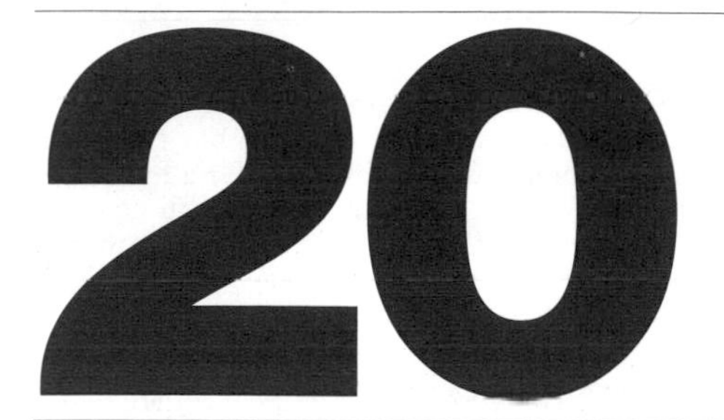

Pulmonary Vasculitis

Alexander C. Chen

OVERVIEW

Pulmonary manifestations of the systemic vasculitides range from mild upper respiratory tract symptoms to devastating alveolar hemorrhage. Although the lungs are infrequently the only organ system involved, respiratory symptoms often prompt patients to seek medical attention. Often, these issues are only part of a larger systemic process, and it is in this context that we address the various systemic vasculitides.

Vasculitis can occur as either a primary or secondary event. **Secondary vasculitis** occurs in the setting of another underlying illness, such as the capillaritis that can be seen in SLE, whereas **primary vasculitis** is a vasculitic syndrome that occurs in the absence of another illness and is usually without identifiable etiology.

Since the original description of the first systemic vasculitis by Kussmaul and Maier in 1866, the nomenclature and classification of these disorders have undergone significant evolution. In 1992, the Chapel Hill Consensus Conference established a standardized method of classification based mainly on histopathologic criteria and on the size of the vessels involved. Furthermore, the discovery of ANCA has significantly influenced the diagnosis and classification of the vasculitides and has provided insight into the possible mechanisms through which these processes progress.

EPIDEMIOLOGY

Primary systemic vasculitides are rare, and epidemiologic studies have been difficult given the changing nomenclature and classification systems. Overall, the frequency of diagnosis has increased over the years, although this may reflect the fact that vasculitic syndromes are being more readily recognized. Giant cell arteritis is the most frequently encountered vasculitis, with an annual incidence of 13 per 1 million adults, followed by rheumatoid arthritis–associated vasculitis (12.5 per million) and then by the small-vessel vasculitides, Wegener's granulomatosis (WG), microscopic polyangiitis (MPA), and Churg-Strauss syndrome (CSS).

WEGENER'S GRANULOMATOSIS

WG is a multisystem disease that affects **small to medium vessels.** Originally described as a variant of polyarteritis nodosa (PAN), the findings of a progressive granulomatous process involving the upper and lower respiratory tract as well as other organ systems led Wegener to believe that he had discovered a unique vasculitic syndrome. Although the **classic Wegener's triad** consisted of necrotizing granulomatous inflammation of the respiratory tract, generalized necrotizing vasculitis of the small arteries and veins, and necrotizing glomerulonephritis, fewer than half of the originally described cases fulfilled these criteria. The evolving process of disease classification and diagnosis has resulted in the 1992 Chapel Hill international consensus statement that WG is a "granulomatous inflammation involving the respiratory tract, and necrotizing vasculitis affecting small to medium-sized vessels."

Clinical Presentation

Before current therapy, the mortality associated with untreated WG was nearly universal, with a mean survival time of 5 mos. WG can occur at any age, but the mean age of onset is approximately 40 yrs. It affects men and women equally and has a predilection for Caucasians. The **initial presentation** is usually insidious, with generalized complaints of malaise, fatigue, weight loss, and upper respiratory symptoms. After this, patients may develop symptoms involving multiple organ systems.

Ear, nose, and throat involvement occurs in up to 99% of cases of WG. Chronic rhinitis, epistaxis, nasal crusting, and chronic sinusitis are commonly reported, and destruction of the nasal cartilage leads to the nasal septal perforation or saddle nose deformity that is associated with the disease. Ulcerations of the oropharynx and gingival hyperplasia also occur, as can the "strawberry" gingival hyperplasia that is rare but pathognomonic of WG.

Tracheobronchial ulcerations, intraluminal inflammatory pseudotumor, and bronchomalacia can occur, resulting in symptoms that can be confused with asthma, and scarring from these lesions can result in **significant airway obstruction.**

Necrotizing granulomas, cavitary lesions, and scattered nodules are the primary **pulmonary** manifestations of WG and are usually clinically insignificant, although mild hemoptysis can occur. Capillaritis in the lung is a result of the generalized vasculitic component of WG and can result in diffuse alveolar hemorrhage with an associated mortality of nearly 50%. This clinical presentation is indistinguishable from that which can occur in Goodpasture's syndrome or in microscopic polyangiitis.

Skin findings in WG include papules, vesicles, palpable purpura, ulcers, or subcutaneous nodules. Leukocytoclastic vasculitis is the most common manifestation and occurs in up to 50% of patients. Other skin lesions such as pyoderma gangrenosum and granulomatous skin lesions, although rare, have been reported.

Nervous system involvement is believed to be secondary to vasculitis of the vasa nervorum and presents most frequently as mononeuritis multiplex. Other possible findings include cranial neuritis, cerebral vasculitis, or granulomatous infiltration, although these occur infrequently.

Renal disease caused by capillaritis can be irreversible if left untreated. The focal segmental necrotizing glomerulonephritis on biopsy can be indistinguishable from that found in microscopic polyangiitis, Goodpasture's syndrome, or SLE. Immunofluorescence microscopy is used to distinguish the former two pauciimmune (little to no immune deposits) glomerulonephritides from Goodpasture's syndrome and the granular pattern of immune deposits in SLE.

Diagnosis

The **diagnosis** of WG is a clinicopathologic one and usually begins with initial lab data and a **chest x-ray (CXR). CBC, serum chemistry panel, urinalysis with microscopy, ESR, and ANCA** should be obtained on all patients with suspected vasculitis. Leukocytosis, anemia, elevations in ESR (~100 mm/hr), and an active urinary sediment with RBCs and RBC casts can all be seen in active small-vessel vasculitis. CXR findings include lung nodules and masses with or without cavitation and, less frequently, pleural effusions, mass lesions, and pleural or mediastinal pseudotumors. **High-resolution CT scanning** has been used for further investigation of abnormalities on CXR and has increased the sensitivity in diagnosing WG in the appropriate clinical setting.

Flexible fiber-optic bronchoscopy is used both to inspect the tracheobronchial tree and to acquire tissue through biopsy to assist in making the diagnosis of WG. Ulcerating tracheobronchitis as well as "cobblestoning" of the mucosa have been described, and secondary scarring as the result of the healing of these lesions can lead to stenosis, airway obstruction, bronchomalacia, and postobstructive pneumonia. Although only approximately 20% of biopsy samples obtained by fiber-optic bronchoscopy may be diagnostic of WG, bronchoscopic findings coupled with the appropriate clinical scenario and lab data can save patients from undergoing an open-lung biopsy.

The **histopathologic hallmarks** of WG are vasculitis, necrosis, and granulomatous inflammation of small and medium vessels such as arterioles, arteries, capillaries, and venules. The lung and the upper respiratory tract offer the highest sensitivity and specificity for biopsy sampling, although size and the presence or absence of concurrent immunosuppressive therapy may affect the diagnostic quality of the specimen. Renal biopsy characteristically shows glomerulonephritis but does not distinguish WG from other small-vessel vasculitides.

ANCA have been identified as possible mechanisms of pathogenesis in the systemic vasculitides. ANCA directed against serine protease 3 cause a cytoplasmic immunofluorescence pattern and have a sensitivity of 28–92% and a specificity as high as 80–100% in WG. Serum ANCA levels have been shown to vary during the course of WG, although serial measurements in patients have not shown reliability in assessing disease course or predicting relapse. See Chap. 19, Diffuse Alveolar Hemorrhage, for more information on ANCA.

Treatment

For prognostic and therapeutic purposes, it is helpful to separate WG into **limited** and **generalized** disease. **Limited disease** has been used to describe cases that do not affect the kidneys and reflects pathology caused mainly by necrotizing granulomas and not by active vasculitis. **Generalized disease** implies pathology marked predominantly by vasculitis and is applicable any time there is evidence of end-organ disease or impending organ failure. The limited phase of WG results in minimal morbidity, is characterized by constitutional symptoms, and is usually marked by modest increases in inflammatory markers such as CRP and ESR. In the generalized vasculitic phase, elevations in CRP and ESR are marked, as are other acute-phase reactants. If left untreated, the limited phase of WG may progress to the generalized phase, although this is not universal.

Therapy for WG is tailored to individual cases and is managed according to disease activity. Treatment for WG can be divided into **remission induction** and **remission maintenance.** The current standard therapy for generalized disease combines the use of **oral cyclophosphamide (2 mg/kg/day)** and **prednisone (1 mg/kg/day).** The prednisone is tapered over the following 2–3 mos after a therapeutic response is achieved, after which it can be discontinued if remission persists. Cyclophosphamide is continued for 3 mos and is then followed by remission maintenance therapy. If the disease relapses, the protocol is reinitiated. Using this regimen, a complete remission rate of 75–93% can be achieved. Although effective, current therapy is not without its drawbacks. Nearly half of patients undergoing cyclophosphamide therapy develop some form of toxicity, including hemorrhagic cystitis, bladder cancer, and myelodysplasia.

For limited disease, **methotrexate (MTX)** has been successfully used and is preferred for its small side effect profile and limited toxicity. A study conducted by the NIH found that a significant complication of MTX and prednisone therapy was *Pneumocystis jiroveci* pneumonia, and therefore, prophylaxis with TMP-SMX is now mandatory. **TMP-SMX** alone has been used with success in treating limited forms of WG but appears to be ineffective in treating generalized disease. TMP-SMX has been shown to significantly reduce the relapse rate when used as adjunctive therapy and therefore is included in most regimens used to treat WG. It is unclear if the antimicrobial or immunomodulatory effects of TMP-SMX are responsible for its activity in treating WG. Remission maintenance for WG is an area of active research. Current regimens consist of MTX alone, although azathioprine has shown promise as well. Other agents such as mycophenolate and leflunomide are currently undergoing investigation.

MICROSCOPIC POLYANGIITIS

Microscopic polyangiitis is a necrotizing vasculitis affecting **small vessels.** Although their clinical courses may be similar, MPA, WG, and PAN are generally distinguished by the lack of granulomatous involvement of the upper respiratory tract in MPA and by the involvement of small vessels only in PAN. This latter distinction is important to establish early on, as disease course and treatment response differ between the two syndromes.

Similar to WG, **MPA** can present at nearly any age, with a mean of approximately 50 yrs. Men and women appear to be affected equally, although some studies suggest a female predominance. The main clinical feature of MPA is renal involvement, with the presence of a rapidly progressive necrotizing glomerulonephritis in nearly 90% of cases. Again, this feature is pathologically indistinguishable from that occurring in other small-vessel vasculitides. Clinical manifestations vary from mild hemoptysis with transient pulmonary infiltrates on CXR to massive hemoptysis and diffuse alveolar hemorrhage. Pulmonary-renal failure may be the initial presentation in fulminant MPA, necessitating hemodynamic and respiratory support as well as hemodialysis. Although MPA has been reported as the most common pulmonary-renal syndrome, cutaneous, peripheral nerve, and GI manifestations may also be present.

Diagnosis

The diagnostic approach to the patient with suspected MPA is similar to that described for the initial evaluation of WG. **Perinuclear ANCA (p-ANCA),** an antibody directed against myeloperoxidase, is found in 80% of patients with microscopic polyangiitis. p-ANCA generates a perinuclear immunofluorescence pattern. See Chap. 19, Diffuse Alveolar Hemorrhage, for more information on ANCA.

Treatment

Relapses are common in MPA, but they are rare in classic PAN, and therefore distinguishing between the two early on can significantly affect the duration of therapy. PAN characteristically affects small and medium muscular arteries and causes renovascular HTN, microaneurysms, and renal infarcts, whereas the capillaritis in MPA yields a rapidly progressive glomerulonephritis that is uncommon in PAN.

Although the success of **remission induction** in MPA remains high, many patients experience disease relapse after therapy is discontinued or during the tapering of remission maintenance. As in WG, **cyclophosphamide** and **oral corticosteroids** are the mainstay of therapy. Relapses are generally milder than the initial presentation, although some may be severe with end-organ damage. Although cyclophosphamide is effective in treating active disease, it has not been shown to prevent relapses. Patients with **mild relapse** may be managed by increasing the dose of oral corticosteroids, whereas major relapse necessitates the reintroduction of initial therapy. In cases of **treatment failure,** plasma exchange may be considered. IV immunoglobulin G has been used in refractory cases with limited success.

CHURG-STRAUSS SYNDROME

CSS is a rare vasculitis affecting small and medium vessels. The hallmarks of CSS are **asthma, hypereosinophilia, and necrotizing vasculitis.**

CSS affects men and women equally and can present at any age. The clinical course has been described in **three phases.** The first consists of a prodrome of allergic rhinitis and asthma, which may last up to 20 yrs, followed by peripheral and tissue eosinophilia, which characterize the second phase. The third phase consists of an extensive vasculitis that can affect the nerve, lung, heart, GI tract, and kidney and can be life-threatening. Although variability has been reported in the order of these phases, the American College of Rheumatology has found them 95% sensitive and specific for CSS when coupled with histopathologic evidence of vasculitis. In the absence of proven vasculitis, the prodromal phase is indistinguishable from typical asthma, and the eosinophilia of the second phase may be confused with eosinophilic pneumonia, Löffler's syndrome, or eosinophilic gastroenteritis.

The unifying pulmonary manifestation in CSS is a history of **asthma,** but **allergic rhinitis, sinusitis,** and **nasal polyps** are also commonly seen. The majority of patients have been treated with oral corticosteroids for symptoms of asthma before the diagnosis of CSS, a feature that can delay the diagnosis. Radiographic findings are widespread and nonspecific, consisting of transient pulmonary infiltrates, peripheral parenchymal infiltrates, cavitating pulmonary nodules, and pleural effusions.

Mononeuritis multiplex is the most distinguishing and common extrapulmonary manifestation of CSS, affecting up to 75% of patients.

Cardiovascular involvement is another common feature and is responsible for a significant proportion of the morbidity and mortality associated with the disease. Manifestations include ECG abnormalities, congestive heart failure, eosinophilic myocarditis, coronary vasculitis, and pericardial effusions resulting in cardiac tamponade.

Renal involvement occurs most commonly as a focal and segmental necrotizing glomerulonephritis and usually does not result in fulminant renal failure.

Abdominal pain is nearly universal in the latter phases and is caused by eosinophilic or vasculitic involvement of the GI tract. Other GI findings include pancreatitis, GI perforation, or hemorrhage.

Cutaneous involvement in CSS is also common and includes purpura, livedo reticularis, and subcutaneous nodules.

Diagnosis

The diagnosis of CSS rests mainly on establishing an **active vasculitis** given the appropriate clinical setting of **asthma** and **hypereosinophilia.** Every effort should be made to obtain tissue before beginning potentially toxic therapy. The utility of ANCA testing is not as well defined in CSS as in WG or MPA, although p-ANCA may be positive in 50% of patients. It is important to note that a positive p-ANCA should be confirmed with ELISA for myeloperoxidase, as other neutrophil antigens resulting in a positive p-ANCA have a low sensitivity in CSS.

The American College of Rheumatology has published the following **criteria** for the diagnosis of CSS once the establishment of vasculitis has been made: asthma, eosinophilia >10% of the total WBC count, mono- or polyneuropathy, migratory pulmonary infiltrates, paranasal sinus abnormality, and extravascular eosinophils. These criteria are 85% sensitive and 99% specific for the diagnosis of CSS when four of the six are positive in the setting of an active vasculitis.

Treatment

Glucocorticoids are the mainstay of treatment of CSS vasculitis. The role of cyclophosphamide and other cytotoxic agents is less clear in CSS than in WG or MPA, although they have been used in addition to corticosteroids in refractory cases and in cases with neurologic or cardiac involvement. Hydroxyurea has been used to treat severe eosinophilia, and despite aggressive therapy, some patients with CSS may remain refractory.

PULMONARY MANIFESTATIONS OF OTHER VASCULITIDES

Giant cell arteritis is a disease of large and medium vessels that predominantly affects the elderly. It is more common among Caucasians and is the most common vasculitis in this population. Respiratory symptoms such as cough, hoarseness, or throat pain may be the presenting symptom in as many as 25% of cases, and diagnostic studies such as pulmonary function tests and CXRs may be normal. Treatment is with prednisone, which usually results in resolution of symptoms.

Takayasu's arteritis has been classically described in young Asian females. The aorta and its major branches are affected, and manifestations include mild pulmonary HTN, fistula formation between pulmonary artery branches and bronchial arteries, and nonspecific inflammatory interstitial lung disease. The diagnosis is best made using CT or magnetic resonance angiography, which demonstrate pulmonary artery stenoses and occlusion in nearly half of all patients. Initial treatment consists of glucocorticoids and immunosuppression, and methotrexate and vascular bypass are options in severe or refractory cases.

Behçet's syndrome is a relapsing multisystem disorder characterized by recurrent oral ulcerations and at least two of the following: genital ulcers, uveitis, cutaneous nodules or pustules, or meningoencephalitis. Cough, fever, dyspnea, and chest pain may be the initial respiratory symptoms, although massive hemoptysis is perhaps the most significant complication.

Immune-complex deposition is believed to be the underlying mechanism in the vasculitis of Behçet's syndrome. Characteristic lung findings include pulmonary artery aneurysms, which result from destruction of the elastic lamina. Erosion of bronchi can result in arterial-bronchial fistulae, producing massive hemoptysis with an associated mortality of nearly 40%. Other manifestations include recurrent venous thrombosis as well as pneumonia and bronchial occlusion.

CT and magnetic resonance angiography have replaced pulmonary angiography in the diagnosis of Behçet's syndrome. Methotrexate, colchicine, chlorambucil, and cyclosporine have all been used with prednisone to treat Behçet's, and the combination of prednisone and azathioprine or cyclophosphamide has been shown to improve pulmonary artery aneurysms. Aspirin at 81 mg/day may be considered for the prevention of recurrent venous thrombosis but should be avoided in any patient with known pulmonary involvement.

Both **SLE and rheumatoid arthritis** are associated with a secondary vasculitis that is believed to be immune complex mediated. Complications of these syndromes include the presence of rheumatoid nodules in rheumatoid arthritis and pulmonary HTN and alveolar hemorrhage that tends to be more severe in SLE and can be the initial disease manifestation. With a mortality >50% in some case series, treatment of alveolar hemorrhage in SLE with the combination of plasmapheresis and pulse-dose cyclophosphamide has met with limited success.

Necrotizing sarcoid granulomatosis is differentiated from sarcoidosis by its extensive vasculitis and necrosis, the paucity for extrapulmonary involvement, and for the radiographic findings of pulmonary masses, nodules, and pleural involvement, which are less commonly seen in sarcoidosis. Well-circumscribed granulomas are prominent in this disease, and the vasculitis may be epithelioid-granulomatous, with histiocytes and multinucleated giant cells reminiscent of giant cell arteritis, or lymphocytic without granuloma formation. The clinical onset of this syndrome is subacute, and patients may complain of nonspecific respiratory symptoms such as cough, dyspnea, or wheezing. Alternatively, the diagnosis is incidental and made radiographically in asymptomatic patients. The prognosis is good, with spontaneous resolution in some cases. Further therapy is similar to that for chronic pulmonary sarcoidosis and consists of oral corticosteroids.

KEY POINTS TO REMEMBER

- Although the lungs are infrequently the only organ system involved in cases of vasculitis, respiratory symptoms are often what prompt patients to seek medical attention. Often, these issues are only part of a larger systemic process.
- The discovery of ANCA has significantly influenced the diagnosis and classification of vasculitides and has provided insight into the possible mechanisms responsible for these diseases.
- WG is classically described as a triad of sinusitis, pneumonitis, and glomerulonephritis, although <50% of cases meet all three criteria.
- The hallmarks of CSS are asthma, hypereosinophilia, and necrotizing vasculitis.

REFERENCES AND SUGGESTED READINGS

Burns A. Pulmonary vasculitis. *Thorax* 1998;53:220–227.

Conron M, Beynon HLC. Churg-Strauss syndrome. *Thorax* 2000;55:870–877.

Franks TJ, Koss MN. Pulmonary capillaritis. *Curr Opin Pulmon Med* 2000;6:430–435.

Guillevin L, Lhote F. Treatment of polyarteritis nodosa and microscopic polyangiitis. *Arthritis Rheum* 1998;41:2100–2105.

Jayne D. Update on the European Vasculitis Study Group trials. *Curr Opin Rheumatol* 2001;13:48–55.

Jeannette JC, Falk RJ, Andrassy K, et al. Nomenclature of systemic vasculitides: proposal of an international consensus conference. *Arthritis Rheum* 1994;37:187–192.

Langford CA. Vasculitis. *J Allergy Clin Immunol* 2003;111[2 Suppl]:S602–612.

Russell KA, Wiegert E, Schroeder DR, et al. Detection of anti-neutrophil cytoplasmic antibodies under actual clinical testing conditions. *Clin Immunol* 2002;103:196–203.

Schwarz MI, Brown KK. Small vessel vasculitis of the lung. *Thorax* 2000;55:502–510.

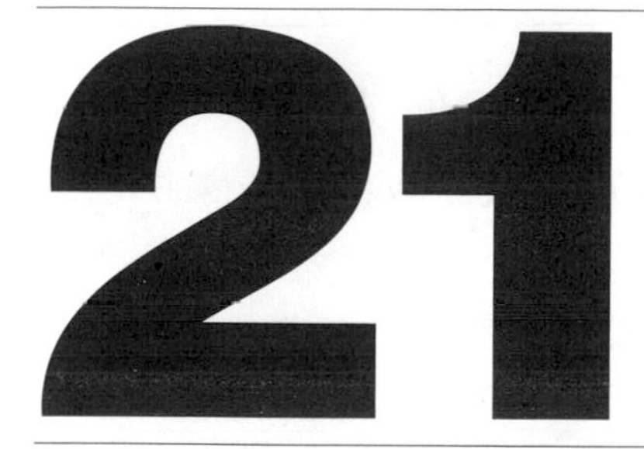

Pulmonary Embolism and Deep Venous Thrombosis

Randy Sasich

RISK FACTORS FOR THROMBOEMBOLISM

Hypercoagulable states, whether inherited or acquired, are the most important single risk factor for thromboembolic disease. Inherited hypercoagulable states are recognized in the range of 25% to >50% of cases of venous thromboembolism (VTE).

The known **inherited risk factors for VTE** include deficiencies of antithrombin, protein C, or protein S, factor V Leiden (clotting factor V with an amino acid substitution that confers a resistance to activated protein C), and the prothrombin G20210A mutation.

Acquired risk factors include increasing age, malignancy, antiphospholipid antibodies (lupus anticoagulant or anticardiolipin antibodies), previous VTE (an independent risk factor itself for additional thrombotic events), surgery or major trauma, pregnancy, oral contraceptives/hormone replacement therapy, and prolonged immobilization.

Other mixed or poorly established risk factors include hyperhomocysteinemia, high levels of factor VIII, IX, or XI, high thrombin activatable fibrinolysis inhibitor, dysfibrinogenemia and high fibrinogen, and activated protein C (APC) resistance in the absence of factor V Leiden. APC resistance is not synonymous with factor V Leiden. Factor V Leiden is simply the most common inherited form of APC resistance. The most common acquired form of APC resistance occurs with oral contraceptive use and in pregnancy.

DIAGNOSIS OF PULMONARY EMBOLISM

The symptoms of an acute pulmonary embolism (PE) are numerous and notoriously nonspecific. A **high level of clinical suspicion** must be maintained in patient populations at risk of PE/DVT to steer the clinical evaluation toward diagnostic studies that can more definitively rule in or rule out pulmonary thromboembolic disease. Fig. 21-1 is one of many proposed algorithms for the diagnosis of PE that exist in the medical literature.

The **most frequent symptoms** are dyspnea (84%), pleuritic chest pain (74%), apprehension (63%), and cough (50%). The classic symptom of hemoptysis occurred in only 22% of patients in one series of angiographically proven PE. Other, less common, symptoms include palpitations, diaphoresis, and, in the case of massive or submassive embolism, syncope.

On **physical exam** of the patient with an acute PE, the most frequent finding is tachypnea (85%). Tachycardia, an increased P_2 component of S_2, and rales occur singly in approximately 50% of patients. In the Urokinase Pulmonary Embolism Trial study, tachypnea (respiratory rate >16/min) was present in 92% of patients. A fever >38°C is present in approximately 20% of cases. As with the presenting symptoms of PE, numerous other signs occur with decreasing frequency and sensitivity, such as pallor, cyanosis, hypotension, neck vein distention, decreased breath sounds, and pleural friction rubs.

The finding of **hypoxemia and/or a widened alveolar-arterial gradient** on ABG analysis is widely, and mistakenly, considered to be nearly uniformly present in the scenario of PE. In one analysis of data collected from the **Prospective Investigation of Pulmonary Embolism Diagnosis (PIOPED)** study of patients with confirmed PE, 25% of the patients with no prior cardiopulmonary disease had a PaO_2 level of >80 mm Hg. Patients with prior cardiopulmonary disease had a PaO_2 >80 mm Hg in 15% of the cases of proven PE. Furthermore, the alveolar-arterial gradient was normal in 11–14% of these 280 patients.

The **D-dimer** is a specific degradation product that forms when cross-linked fibrin from a thrombus undergoes endogenous fibrinolysis. Two types of tests exist for detec-

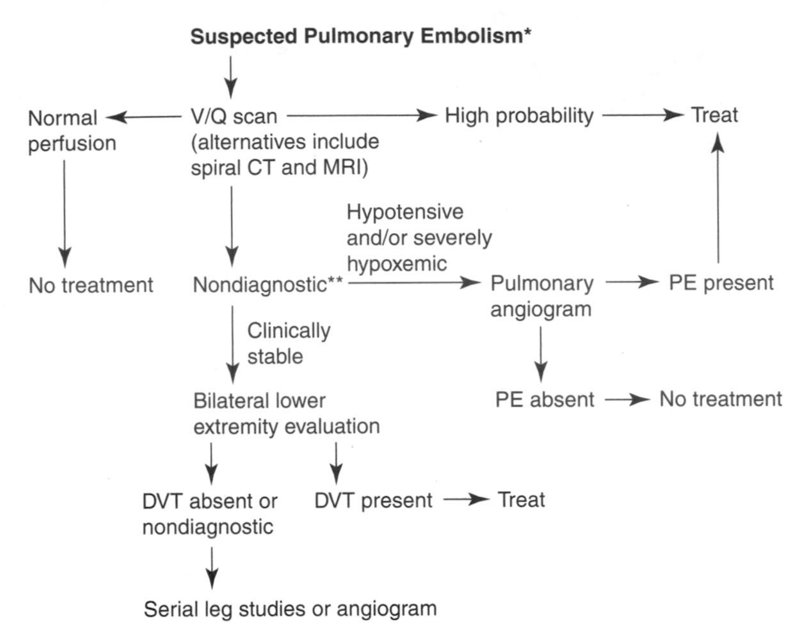

FIG. 21-1. Diagnosis of pulmonary embolism (PE). *When PE is suspected and the risk of bleeding is deemed low, it is appropriate to begin anticoagulation while diagnostic testing is underway. **Patients with low-probability V/Q scans and low clinical suspicion are unlikely to have PE. Others require further evaluation. DVT, deep venous thrombosis. From Tapson VF, Carroll BA, Davidson BL, et al. The diagnostic approach to acute venous thromboembolism clinical practice guideline. American Thoracic Society. *Am J Respir Crit Care Med* 1999;160:1043–1066, with permission.

tion of D-dimer product in the blood: a rapid latex agglutination test and an ELISA. The ELISA has a far greater sensitivity than the latex agglutination test and is the test of choice. Currently, the test's utility lies in its **high negative predictive value** in patients with a low clinical suspicion for PE. The most recent American Thoracic Society guideline on the diagnostic approach to VTE does not recommend the use of the D-dimer as part of the standard PE or DVT diagnostic algorithm.

Approximately 70% of patients without prior cardiac or pulmonary disease presenting with acute PE have changes on ECG. **Tachycardia and ST segment depression** are the most common findings (44% and 50% respectively) but are nonspecific. The classic $S_1Q_3T_3$ (an S-wave in lead I and a Q wave and T wave inversion in lead III) is a specific sign of right heart strain but is not diagnostic of acute PE. In one study, an $S_1Q_3T_3$ pattern or a new (complete or incomplete) right-bundle-branch block was present in 9 of 47 patients with angiographically documented PE. Other ECG findings include atrial flutter or fibrillation, right axis deviation, RV hypertrophy, or a pseudoinfarction pattern.

Most authorities on **chest x-ray findings** in PE claim that the majority of patients with PE have an abnormal film. Most of these abnormal findings, such as atelectasis and small pleural effusions, are subtle and very nonspecific. The **Westermark sign,** an area of lucency in the lung on radiograph representing hypovolemia distal to the embolism occlusion, is one of the classic findings of acute PE but occurs only rarely. In one study of 383 patients with angiographically proven PE, only 6% had this sign. Hampton's hump is another rare classic finding that describes a rounded or wedge-shaped infiltrate, often near the diaphragm, that is thought to represent an area of infarction in the lung.

Massive or submassive PE can cause acute RV dysfunction. Complicating the use of echocardiograms in the diagnosis is the not infrequent concomitant preexisting cardiopulmonary disease in patients presenting with acute PE. A study by Kasper et al. showed that dilation of the right pulmonary artery and RV were the most frequent, although nonspecific, findings. Of note, 19% of these patients with PE documented by angiography, V/Q scan, or autopsy had a normal echocardiogram.

The **V/Q scan** is a technique in which the patient first inhales ^{133}Xe to evaluate uniformity of ventilation of the lungs, and then ^{99m}Tc (usually attached to macroaggregated albumin) is embolized into the lung vasculature to evaluate lung perfusion. The PIOPED study was instrumental in standardizing the interpretation of matched and unmatched ventilation and perfusion defects in the V/Q scan, data on which the likelihood of PE is based. With pulmonary angiography or autopsy as the gold standard, the sensitivity and specificity of low-probability, high-probability, or indeterminate V/Q scans were determined. These were combined with a clinician's pretest suspicion (percentages representing low, medium, or high likelihood) of PE based on clinical assessment. The results showed the need for further testing in patients with intermediate-probability V/Q results, especially those with high or medium clinical suspicion. Furthermore, patients with low-probability V/Q scans and a high clinical suspicion were proved to have a PE in 40% of the cases. In summary, **low-probability** or **normal V/Q scans** along with low-probability pretest suspicion are usually adequate to rule out acute PE. Similarly, **high-probability V/Q scans** are usually diagnostic of PE. All other cases require further workup, which usually involves a U/S study of the lower extremities (see below) to document the presence of deep venous thrombosis (DVT). Positive U/S studies provide a surrogate marker for the existence of acute PE based on a documented source of thromboembolism in concert with symptoms suggesting pulmonary complications.

Spiral volumetric computed tomography (SVCT or helical CT) is a relatively new imaging technology that uses contrast dye injected into peripheral or central veins to visualize the pulmonary arteries to the segmental level but not into the smaller subsegmental branches. Multiple studies have looked at the sensitivity and specificity of CT scan for the diagnosis of PE, and reviews have shown that both are approximately 90%. The limitations of SVCT are its poor resolution in the subsegmental branches and inter- and intraobserver variability at centers where experience is limited.

In general, a normal finding on SVCT should not be considered to rule out a PE. Nor should it be thought of as a more diagnostic study than the V/Q scan, but rather as another choice in initial imaging studies in the diagnostic algorithm. Additional studies, including PIOPED II, are awaited to clarify further the role of SVCT in the diagnosis of venous thromboembolic disease.

Pulmonary angiography is considered the gold standard for documentation of PE, but similar to all studies, it, too, can be nondiagnostic. Complications documented from the PIOPED trial included renal failure requiring dialysis (0.3%), severe groin bleeding (0.2%), and death (0.5%). Despite its risks, it is considered necessary when a definitive diagnosis is essential.

DIAGNOSIS OF DEEP VENOUS THROMBOSIS

Fig. 21-2 shows the American Thoracic Society guidelines for the evaluation of lower-extremity DVT. Like the signs and symptoms of PE, the clinical symptoms and exam findings of a DVT (i.e., erythema, warmth, pain/tenderness, swelling, and a palpable cord) are of relatively poor sensitivity and specificity and should be used to suggest to the examiner the need for further diagnostic testing.

The classic **Homan's sign,** pain in the calf on forced dorsiflexion of the foot, has a sensitivity of only 13–48% and a specificity of 39–84%. The most sensitive exam finding, swelling in the affected leg, has a sensitivity ranging from 35% to 97% and specificity between 8% and 88%. However, unilateral leg swelling exists in <10% of patients with DVT.

Compression U/S for diagnosing DVT is done by examining the compressibility of the deep veins of the lower extremity. Veins with thrombus are less compressible than veins without a thrombus. Doppler imaging of venous flow is also done for added information about the patency of the vein being imaged.

Contrast venography is the gold standard for the diagnosis of DVT and is considered to be 100% sensitive and specific. Its main disadvantages include its invasiveness and potential complications from the administration of IV contrast dye, such as hypersensitivity reactions and nephrotoxicity. If initial testing with plethysmography or U/S is nondiagnostic, contrast venography should be performed. MRI may be a viable substitute for venography.

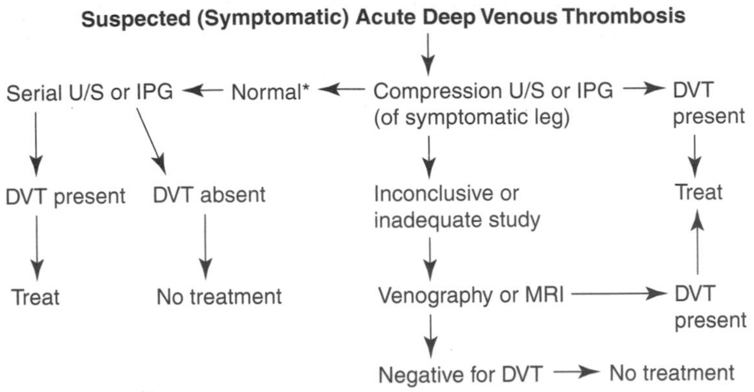

Suspected (Symptomatic) Acute Deep Venous Thrombosis

Serial U/S or IPG ← Normal* ← Compression U/S or IPG (of symptomatic leg) → DVT present → Treat

Serial U/S or IPG → DVT present → Treat

Serial U/S or IPG → DVT absent → No treatment

Compression U/S or IPG → Inconclusive or inadequate study → Venography or MRI → DVT present → Treat

Venography or MRI → Negative for DVT → No treatment

FIG. 21-2. American Thoracic Society guidelines for the evaluation of lower-extremity deep venous thrombosis (DVT). *Because the sensitivity for U/S or impedance plethysmography (IPG) for calf DVT is lower than that for proximal DVT, three studies over 7–14 days (IPG) or one to two studies over 5–7 days (U/S) are needed to detect proximal extension. If iliac thrombosis is suspected, then venography (or MRI) should be undertaken. Adapted from Tapson VF, Carroll BA, Davidson BL, et al. The diagnostic approach to acute venous thromboembolism clinical practice guideline. American Thoracic Society. *Am J Respir Crit Care Med* 1999;160:1043–1066, with permission from the publishers.

MRI can be performed in the evaluation of lower-extremity DVT. In addition to imaging information of the deep veins of the leg and thigh, the deep pelvic veins are also effectively imaged. Multiple studies have been done comparing MRI to venography and have shown results of sensitivity and specificity at or very near 100%.

EVALUATION OF THROMBOPHILIA

As mentioned, a significant portion of patients presenting with VTE have an inherited hypercoagulable disorder. Obviously, not every patient diagnosed with a VTE should undergo every test available to identify inherited thrombophilia states. The issue of whom to test and what to test for is a common one in the workup of a patient with a new or recurrent DVT or PE.

A recent consensus statement by the College of American Pathologists states that **testing** is appropriate in patients with (a) a history of recurrent VTE; (b) VTE before the age of 50 yrs; (c) unprovoked VTE at any age; (d) VTE at unusual sites (e.g., cerebral, mesenteric, portal, hepatic); (e) VTE patients with a positive family history; or (f) VTE secondary to pregnancy, oral contraceptives, or hormone replacement therapy. Testing for thrombophilia is controversial in a first, provoked (history of a predisposing factor) VTE in patients aged >50 yrs, VTE associated with active cancer, or in patients with an intravascular device. Testing is also not recommended in VTE associated with selective estrogen receptor modulators such as tamoxifen.

If the decision is made to **test the patient for thrombophilia,** then the following tests should be ordered: (a) test for factor V Leiden (an activated protein C resistance assay can be used as an initial test); (b) functional protein C and S (cannot be assessed while patient is on a coumarin derivative such as warfarin because it lowers the levels of protein C and S); (c) functional antithrombin (cannot be measured while the patient is on heparin); and (d) prothrombin G20210A mutation. Anticardiolipin antibody and lupus anticoagulant testing is also appropriate, especially if the VTE is associated with an autoimmune disease. Testing selected patients for homocysteine levels is currently controversial.

TREATMENT OF VENOUS THROMBOEMBOLIC DISEASE

The mainstays of **therapy for DVT/PE** are antithrombotic regimens of a mechanical nature (compression stockings, pneumatic compression devices), anticoagulant drug ther-

TABLE 21-1. WEIGHT-BASED NOMOGRAM FOR IV HEPARIN DOSING

aPTT	Dose change (U/kg/hr)	Additional action	Next aPTT (hrs)
<35 (<1.2 × mean normal)	+4	Rebolus with 50 IU/kg	6
35–45 (1.2–1.5 × mean normal)	+2	Rebolus with 40 IU/kg	6
46–70 (1.5–2.3 × mean normal)	0	0	6
71–90 (2.3–3.0 × mean normal)	–2	0	6
>90 (>3.0 × mean normal)	–3	Stop infusion × 1 h	6

Heparin, 25,000 IU in 250 mL D_5W.
Initial dosing: loading, 80 IU/kg; maintenance infusion: 18 IU/kg/hr (aPTT in 6 hrs).
During the first 24 hrs, repeat aPTT q6h. Thereafter, monitor aPTT once every morning unless outside therapeutic range.
Adapted from Hyers TM, Agnelli G, Hull RD, et al. Antithrombotic therapy for venous thromboembolic disease. *Chest* 2001;119[1 Suppl]:176S–193S.

apy [heparin, low-molecular-weight heparin (LMWH), and warfarin], direct thrombin inhibitors (hirudin and danaparoid), or thrombolytic agents (streptokinase, urokinase).

Proximal DVT and PE should be considered different manifestations of the same disease. The majority of patients with proximal DVT also have PE, and vice versa. The only major difference is that patients with PE are nearly four times more likely (1.5% vs 0.4%) to die of recurrent VTE in the next year than patients who are treated for DVT alone.

Heparin is a glycosaminoglycan that is commercially prepared from the gut mucosa of animals and has a molecular weight of 5000–30,000 d. It has been shown in numerous studies to be effective treatment for DVT/PE. Current recommendations for initial **treatment of venous thromboembolic disease** from the Sixth American College of Chest Physicians (ACCP) Consensus Conference on Antithrombotic Therapy involve initiation of heparin at a 5000 U IV bolus when DVT/PE is suspected and no contraindications exist. A CBC, aPTT, and PT level should be checked at the start of therapy. After diagnostic testing for confirmation, warfarin should be initiated on day 1 at 5 mg PO, and heparin continued until the INR is >2.0. A platelet count should be checked between days 3 and 5 to look for heparin-induced thrombocytopenia.

A weight-based nomogram for IV heparin dosing is reproduced in Table 21-1.

LMWH has a mean molecular weight of 4000–5000 d. It is dosed qd–bid by body weight via SC injection. Unlike unfractionated heparin, LMWH is renally cleared, and caution should be used in patients with creatinine clearances of <30 mL/min.

Multiple randomized clinical trials have convincingly demonstrated that LMWH is at least as safe and effective as unfractionated heparin in the initial treatment of patients with thromboembolic disease. Several potential benefits exist in using LMWH over unfractionated heparin. Metaanalyses (most individual studies are not in support) have suggested lower rates of recurrence and less bleeding in addition to a small survival benefit in patients with cancer. In appropriate patients, home treatment with LMWH appears to have a cost saving by eliminating or shortening hospital stay. Current recommendations from the Sixth ACCP Consensus Conference on Antithrombotic Therapy are for the **use of LMWH** over unfractionated heparin **in initial treatment.**

Warfarin is the predominant coumarin in use in North America and acts by inhibiting the vitamin K–dependent coagulant proteins II, VII, IX, and X. The optimum intensity of therapy has been determined in multiple studies to be an **INR between 2.0 and 3.0.** Recent data suggest that aiming for a specific INR (e.g., 2.5 instead of anywhere between 2 and 3) may decrease the risk of over- or underanticoagulating patients. Higher INR levels are sometimes advocated in hypercoagulable states such as the antiphospholipid syndrome (2.5–3.5).

The general recommendations for **duration of therapy** are for 3–6 mos in first-event patients with reversible or time-limited risk factors such as surgery, trauma, immobilization, or estrogen use. At least 6 mos of therapy is advised in patients with an idiopathic first event, and 12 mos to lifetime is recommended in patients with recurrent VTE or a first event with an inherited thrombophilia, cancer, or antiphospholipid antibodies. In all cases, it should be realized that these are guidelines, and the exact duration of therapy for many patients, in light of individual bleeding risks and specific thrombophilic states, is unknown.

A recent randomized, placebo-controlled study by the **Prevention of Recurrent Venous Thromboembolism (PREVENT)** investigators examined the use of long-term, low-intensity warfarin (target INR of 1.5–2.0) in 508 patients with idiopathic VTE. The patients were followed for a mean of 2.1 yrs, with the treatment group having a 48% reduction in the composite endpoint of recurrent VTE, major hemorrhage, or death. The reduction in the risk of recurrent VTE was between 76% and 81%. A statistically insignificant increase in major hemorrhage ($p = .25$) occurred in the warfarin group (five patients) compared to placebo (two patients).

The indication for use of **thrombolytics** for thromboembolic disease is plagued by a lack of evidence regarding mortality benefit in light of the confirmed effectiveness of heparin and warfarin therapy and the concerns over excessive bleeding in patients treated with thrombolytic agents. Some authorities argue for its use only in PE causing shock, whereas others have argued for its use in patients with PE and RV dysfunction.

A recent randomized, placebo-controlled, multicenter trial of patients with submassive PE (RV dysfunction and pulmonary HTN without arterial hypotension or shock) compared a 100-mg infusion of alteplase over a 2-hr period with heparin to heparin alone. The authors found a threefold increase in the combined endpoint of risk of death and treatment escalation with the use of heparin only (no statistical difference was found in mortality alone).

Inferior vena cava (IVC) filters are "sieve" or "net" devices placed (under fluoroscopic or U/S guidance) into the IVC with the intention of preventing the migration of DVT from the pelvis or lower extremities to the central venous circulation and heart. IVC filters have an accepted indication in the treatment of venous thromboembolism when an absolute contraindication to anticoagulation exists, such as active hemorrhage, severe thrombocytopenia, or a documented failure of antithrombotic therapy (a new or recurrent PE or DVT while properly anticoagulated). Interestingly, despite widespread use of IVC filters, only a single randomized trial studying their effectiveness exists. This trial, by Decousous et al., found no difference in early or late survival in patients with a first episode of VTE after a 2-yr followup.

PREVENTION OF VENOUS THROMBOEMBOLISM

Primary prophylaxis for patients at risk for thromboembolic disease—whether in the perioperative setting, as an outpatient, or as a medical inpatient—is an important part of proper patient care. The often clinically silent nature of DVT makes identifying at-risk patients and applying effective anticoagulation critical.

Numerous studies of **antithrombotic prophylaxis** with well-documented benefit exist for surgical patients with burns or trauma and for those undergoing general, orthopedic, gynecologic/urologic, or neurosurgical procedures. The reader is referred to the Sixth ACCP Consensus Conference on Antithrombotic Therapy, Prevention of Venous Thromboembolism [*Chest* 2001;119(1 Suppl):132S–175S] for specific recommendations in these patients.

Most patients hospitalized with **acute myocardial infarction** are treated with combinations of antiplatelet and antithrombotic drugs for their primary diagnosis, making prophylaxis unnecessary. Without this treatment, the overall incidence of DVT is approximately 24%. Current data show benefit with unfractionated heparin at low dose (5000 U bid or tid, and 7500 U bid) or full anticoagulation. The utility of thrombolytics and LMWH is unknown. Mechanical devices such as compression stockings or sequential compression devices may be of benefit when anticoagulation is contraindicated.

Cancer is in itself an acquired hypercoagulable state, and its treatment with chemotherapy and indwelling venous catheters further increases the risk of thromboembolic disease. Cancer patients have three times the risk of fatal PE during a given surgical procedure than their cohorts without cancer undergoing a similar procedure.

A specific indication for low-dose anticoagulation (warfarin, 1 mg PO qd or LMWH) exists for patients with **chronic indwelling venous catheters.**

When the results from multiple studies are pooled, **stroke patients** have a DVT incidence of 55%, and approximately 5% of early deaths after stroke are attributed to PE. The current recommendation from the Sixth ACCP Consensus Conference on Antithrombotic Therapy, Prevention of Venous Thromboembolism is for the routine use of low-dose unfractionated heparin (LDUH), LMWH, or the heparinoid danaparoid.

Critically ill patients often have multiple risk factors for VTE and are often subjected to prolonged immobilization. One double-blind trial of medical ICU patients used duplex scanning every 72 hrs until discharge from the unit and found DVT in 31% of the control patients.

A study by Ibrahim et al. of 110 **ICU patients** requiring prolonged mechanical ventilation (>7 days) showed that despite prophylaxis, nearly 25% developed DVT. Furthermore, those patients with documented DVT by duplex U/S had a statistically greater frequency of PE during their hospitalization (11.5% vs 0.0%; $p = .012$).

A large number of studies in **general medical patients** exist using either LDUH or LMWH to compare VTE rates and mortality in hospitalized patients on general medical wards. LDUH or LMWH is recommended in these patients, as the rate of DVT without prophylaxis is approximately 16%. One metaanalysis of randomized trials comparing LMWH to LDUH showed no significant difference in thromboembolic events or death but did show that LMWH was associated with a 52% lower incidence of major bleeding.

UPPER-EXTREMITY DEEP VENOUS THROMBOSIS

Upper-extremity DVT (UEDVT) was previously thought to be less clinically significant than other forms of DVT. It is now known that UEDVT is a **significant contributor to PE** and requires attention to diagnosis and treatment. PE has been estimated to be present in up to one-third of patients who have an UEDVT.

UEDVT can be divided into primary and secondary causes. **Secondary UEDVT** occurs with the use of catheters, pacemakers, and the like and is increasing with the increased use of these devices. Cancer patients may also present with a secondary UEDVT. **Primary UEDVT** is rare and can occur in young or otherwise healthy athletes as an *effort thrombosis* (Paget-Schroetter syndrome) or in the setting of an inherited thrombophilia such as factor V Leiden.

The **presenting signs and symptoms** of UEDVT are supraclavicular fullness, arm and hand edema, extremity cyanosis, a palpable cord, and dilated cutaneous veins. Similar to lower-extremity DVT, these findings are nonspecific. Diagnosis uses modalities similar to those used in lower-extremity DVT and includes initial use of duplex U/S, with contrast venography or MRI being used in nondiagnostic cases. Treatment of UEDVT is largely the same as in lower-extremity DVT with the exception of improved outcome and decreased morbidity in young, healthy patients with primary UEDVT treated with catheter-directed thrombolysis. Patients with a mandatory central venous catheter can also be treated with thrombolytics.

KEY POINTS TO REMEMBER

- Inherited risk factors for VTE include deficiencies of antithrombin, protein C, or protein S, factor V Leiden, and the prothrombin G20210A mutation.
- Acquired risk factors include increasing age, malignancy, antiphospholipid antibodies, previous VTE, surgery or major trauma, pregnancy, oral contraceptives/hormone replacement therapy, and prolonged immobilization.
- The most frequent symptoms of PE are dyspnea, pleuritic chest pain, apprehension, and cough.
- Contrast venography is the gold standard for the diagnosis of DVT. Pulmonary angiography remains the gold standard for diagnosis of PE.
- The mainstays of therapy for DVT/PE are antithrombotic regimens using anticoagulant drug therapy. Thrombolytic therapy is rarely indicated and is used only in an ICU setting.

- The presenting signs and symptoms of UEDVT are supraclavicular fullness, arm and hand edema, extremity cyanosis, a palpable cord, and dilated cutaneous veins.

REFERENCES AND SUGGESTED READINGS

Bounameaux H, Schneider PA, Reber G, et al. Measurement of plasma D-dimer for diagnosis of deep venous thrombosis. *Am J Clin Pathol* 1989;91:82–85.

Dalen J. Pulmonary embolism: what have we learned since Virchow? Natural history, pathophysiology, and diagnosis. *Chest* 2002;122:1440–1456.

Decousus H, Leizorovitz A, Parent F, et al. A clinical trial of vena cava filters in the prevention of pulmonary embolism in patients with proximal deep-vein thrombosis: Prevention du Risque d'Embolie Pulmonaire par Interruption Cave Study Group. *N Engl J Med* 1998;338:409–415.

Dupas B, El Khouri D, Curter C, et al. Angiomagnetic resonance imaging of iliofemorocaval venous thrombosis. *Lancet* 1995;346:17–19.

Geerts WH, Heit JA, Clagett GP, et al. Prevention of venous thromboembolism. *Chest* 2001;119[1 Suppl]:132S–175S.

Girard P, Stern J, Parent F. Medical literature and vena cava filters: so far so weak. *Chest* 2002;122:963–967.

Gould MK, Dembitzer AD, Doyle RL, et al. Low-molecular-weight heparins compared with unfractionated heparin for the treatment of acute deep venous thrombosis. *Ann Intern Med* 1999;130:800–809.

Greengard JS, Eichinger S, Griffin JH, Bauer KA. Brief report: variability of thrombosis among homozygous siblings with resistance to activated protein C due to an arg→gln mutation in the gene for factor V. *N Engl J Med* 1994;331:1559–1562.

Hull RD, Pineo GF. Clinical features of deep venous thrombosis. In: Hull RD, Raskob GE, Pineo GF, eds. *VTE: an evidence-based atlas.* Armonk, NY: Futura, 1996:87–91.

Hyers TM, Agnelli G, Hull RD, et al. Antithrombotic therapy for venous thromboembolic disease. *Chest* 2001;119[1 Suppl]:176S–193S.

Ibrahim EH, Iregui M, Prentice D, et al. Deep venous thrombosis during prolonged mechanical ventilation despite prophylaxis. *Crit Care Med* 2002;30:771–774.

Kakkar AK, Williamson RCN. Prevention of VTE in cancer patients. *Semin Thromb Hemost* 1999;25:239–243.

Kasper W, Meinertz T, Henkel B, et al. Echocardiographic findings in patients with proved pulmonary embolism. *Am Heart J* 1986;112:1284–1290.

Konstantinides S, Geibel A, Heusel G, et al. Management Strategies and Prognosis of Pulmonary Embolism-3 Trial Investigators. Heparin plus alteplase compared with heparin alone in patients with submassive pulmonary embolism. *N Engl J Med* 2002;347:1143–1150.

Kupfer Y, Anwar J, Senenvirante C, et al. Prophylaxis with subcutaneous heparin significantly reduces the incidence of deep venous thrombosis in the critically ill [abstract]. *Am J Respir Crit Care Med* 1999;159[Suppl]:A519.

Lane AD, Mannucci PM, Bauer AK, et al. Inherited thrombophilia: part 2. *Thromb Haemost* 1996;76:824–834.

Manganelli D, Palla A, Donnamaria V, Giuntini C. Clinical features of pulmonary embolism: doubts and certainties. *Chest* 1995;107[1 Suppl]:25S–32S.

Martinelli I. Risk factors in venous thromboembolism. *Thromb Haemost* 2001;86:395–403.

Mismetti P, Laporte-Simitsidis S, Tardy B, et al. Prevention of VTE in internal medicine with unfractionated or low-molecular-weight heparins: a meta-analysis of randomized clinical trials. *Thromb Haemost* 2000;83:14–19.

THe PIOPED Investigators. Value of the ventilation/perfusion scan in acute pulmonary embolism. Results of the prospective investigation of pulmonary embolism diagnosis (PIOPED). *JAMA* 1990;263:2753–2759.

Rathbun SW, Raskob GE, Whitsett TL. Sensitivity and specificity of helical computed tomography in the diagnosis of pulmonary embolism: a systematic review. *Ann Intern Med* 2000;132:227–232.

Ridker PM, Goldhaber SZ, Danielson E, et al. Long-term, low-intensity warfarin therapy for the prevention of recurrent venous thromboembolism. *N Engl J Med* 2003;348:1425–1434.

Siragusa S, Cosmi B, Piovella F, et al. Low-molecular-weight heparins compared with unfractionated heparin in the treatment of patients with acute venous thromboembolism: results of a meta-analysis. *Am J Med* 1996;100:269–277.

Stein PD. *Pulmonary embolism*. Baltimore, MD: Williams & Wilkins, 1996:34.

Stein PD, Goldhaber SZ, Henry JW. Alveolar-arterial oxygen gradient in the assessment of acute pulmonary embolism. *Chest* 1995;107:139–143.

Stein PD, Terin ML, Hales CA, et al. Clinical, laboratory, roentgenographic, and electrocardiographic findings in patients with acute pulmonary embolism and no pre-existing cardiac or pulmonary disease. *Chest* 1991;100:598–603.

Stein PD, Willis PW III, DeMets DL, Greenspan RH. Plain chest roentgenogram in patients with acute pulmonary embolism and no preexisting cardiac or pulmonary disease. *Am J Noninvas Cardiol* 1987;1:171–176.

Szucs MM, Brooks HL, Grossman W, et al. Diagnostic sensitivity of laboratory findings in acute pulmonary embolism. *Ann Intern Med* 1971;74:161–166.

Tapson VF, Carroll BA, Davidson BL, et al. The diagnostic approach to acute venous thromboembolism clinical practice guideline. American Thoracic Society. *Am J Respir Crit Care Med* 1999;160:1043–1066.

The urokinase pulmonary embolism trial. A national cooperative study. *Circulation* 1973;47[2 Suppl]:II1–108.

Van Cott EM, Laposata M, Prins MH. Laboratory evaluation of hypercoagulability with venous or arterial thrombosis. College of American Pathologists Consensus Conference XXXVI: Diagnostic Issues in Thrombophilia. *Arch Pathol Lab Med* 2002;126:1281–1295.

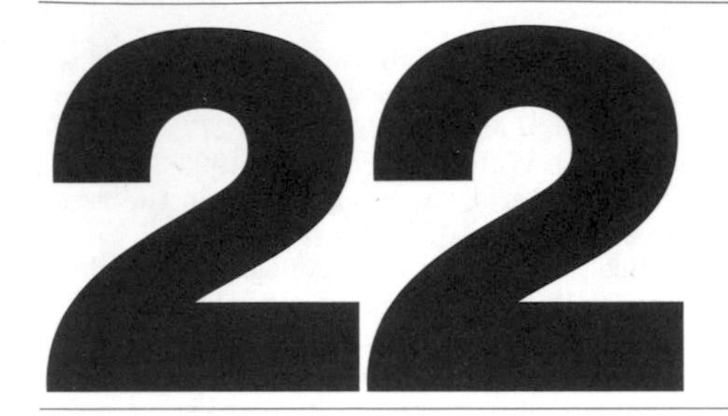

Pulmonary Hypertension

Murali Chakinala and
Dan Schuller

INTRODUCTION

Pulmonary HTN (PH) is commonly encountered during the evaluation of patients with symptoms suggesting respiratory disease. This chapter first discusses unique features of the pulmonary circulation and then provides a definition of PH. A classification scheme for PH is then introduced, with emphasis on **pulmonary arterial HTN (PAH).** Last, attention is directed toward the diagnostic evaluation and specific management of PAH.

DEFINITION OF PULMONARY HYPERTENSION

The pulmonary circulation has distinguishing features compared to other circulatory systems. The lungs are the only organs to receive blood from the low-pressure RV. In addition, the entire cardiac output is pumped through the pulmonary circulation during each minute. To accommodate such large volumes of blood while maintaining low pressure, the pulmonary circulation has tremendous capacitance owing to an immense network of capillaries with a vast combined surface area. Finally, the pulmonary circulation is able to autoregulate blood away from diseased regions of the lung, thus minimizing V/Q mismatch. As vascular capacitance diminishes and the total vascular surface area is reduced, high pressures are prone to develop.

PH is defined as a **mean pulmonary artery pressure (PAP) >25 mm Hg at rest or >30 mm Hg with exercise.** Pressures are most reliably measured invasively via a pulmonary artery catheter (PAC). Alternatively, pulmonary artery systolic pressure (PASP) can be estimated noninvasively by transthoracic echocardiography, whereby a PASP >40 mm Hg is considered abnormal.

The true basis of PH is **increased pulmonary vascular resistance (PVR),** which is related to the pressure difference across the pulmonary circuit and the cardiac output. The normal range for PVR is 20–120 dynes-sec-cm^{-5}. Meanwhile, the resistance due to the pulmonary circuit is represented by the total pulmonary resistance.

Classification

Once PH has been established, two important questions must be answered. **Is the PH acute or chronic? Acute PH** can develop coincident with numerous acute respiratory conditions, including pneumonia, pulmonary embolism, adult respiratory distress syndrome, and cardiogenic pulmonary edema. Generally, PAPs are only modestly elevated in these situations. **Chronic PH** develops with a myriad of conditions and may display severely elevated PAPs, often with secondary changes in RV morphometry (dilatation) and/or function (hypokinesis). If PH is initially detected during an acute respiratory illness, reassessment of the PAP is advised several weeks after resolution of the acute respiratory condition and before pursuing an exhaustive evaluation of chronic PH.

Is PH originating from the postcapillary or the precapillary vessels? Answering this question not only differentiates chronic forms of PH into two major categories (Fig. 22-1) but also directs the diagnostic evaluation and therapeutic options. Postcapillary or pulmonary venous HTN represents a frequent cause of PH and is overwhelmingly due to left-sided heart disease. Abnormalities restricting left ventricular filling, such as mitral stenosis and severe left ventricular hypertrophy, are particularly asso-

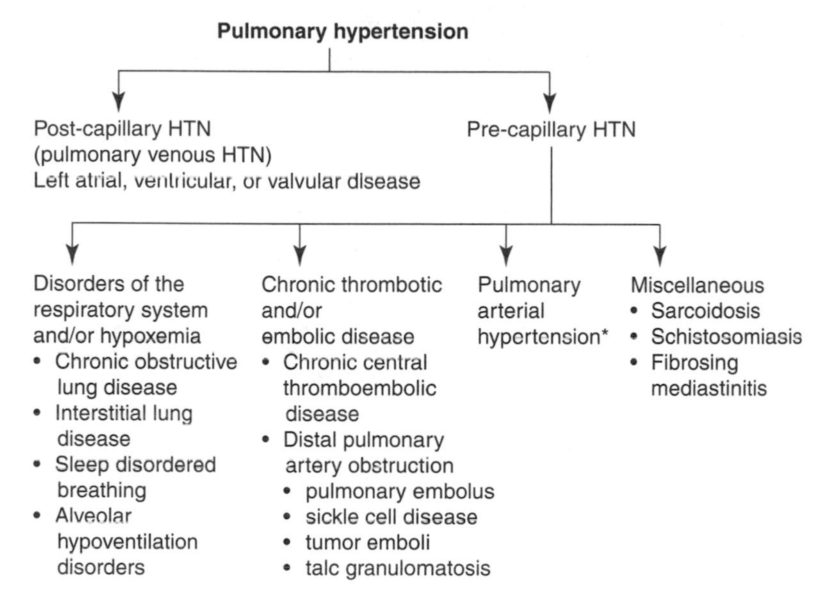

FIG. 22-1. Classification of pulmonary HTN. Modified from the WHO executive summaries on pulmonary hypertension (1998, 2003). *See Table 22-1 for causes of pulmonary arterial hypertension. Adapted from Rich S, ed. Executive summary from the World Symposium on Primary Pulmonary Hypertension 1998. Evian, France, September 6–10, 1998, cosponsored by the World Health Organization.

ciated with PH. PH is not independently related to the degree of left ventricular dysfunction, as quantified by depressed ejection fraction.

Precapillary PH represents a large, heterogeneous group of disorders (Fig. 22-1) that can be further divided into the following categories: (a) pulmonary arterial HTN (PAH), (b) PH secondary to disorders of the respiratory system and/or hypoxemia, (c) PH secondary to chronic thrombotic and/or embolic disease, and (d) PH secondary to disorders directly affecting the vasculature. PAH (Table 22-1) represents a unique class of disorders with unifying vascular pathology but diverse triggers.

The distinction between postcapillary and precapillary PH can often be made by a history of chronic left-sided cardiac disease or relevant findings during echocardiography (e.g., left atrial disease, left ventricular dysfunction, mitral valve disease). When an explanation for chronic PH cannot be ascertained from the echocardiogram, a more comprehensive evaluation is necessary, particularly for causes of PAH.

EVALUATION

History

Dyspnea is the most often reported symptom for patients with PH, particularly dyspnea with exertion. Symptoms that reflect more advanced disease and secondary RV dysfunction include fatigue, syncope, peripheral edema, and chest pain. Symptoms related to underlying primary diseases [e.g., chronic cough (interstitial lung disease, or ILD), dysphagia (esophageal dysmotility associated with scleroderma), snoring and excessive daytime sleepiness (obstructive sleep apnea), and bleeding tendencies (cirrhosis)] must be pursued with a thorough review of systems.

Past medical history relevant to several organ systems, including the respiratory, cardiovascular, hepatic, rheumatologic, and hematologic systems, must be exhaustively explored. Particular emphasis should be placed on prior cardiac conditions,

TABLE 22-1. PULMONARY ARTERIAL HYPERTENSION (PAH)

Idiopathic PAH
Familial PAH
PAH associated with
- Drug and toxins (anorexigenics)
- Collagen vascular disease (systemic sclerosis > mixed connective tissue disease > SLE)
- Portal HTN
- HIV infection
- Congenital systemic to pulmonary shunts
- Other: hereditary hemorrhagic telangiectasia, thyroid disorders, hemoglobinopathies

PAH associated with significant venous or capillary involvement
- Venoocclusive disease
- Pulmonary capillary hemangiomatosis

including myocardial infarction, congestive heart failure, arrhythmias, rheumatic heart disease, other valvular heart disease, and congenital heart disease.

Social history should focus on prior or current tobacco and alcohol use, as well as illicit or recreational drug use, particularly cocaine or crack. Risk factors for exposure to HIV may disclose an unexpected etiology for PH. Careful medication history to document the use of current or past drugs linked to the development of PH (e.g., aminorex, fenfluramine, dexfenfluramine, contaminated L-tryptophan) is also necessary. Finally, family history should also be explored, as 10% of idiopathic PAH (IPAH) cases have a genetic basis.

Physical Exam

Although a thorough physical exam to corroborate or refute suspicions of underlying medical problems should be performed (e.g., emphysema, ILD, scleroderma, cirrhosis, and congestive heart failure), particular attention should be directed toward the **cardiopulmonary exam.** Auscultatory exam of the heart may reveal an accentuated S_2 sound with a prominent P_2 component, systolic ejection murmur at left lower sternal border due to tricuspid regurgitation, and diastolic decrescendo murmur along the left sternal border due to pulmonary insufficiency. Additional cardiac findings, including continuous murmurs or rumbles and fixed-split S_2, may suggest an underlying congenital cardiac defect. As PH worsens and right heart failure ensues, resting tachycardia, S_3 gallop, elevated jugular venous pulsation of the neck, hepatomegaly, ascites, peripheral edema, diminished peripheral pulses, and cyanosis occur. Digital clubbing indicates underlying conditions such as ILD, bronchiectasis, or congenital heart disease.

Laboratory Studies

Essential lab studies for the evaluation of unexplained PH mirror the studies of a general medical evaluation: CBC, indices of renal function (BUN, creatinine), liver transaminases (ALT, AST), liver function studies (albumin, bilirubin), and coagulation studies (PTT and PT). Prerenal pattern of renal dysfunction (BUN elevation >> creatinine elevation) in conjunction with passive congestion of the liver (elevated bilirubin and PT) is a harbinger of advanced right heart failure and low cardiac output. Additionally, screening for collagen vascular disease with ANA, anticentromere antibody, rheumatoid factor, anti-scl-70 antibody, antiribonucleoprotein antibody, and ESR should be completed. Thyroid studies (thyrotoxicosis), hemoglobin electrophoresis (sickle cell disease), HIV serology, hepatitis serologies (cirrhosis), antiphospholipid antibody, or anticardiolipin antibody (hypercoagulable state or recurrent thromboemboli) should also be performed if clinical suspicion exists.

Radiographic Imaging

Features indicative of PH on **chest radiography** are enlarged central pulmonary arteries on frontal views (pulmonary artery transverse diameter >17 mm for men and >15 mm for women) and RV enlargement on lateral exam. When PAPs reach systemic levels, pulmonary artery calcifications can be seen. Obliteration of distal pulmonary arteries leads to tapering of vessels in the peripheral third of the lung parenchyma, referred to as *pruning*, and is classically seen in IPAH. In contrast, patients with congenital heart disease and left-to-right shunts who maintain a chronic high-flow state display enlarged pulmonary arteries throughout the lung parenchyma. Chest radiography should also be reviewed for underlying cardiopulmonary diseases, including ILD, emphysema, or congestive heart failure.

V/Q scans provide an easy and sensitive screen for the detection of chronic thromboembolic disease. Even though patients with PH due to nonembolic processes, such as IPAH, can illustrate a mottled perfusion pattern owing to subsegmental defects, larger or segmental perfusion defects are more concerning for thromboembolic disease and should be further evaluated with pulmonary angiography.

Pulmonary Function Testing

Routine spirometry with and without bronchodilators should be inspected for evidence of underlying obstructive lung disease (i.e., forced expiratory volume over 1 sec/forced vital capacity <70%). Measurement of lung volumes may provide a valuable clue for **ILD** (i.e., reduced total lung capacity, vital capacity, and residual volume). DLCO, which measures the ability of gas to traverse from the alveolar space into the vascular compartment, is reduced in a variety of circumstances other than PH, including ILD, emphysema, previous pulmonary resection, or pulmonary edema, but normal or elevated DLCO results point away from PH as the cause of a patient's symptoms. The **ABG** most reliably detects arterial hypoxemia, which contributes to pulmonary arterial vasoconstriction. Significant resting hypoxemia in patients with PH should raise the suspicion of a right-to-left shunt, severely reduced cardiac output with reduced mixed-venous oxygen levels, or underlying pulmonary disease (e.g., ILD or emphysema). **Ambulatory pulse oximetry** is a sensitive marker of PH, as many patients can maintain normal oxyhemoglobin levels at rest but desaturate with exertion. The 6-min walk test is widely used to titrate supplemental oxygen flow rates and place patients into functional classifications (I, II, III, or IV) (Table 22-2), which is a strong predictor of long-term survival in IPAH. Although cardiopulmonary exercise testing may be useful for patients with unexplained dyspnea or exercise limitations, it should be ***avoided*** in patients with known PH because risks to the patient may outweigh the little additional information provided. The classic findings for patients with IPAH are normal spirometry, minimally reduced total lung capacity (~75%), significant reduction of DLCO, normal resting PaO_2, and exercise-induced hypoxemia.

Electrocardiography

RV enlargement is suspected by the presence of an R wave in lead V_1 or an S wave in lead V_6. RV strain appears as a triad of S wave in lead I, Q wave in lead III, and inverted T wave in lead III. Other potential findings in cases of PH include right atrial enlargement

TABLE 22-2. WHO FUNCTIONAL CLASSIFICATION

Class I: No limitation of physical activity. Ordinary physical activity does not cause undue dyspnea, fatigue, chest pain, or near syncope.

Class II: Slight limitation of physical activity. Comfortable at rest. Ordinary activity causes undue dyspnea, fatigue, chest pain, or near syncope.

Class III: Marked limitation of physical activity. Comfortable at rest. Less than ordinary activity causes undue dyspnea, fatigue, chest pain, or near syncope.

Class IV: Unable to carry out any physical activity without symptoms. Dyspnea and/or fatigue may be at rest. Discomfort is increased by any physical activity.

and right bundle branch block. Prior myocardial infarction or left ventricular hypertrophy, as a hint of diastolic dysfunction, may also provide clues to the etiology of PH.

Echocardiography

As mentioned before, echocardiography is an invaluable tool for noninvasive measurement of PAPs. For a multitude of reasons, noninvasive measurements of PAPs may differ from invasive measurements by 10–20 mm Hg. Invasive measurement with a PAC should be performed if echocardiography does not corroborate a clinical suspicion of PH.

Nevertheless, echocardiography provides additional information on chamber sizes, biventricular function, and valvular competence, making it an essential study in the initial evaluation of PH. In addition, agitated saline contrast studies and Doppler evaluations can identify intracardiac shunts (e.g., ostium secundum defect, patent foramen ovale).

Additional Studies

When suggested by other clinical findings, **high-resolution CT of the chest, pulmonary angiography, and polysomnography** should be performed to complete the evaluation of PH. Because high-resolution CT is the most sensitive radiographic study for the detection of ILD and is also abnormal in pulmonary venoocclusive disease (i.e., prominent septal markings in the distal lung parenchyma), it provides invaluable information in certain patients. In addition, mediastinal images may demonstrate abnormalities causing PH from extrinsic compression owing to lymphadenopathy, tumors, or fibrosing mediastinitis. The diagnosis of chronic thromboembolic disease should be pursued with pulmonary angiography if V/Q scan or helical CT is suggestive. Although pulmonary angiography is riskier in patients with moderate to severe PH, it can be safely performed with low-volume injections of nonionic contrast. However, pulmonary angiography should be avoided in the setting of severe RV pressure elevations (RV end-diastolic pressure >20). Patients with significant proximal thromboembolic disease (i.e., fourth-generation artery or more proximal) may be candidates for pulmonary thromboendarterectomy at specialized centers. Meanwhile, all-night polysomnogram should be pursued when features of obstructive sleep apnea or the obesity-hypoventilation syndrome are uncovered, such as excessive snoring, poor sleep efficiency, excessive daytime sleepiness, and obese body habitus.

At the conclusion of the above workup, a patient's PH should be classifiable as postcapillary, precapillary, or mixed in origin. In the majority of cases with a postcapillary etiology, therapy should be directed toward optimizing cardiac function and correcting reversible causes. Treatment for pulmonary venoocclusive disease is limited to lung transplantation. If PH is originating from precapillary vessels and related to an underlying disorder of the respiratory system, chronic thromboembolic disease, or disorder directly affecting the vasculature, effort should be focused on optimizing treatment of the underlying condition. In addition, avoidance of hypoxemia with the use of supplemental oxygen is advised. Patients with PAH and primary arterial pathology should undergo right-heart catheterization to dictate therapy for their vascular disease.

Right-heart catheterization serves several purposes during the evaluation and management of patients with PAH. First, definitive documentation of PH can be made and the severity graded by **mean PAP:** mild (26–35 mm Hg), moderate (36–45 mm Hg), and severe (>45 mm Hg). Second, **assessments of RV function** by measurement of RV end-diastolic pressure, right atrial pressure (RAP), and cardiac index correlate with survival. Third, indicators of left-sided heart disease (e.g., elevated pulmonary artery occlusion pressure or large "v" waves in the pulmonary artery occlusion pressure tracing indicative of mitral regurgitation) and left-to-right intracardiac shunts (abnormal step-up during successive oxygen saturation measurements) can be investigated. Fourth, an acute vasodilator challenge can be performed to guide the choice of therapeutic agent. After a PAC has been placed into the pulmonary artery and baseline hemodynamic measurements recorded, including PASP, pulmonary artery diastolic pressure, cardiac output, RAP, and PVR, a **short-acting vasodilator** (e.g., IV adenosine, IV epoprostenol, or inhaled nitric oxide) is administered. After each dose administration, PAP and cardiac index measurements are repeated; this sequence continues until there is a significant vasodilatory response (≥ 10 mm Hg drop of the mean PAP and a concluding mean PAP <40 mm Hg with stable or improved cardiac output) or a significant side effect occurs [systemic hypotension (SBP <90 mm Hg), decrease in cardiac output, increase in PAP or RAP, or decrease in oxygen saturation]. If neither response occurs after several administrations of the vasodilator, the patient is classified as a nonresponder. Patients who are **responders** to acute vasodilator administration should then be offered a trial of oral calcium channel blockers, whereas nonresponders or those who have an unfavorable side effect should be considered for alternative therapies, such as bosentan or epoprostenol.

THERAPY FOR PULMONARY ARTERIAL HYPERTENSION

Vasodilators/"Vasomodulators"

The choice of vasodilator in PAH is determined by the response to acute vasodilator challenge and the patient's functional class (Fig. 22-2).

Calcium channel blockers, such as nifedipine and diltiazem, are indicated for patients established as responders to acute vasodilator challenge. Owing to poor tolerance and the risk of circulatory collapse, these oral agents should not be used in the setting of severe right heart failure (mean RAP >20 mm Hg). If there are no contraindications to calcium channel blocker, these patients should be moved to a closely monitored environment for initiation of the oral agent. The choice of calcium channel blocker is determined by various concomitant factors—for example, tachycardia (use diltiazem), ventricular dysfunction, atrioventricular conduction disturbances, or Raynaud's phenomenon from peripheral vasoconstriction (use nifedipine). Owing to drug half-lives and the potential for systemic hypotension and negative inotropy, these oral drugs should be initiated with a PAC in place. Successive hourly doses of the calcium channel blocker (e.g., nifedipine, 20 mg PO, or diltiazem, 60 mg PO) should be administered, with hemodynamic measurements performed before each additional dose. This sequence should continue for a maximum of 10 doses, unless there is a significant vasodilator response (as outlined in the previous section on additional studies) or significant side effect (bradycardia, systemic hypotension, decreased cardiac output, increased PAP or RAP, or decreased oxyhemoglobin saturation). Once a significant vasodilator response to calcium

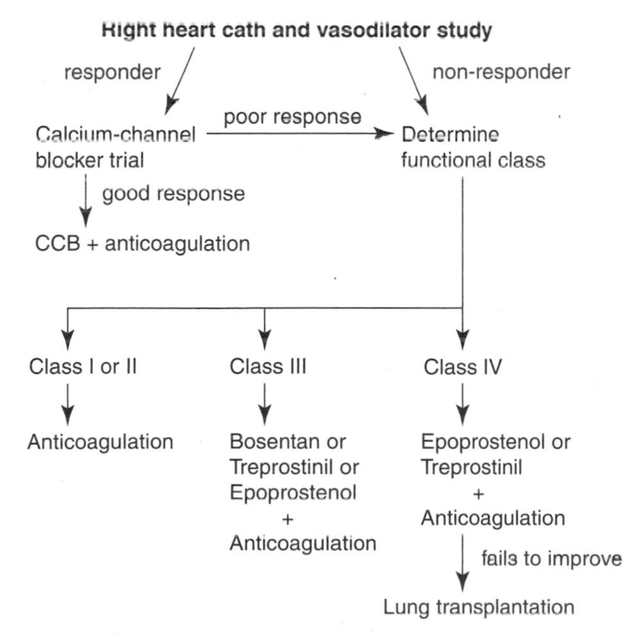

FIG. 22-2. Determination of therapy for pulmonary arterial hypertension based on vasodilator challenge. CCB, calcium channel blocker.

channel blocker therapy has been confirmed, patients should be started on a modest dose q8h (nifedipine) or q6h (diltiazem). To avoid orthostasis and intolerance, the drug should be escalated gradually over several weeks to a maximally tolerated dosage, typically nifedipine, 240 mg/day, or diltiazem, 720 mg/day. If patients report increased fatigue and dyspnea after beginning calcium channel blocker therapy, bradycardia, systemic hypotension, worsened hypoxemia, and aggravated ventricular dysfunction should be considered. Patients who can tolerate high-dose calcium channel blockers and demonstrate early subjective and objective improvements have excellent long-term survival with improved exercise tolerance, hemodynamics, and functional classification.

Patients unresponsive to acute vasodilator challenge, intolerant of calcium channel blocker therapy, or who progress despite calcium channel blocker therapy should be considered for **oral bosentan** (functional class III–IV), **SC treprostinil** (functional class II–IV), or **IV epoprostenol therapy** (functional class III–IV) (see Fig. 22-2). Patients in New York Heart Association class I should be **anticoagulated** and closely monitored for disease progression.

As the first available endothelin-receptor antagonist, bosentan has been shown to improve exercise capacity, functional classification, and time to clinical deterioration in various forms of PAH. **Bosentan** binds to endothelin receptors type A and B and antagonizes the effects of their natural ligand endothelin-1, which is a potent vasoconstrictor and smooth-muscle mitogen that has been implicated in the pathogenesis of PAH. Oral bosentan (initially 62.5 mg PO bid ×4 wks titrated to a maximum of 125 mg PO bid) is generally well tolerated, with the main potential toxicity being elevation of hepatic enzymes in a minority of cases. Owing to its ease of delivery, it is often the first option for patients with PAH in functional class III.

Functional class IV patients who are more tenuous should receive **epoprostenol.** Because of its short half-life (1–2 mins) and gastric inactivation, epoprostenol is infused continuously via a chronic indwelling catheter, typically a double-lumen Hickman catheter in the subclavian vein site. Chronic epoprostenol therapy requires meticulous care of the catheter and ambulatory infusion pump, daily preparation of the infusion, and manual dexterity. This commitment not only requires supreme compliance but also major lifestyle modifications. These issues should be clearly discussed with patients before initiating therapy. If the patient is willing to invest the time and commitment to chronic therapy, epoprostenol should be initiated at low infusion rates (2–5 ng/kg/min) and closely monitored for hypotension or hypoxemia. The majority of patients tolerate initiation quite well except for annoying drug-related side effects including jaw pain, headache, nausea, diarrhea, and musculoskeletal pain. As side effects wane, the infusion rate is increased on an outpatient basis. The typical therapeutic range for epoprostenol is 20–50 ng/kg/min. Bacterial infections at the catheter insertion site or in the bloodstream are not infrequent complications of the indwelling catheters and warrant meticulous care as well as prompt antimicrobial therapy and possible replacement of the catheter. Despite the cumbersome nature of the therapy and its drawbacks, short-term and long-term survival, exercise tolerance, hemodynamics, and functional classification are significantly improved for patients with chronic epoprostenol therapy, even for those who lack response to acute vasodilator challenge. Although the bulk of experience is in the IPAH population, epoprostenol has also been successfully used with other PAH-related conditions.

A subcutaneous prostacyclin analogue **(treprostinil)** is also available and obviates the need for an indwelling catheter; however, administration has been hampered in some cases by pain at the site of drug infusion. Nevertheless, treprostinil is an acceptable treatment for patients in functional class II–IV. Inhaled analogues of prostacyclin are in varying stages of development and may have unique indications in the future, thus obviating the need for IV therapy in some patients.

Anticoagulation

In situ thrombosis has been shown to be a significant contributor to the pathogenesis of IPAH. In addition, retrospective and prospective evidence suggests improved survival for IPAH patients with chronic anticoagulation. All PAH patients without contraindications to anticoagulation should receive warfarin, with a **target INR of ~2.** Although survival improvement with anticoagulation has not been studied in other conditions of PAH, anticoagulation can be considered if there are no contraindications, especially for the prevention of catheter-related thromboemboli with chronic epoprostenol infusion. Short-term discontinuation of warfarin for invasive procedures does not mandate the need for IV anticoagulant therapy.

Diuretics

When significant RV dysfunction develops, patients are afflicted with significant peripheral edema and ascites. To address these symptoms, diuretics are prescribed on a chronic basis. **Loop diuretics,** such as furosemide (Lasix) or bumetanide, are often combined with other diuretic classes, such as thiazides or aldosterone receptor antagonists, for more effective therapy. Unlike the setting of left ventricular dysfunction, patients with RV dysfunction are extremely **preload dependent** and must be diuresed carefully, avoiding overzealous fluid removal that can precipitate circulatory collapse. In conjunction with a stable regimen of diuretics, patients with significant right heart failure should be advised to **limit daily fluid intake** to no more than 2 L in addition to limiting their sodium intake.

Inotropes

Limited benefit of **digoxin** has been shown with IPAH. In the absence of contraindications, such as severe renal dysfunction or arrhythmias, digoxin can be instituted for significant RV dysfunction. In general, IV inotropes should be avoided in the setting of ventricular compromise associated with severe afterload (i.e., elevated PVR) because of limited benefit as well as significant deleterious effects, including arrhythmogenesis, increased myocardial oxygen demand, and myocardial ischemia.

Oxygen

In all cases of PH, hypoxemia further augments the PVR through hypoxic vasoconstriction. Patients should be provided with supplemental oxygen to maintain **oxyhemoglobin saturations >90%.** To achieve this goal throughout the day, monitoring of oxyhemoglobin saturation should be performed at rest, with exertion, and during sleep to optimally titrate the oxygen flow rate.

General Measures

In addition to the above specific therapies, several general measures should not be overlooked. Patients with significant PH should receive an annual **influenza vaccination** and a **pneumococcal vaccination** (Pneumovax) q5yrs because of their limited tolerance to respiratory infections. Ongoing **tobacco use** should be strongly admonished. Patients should **avoid over-the-counter decongestants,** which have sympathomimetic properties that exacerbate PH. Although physical conditioning is important, more strenuous activity may be deleterious due to a limited ability to augment cardiac output. Therefore, patients can be encouraged to perform **graduated exercises** with minimal aerobic requirements (with supplemental oxygen, if needed) but avoid more strenuous physical activities. Patients also should be cautioned against deep Valsalva maneuvers that can decrease venous blood return to the heart and further compromise cardiac output. Treatment for constipation and persistent coughing should be offered; patients should be advised to avoid lifting objects >20 lbs.

Atrial Septostomy

Patients with **medically refractory right heart failure,** including syncope, ascites, and peripheral edema, may be candidates for an atrial septostomy. In these advanced cases, a small atrial septal defect is created percutaneously in the fossa ovalis of the atrial septum, creating a new right-to-left shunt. Even though arterial oxygenation suffers by the creation of the intracardiac shunt, total oxygen delivery may increase owing to augmentation of cardiac output:

$$\text{Oxygen delivery} = [(\text{Hgb} \times 1.34) \times \text{arterial oxygen saturation } (\text{SaO}_2) + (\text{PaO}_2 \times 0.0031)] \times \text{CO} \times 10$$

$$(\downarrow)\ \text{SaO}_2 \text{ but } (\uparrow)\ \text{CO}$$

When done appropriately by specialized centers, significant symptom relief (decreased fatigue, syncope, ascites, peripheral edema), hemodynamic improvement (augmented cardiac output and improved renal perfusion), and possible survival benefits may be realized. However, negative outcomes, including procedure-related mortality, refractory hypoxemia, and lack of hemodynamic improvement, are also possible. Therefore, atrial septostomy should be reserved for the medically refractory cases as a bridge to transplantation, before the onset of extreme right heart failure (e.g., RAP <20 and cardiac index >1.5) and severe resting hypoxemia (oxyhemoglobin saturation <90%).

Organ Transplantation

The advances in medical therapy have at least temporarily reduced the number of lung and heart-lung transplants performed for IPAH to the minority of people who are intolerant or refractory to medical therapy. If patients do not stabilize with epoprostenol and no contraindications to transplantation exist, isolated **single** or **bilateral lung transplantation** can be performed, as RV function improves within months of surgery. IPAH is a significant negative predictor of 1-yr mortality after transplantation owing to the compromised cardiac status and poor tolerance to early postop complications. If patients survive the first 3 mos, long-term survival (60% at 3 yrs, 45% at 5 yrs, and 20% at 10 yrs) equalizes with other transplanted conditions, such as COPD and idiopathic pulmonary fibrosis. Consideration of lung transplantation for PAH related to connective tissue disorders is predicated by the degree of other end-organ damage from the underlying disorder. **Heart-lung transplantation** is generally reserved for patients with PH secondary to complex congenital heart defects that cannot be repaired at the time of transplantation. **Liver transplantation** can abolish mild cases of portal-pulmonary HTN (mean PAP <35 mm Hg); patients with more advanced and irreversible vascular disease do poorly after liver transplantation.

Future Therapies

Future therapies for PAH remain promising as its pathogenesis is further elucidated. New classes of drugs, phosphodiesterase inhibitors and serine elastase inhibitors, are in varying stages of development. More ambitious therapies, such as chronic nitric oxide inhalation and gene therapy, may eventually be implemented, but significant roadblocks exist.

KEY POINTS TO REMEMBER

- PH is defined as a mean PAP that exceeds 25 mm Hg at rest or 30 mm Hg with exercise. A PASP >40 mm Hg is considered abnormal.
- Dyspnea is the most often reported symptom for patients with PH, particularly dyspnea with exertion.
- Features indicative of PH on chest radiography are enlarged central pulmonary arteries on frontal views and right ventricular enlargement on lateral examination. When PAPs reach systemic levels, pulmonary artery calcifications can be seen.
- In all cases of PH, hypoxemia further augments the PVR through hypoxic vasoconstriction. Patients should be provided with supplemental oxygen to maintain oxyhemoglobin saturations above 90%.

REFERENCES AND SUGGESTED READINGS

Badesch DB, Tapson VF, McGoon MD, et al. Continuous intravenous epoprostenol for pulmonary hypertension due to the scleroderma spectrum of disease: a randomized, controlled trial. *Ann Intern Med* 2000;132(6):425–434.

Channick RN, Simonneau G, Sitbon O, et al. Effects of the dual endothelin-receptor antagonist bosentan in patients with pulmonary hypertension: a randomized placebo-controlled trial. *Lancet* 2001;358:1119–1123.

D'Alonzo GE, Barst RJ, Ayres SM, et al. Survival in patients with primary pulmonary hypertension: results from a national prospective registry. *Ann Intern Med* 1991;115:343–349.

Enriquez-Sarano M, Rossi A, Seward JB, et al. Determinants of pulmonary hypertension in left ventricular dysfunction. *J Am Coll Cardiol* 1997;29(1):153–159.

Fuster V, Steele PM, Edwards WD, et al. Primary pulmonary hypertension: natural history and the importance of thrombosis. *Circulation* 1984;70(4):580–587.

Hinderliter AL, Willis PW 4th, Barst RJ, et al. Effects of long-term infusion of Prostacyclin (epoprostenol) on echocardiographic measures of right ventricular structure and function in primary pulmonary hypertension. *Circulation* 1997;95:1479–186.

Hosenpud JD, Bennett LE, Keck BM, et al. The registry of the International Society for Heart and Lung Transplantation: Eighteenth Official Report–2001. *J Heart Lung Transplant* 2001;20:805–815.

Krowka MJ, Frantz RP, McGoon MD, et al. Improvement in pulmonary hemodynamics during intravenous epoprostenol (Prostacyclin): a study of 15 patients with moderate to severe portopulmonary hypertension. *Hepatology* 1999;30:641–648.

McLaughlin VV, Genthner DE, Panella MM, Rich S. Reduction in pulmonary vascular resistance with long-term epoprostenol (Prostacyclin) therapy in primary pulmonary hypertension. *N Engl J Med* 1998;338(5):273–277.

Miyamoto S, Nagaya N, Satoh T, et al. Clinical correlates and prognostic significance of six-minute walk test in patients with primary pulmonary hypertension. *Am J Respir Crit Care Med* 2000;1661:487–492.

Rich S, ed. Executive summary from the World Symposium on Primary Pulmonary Hypertension 1998. Evian, France, September 6–10, 1998, cosponsored by the World Health Organization.

Rich S, Brundage BH. High-dose calcium channel-blocking therapy for primary pulmonary hypertension: evidence for long-term reduction in pulmonary artery pressure and regression of right ventricular hypertrophy. *Circulation* 1987;76(1):135–141.

Rich S, Dodin E, McLaughlin VV, et al. Usefulness of atrial septostomy as a treatment for primary pulmonary hypertension and guidelines for its application. *Am J Cardiol* 1997;80(3):369–371.

Rich S, Kaufmann E, Levy PS, et al. The effect of high doses of calcium channel blockers on survival in primary pulmonary hypertension. *N Engl J Med* 1992;327 (2):76–81.

Rich S, Seidlitz M, Dodin E, et al. The short-term effects of digoxin in patients with right ventricular dysfunction from pulmonary hypertension. *Chest* 1998;144 (3):787–792.

Rothman A, Sklansky MS, Lucas VW, et al. Atrial septostomy as a bridge to lung transplantation in patients with severe primary pulmonary hypertension. *J Am Coll Cardiol* 1999;84(6):682–686.

Rubin LJ, Badesch DB, Barst RJ, et al. Bosentan therapy for pulmonary arterial hypertension. *N Engl J Med* 2002;346(12):896–903.

Simmoneau G, Barst RJ, Galie N, et al. Continuous subcutaneous infusion of treprostinil, a prostacyclin analogue, in patients with pulmonary arterial hypertension: a double-blind, randomized, placebo-controlled trial. *Am J Respir Crit Care Med* 2002;165(6):800–804.

Zuckerman DA, Sterling KM, Oser RF, et al. Safety of pulmonary angiography in the 1990s. *J Vasc Interv Radiol* 1996;7(2):199–205.

23 Pleural Diseases

Latha Sivaprasad and
Adrian Shifren

INTRODUCTION

The pleural lining is a serous membrane covering the lung parenchyma, chest wall, diaphragm, and mediastinum. The pleural membrane covering the surface of the lung is known as the visceral pleura, whereas the parietal pleura covers the remaining mentioned structures. In between the visceral and parietal pleura is the pleural space, a potential space that contains a thin layer of fluid (approximately 0.15 mL/kg/pleural space)—usually around 10 mL in each pleural space. The parietal pleura secretes approximately 2400 mL of fluid daily, which is reabsorbed by the visceral pleura.

PLEURAL EFFUSIONS

More than 1 million cases of **pleural effusion** occur annually in the United States. Symptoms of an effusion include dyspnea and pain. The pain may be induced by deep breathing, coughing, sneezing, or body movement. Because of the shared lower intercostal nerve supply to the abdominal wall, chest, and diaphragm, referred pain in the abdomen is possible. Pain in the shoulder region may occur secondary to irritation of afferent nerve fibers from the phrenic nerves that supply the central diaphragm.

Localizing the Effusion

A pleural effusion may present with a combination of decreased expansion of the affected hemithorax on inspiration, stony dullness to percussion, and decreased or absent breath sounds on auscultation.

On a posteroanterior chest film, fluid in the pleural space can be seen as blunting of the costophrenic angle or blurring of the diaphragmatic margin if **>200–500 mL** is present (depending on the size of the patient). A lateral decubitus film of the affected side can reveal an effusion of approximately 100 mL. A lateral decubitus film also allows assessment of whether the effusion is free flowing or loculated.

A CT scan can better visualize fluid in the paraspinous regions, anterior mediastinum, and apical regions of the thorax. In addition, the extent of the effusion can be defined and loculations can be characterized.

U/S can be used to locate small amounts of loculated fluid for diagnostic purposes, to drain pus or blood, or to aid in needle biopsy.

Differentiating a Transudate from an Exudate

Differentiation of a transudate from an exudate helps evaluate the underlying etiology of the effusion and facilitates the management of the effusion. **Transudates** result primarily from fluid shifts that occur as a result of changes in the hydrostatic and oncotic pressures of the circulation. The causes are usually limited (Table 23-1). **Exudates** are more complex because they are primarily the result of inflammation of the pleura or underlying lung tissue. The causes are more numerous (see Table 23-1), and they usually require a more extensive investigation to guide management.

The current standards for differentiating a transudate from an exudate are defined by **Light's criteria** (Table 23-2). These criteria compare the levels of **protein** and **lac-**

TABLE 23-1. CAUSES OF PLEURAL EFFUSION

Exudate	Transudate
Infections (parapneumonic effusions/empyema)	Increased hydrostatic pressure
Bacteria	Congestive heart failure
TB	Constrictive pericarditis
Fungi	Superior vena caval obstruction
Parasites	Decreased oncotic pressure
Viruses	Cirrhosis
Mycoplasma	Nephrotic syndrome
Neoplasms	Hypoalbuminemia
Metastatic carcinoma	Peritoneal dialysis
Lymphoma	Miscellaneous
Leukemia	Acute atelectasis
Mesothelioma	Subclavian catheter misplacement
Bronchogenic carcinoma	Myxedema
Chest wall tumors	Idiopathic
Intraabdominal disease/GI	
Abdominal surgery	
Pancreatitis	
Meigs' syndrome (benign ovarian fibroma)	
Intrahepatic abscess	
Incarcerated diaphragmatic hernia	
Subdiaphragmatic abscess	
Esophageal rupture	
Endoscopic variceal sclerotherapy	
Hepatitis	
Collagen-vascular diseases	
Systemic lupus erythematosus	
Rheumatoid arthritis	
Drug-induced lupus	
Sjögren's syndrome	
Wegener's granulomatosis	
Churg-Strauss syndrome	
Immunoblastic lymphadenopathy	
Drug-induced pleural disease	
Nitrofurantoin	
Dantrolene	
Methysergide	
Bromocriptine	
Procarbazine	
Amiodarone	
Pulmonary infarction	

(*continued*)

TABLE 23-1. (*continued*)

Exudate
Miscellaneous
Dressler's syndrome (post-cardiac injury)
Sarcoidosis
Uremia
Yellow nail syndrome (lymphedema)
Trapped lung
Radiation therapy
Electrical burns
Iatrogenic injury
Ovarian hyperstimulation syndrome
Chronic atelectasis
Asbestos exposure
Familial Mediterranean fever
Urinoma (urinary tract obstruction)
Idiopathic
Lipid laden
Chylous
Pseudochylous
Hemothorax
Penetrating injury
Iatrogenic
Spontaneous pneumothorax
Metastatic cancer

tate dehydrogenase in the effusion with those in the patient's serum to determine whether inflammation or fluid shift is responsible for the effusion. If even one of the three Light's criteria is met, the effusion is defined as an exudate.

TABLE 23-2. CRITERIA FOR DEFINING AN EFFUSION

Light's criteria	Heffner criteria
Pleural fluid protein to serum protein ratio of >0.5	Pleural fluid protein >2.9 g/dL
Pleural fluid LDH to serum LDH ratio of >0.6	Pleural fluid cholesterol >45 mg/dL
Pleural fluid LDH >2/3 serum upper limit of normal	Pleural fluid LDH >45% of upper limits of normal serum value

LDH, lactate dehydrogenase.
Adapted from Clinical manifestations and useful tests. In: Light RW. *Pleural diseases*, 4th ed. Baltimore: Lippincott Williams & Wilkins, 2001:42–86; and Heffner JE, Brown LK, Barbieri CA. Diagnostic value of tests that discriminate between exudative and transudative pleural effusions. *Chest* 1997;111:970–980.

Recently, a new set of criteria developed by **Heffner** compared favorably to Light's criteria in a study using both to differentiate between transudates and exudates. These criteria are useful in that they do not require a serum sample for comparison. As with Light's criteria, if even one of the Heffner's criteria is met, the effusion is defined as an exudate (see Table 23-2).

Despite the large number of etiologies for exudative pleural effusions, the pleural fluid findings often point to a specific cause of effusion, with certain findings suggesting certain etiologies that help guide management (Table 23-3).

Thoracentesis

After localizing the effusion, the pleural fluid should be sampled to **define the effusion** as a transudate or exudate. Position the patient sitting up on the side of the bed leaning forward over a table. Clean and drape the patient in a sterile fashion. Using aseptic technique, percuss posteriorly in the midscapular line to one interspace below the upper limit of the dullness, staying above the level of the diaphragmatic pleura. For a diagnostic pleural tap, a 21-ga needle attached to a 20-mL syringe can be used to aspirate fluid. For therapeutic pleural taps, special kits are commercially available for the removal of large volumes of fluid. The needle is inserted under suction perpendicular to the skin and over the top surface of the rib below the interspace chosen. This technique minimizes the chance of lacerating an intercostal artery that runs in the intercostal groove on the undersurface of the rib above a given interspace.

The requisite amount of fluid is then removed by suction. Removing >1.5 L of fluid increases the risk of **reexpansion pulmonary edema.** This reexpansion may be related to the rate of lung reexpansion after fluid drainage and the duration and severity of the underlying lung collapse before drainage. The underlying mechanism is not totally clear but may be related to excess free radical formation leading to increased microvascular permeability. Once the procedure is complete, the needle is removed and the wound cleaned and dressed. A chest x-ray (CXR) should always be obtained after a thoracentesis to rule out a complicating pneumothorax.

Please note: Reading the above text is no substitute for being taught how to perform a thoracentesis. Under no circumstances should this procedure be attempted without formal teaching and supervision of the procedure by a physician skilled at thoracentesis.

Treatment

If the fluid meets the criteria for a transudate, treatment of the underlying cause is appropriate and further investigation is unnecessary. Symptomatic treatment may involve drainage of the effusion.

If the fluid meets any of the criteria for an exudate, the patient needs to be evaluated for an underlying cause. Treatment of the cause often, but not always, leads to resolution of the effusion. Symptomatic treatment may involve drainage of the effusion and even pleurodesis to prevent reaccumulation of fluid. See specific effusion types below for more detailed therapy.

PARAPNEUMONIC EFFUSIONS AND EMPYEMA

Parapneumonic effusions and empyemas are specific types of **exudative pleural effusions** due to infection adjacent to or in the pleural space, respectively. They are most frequently due to extension of infection from an underlying **pneumonia.** Hence, risk factors for empyema are similar to those for pneumonia.

One of the most common causes of empyema is **aspiration.** Patients at the highest risk for aspiration include those with poor dentition, alcohol abuse, seizure disorder, and absent gag reflex (e.g., comatose patients, patients with altered mental status, and patients undergoing general anesthesia). The infections are usually polymicrobial and include *Bacteroides, Fusobacterium,* and *Peptostreptococcus* species. One should always consider methicillin-resistant *Staphylococcus aureus* and *Mycobacterium tuberculosis* as potential pathogens in any pulmonary infection.

Another common cause of empyema is **penetrating chest injury,** which includes both trauma and iatrogenic injury. Empyema may be caused by contamination of the

TABLE 23-3. HELPFUL FEATURES OF EXUDATIVE EFFUSIONS

Etiology	Biochemical features	Other clues
Malignancy (bronchogenic, breast, and lymphoma most common)	GB/GT, positive cytology	Needle biopsy or thoracoscopy could help with diagnosis, usually effusion is symptomatic, other systemic clues of cancer, larger volume tap does not improve yield
Pulmonary infarction	Careful—can be transudative or exudative, PF is bloodstained	Dyspnea common
TB	PF is lymphocytic, +AFB stain of PF (very rare). ADA level may be elevated in PF	Relatively uncommon, weight loss, dyspnea, pleuritic pain, +PPD Needle biopsy could reveal granulomas—more helpful than culture
Connective tissue disease	+ANA in PF Usually lymphocytic Decreased PF complement and increased immune complexes Rheumatoid pleuritis—grossly green Wright's stain could detect LE cells	Support of serum lab tests, physical exam (e.g., rheumatoid nodules, sclerodactyly)
Pancreatitis	Increased amylase in PF	
Intraabdominal abscess	PF is mostly PMNs	
Meigs' syndrome	—	Ascites, ovarian tumor
Yellow nail syndrome	—	Yellow nails, lymphedema
Drug-related	PF is usually eosinophilic	Drug history
Chylothorax	Milky fluid, triglyceride level >110 mg/dL	Recent trauma, usually a large and symptomatic effusion, lymphangiogram or mediastinal CT could be helpful
Hemothorax	PF is GB Hct of PF is >50% of peripheral blood	Recent trauma, rupture of tumor of blood vessel
Mesothelioma	Hyaluronic acid concentration >0.8 mg/dL (nonspecific)	Asbestos exposure, pleural thickening, thoracoscopic or open pleural biopsy may be needed

ADA, adenosine deaminase; ANA, antinuclear antibody; GB, grossly bloody; GT, grossly turbid; LE, lupus erythematosus; PF, pleural fluid; PMN, polymorphonuclear neutrophil.

TABLE 23-4. CLASSIFICATION AND MANAGEMENT OF EMPYEMA

Size on CXR	Microbiology	Chemistry	Drainage
Small (<10 mm on lateral decubitus film) and free flowing	Too small to tap	Too small to tap	None
Moderate (>10 mm but <1/2 of the affected hemithorax) and free flowing	Negative Gram's stain *and* negative culture	pH ≥ 7.2	None
Large (>1/2 of the affected hemithorax) and free flowing *or* loculated effusion	Positive Gram's stain *or* positive culture *or* frank pus	pH <7.2	Chest tube ± fibrinolytics

Adapted from Colice GL, Curtis A, Deslauriers J, et al. Medical and surgical treatment of parapneumonic effusions: an evidence-based guideline. *Chest* 2000;118(4):1158.

traumatic wound or inadequate skin preparation before medical procedures such as chest tube placement or thoracentesis. The microbiologic organisms involved are usually skin flora such as *S. aureus* or *S. epidermis.*

Thoracentesis is the only way to confirm that an effusion is an empyema. Pleural tap should be done immediately once empyema is considered. If the fluid is grossly purulent, the diagnosis is established. If the fluid is not purulent, then the most important investigations needed include pleural fluid pH, glucose, and lactate dehydrogenase. These studies help categorize parapneumonic effusions as simple or complicated and define the choice of therapy for the effusion. Gram's stain and cultures of pleural fluid (for both aerobes and anaerobes) should be obtained on any samples whether they are purulent or not.

The current classification of parapneumonic effusions and empyemas is presented in Table 23-4. This classification is very useful because it guides the therapy of these specific effusions. All patients being treated for empyema or parapneumonic effusions should receive **antibiotics.**

CHYLOTHORAX

Chylothorax is defined as the presence of chyle within the pleural space. Because chyle is both bacteriostatic and nonirritating, symptoms resulting from pleural inflammation and infection are most unusual. Chyle contains large amounts of **fat, protein, and lymphocytes,** which accounts for the nutritional and immunologic deficiencies observed with more chronic chylous effusions.

There are three **basic mechanisms** whereby chyle can accumulate within the pleural space. These include leakage from the thoracic duct, obstruction of pleural lymphatics, and transdiaphragmatic passage of a chylous ascites.

The four major grouped **causes** of chylothorax are tumors (50% of all cases), trauma (25% of all cases), idiopathic (15% of all cases), and other (the remaining 10%) (Table 23-5).

Lymphomas, as a group, are the most common cause of pleural chyle collections and are therefore the most common source of chylothorax overall. Approximately 75% of all chylous effusions related to malignant tumors are due to lymphomas. Therefore, any nontraumatic chylous effusion without an obvious cause should be thoroughly evaluated to exclude the possibility of a lymphoma.

Iatrogenic trauma is more common than noniatrogenic trauma as a cause of chylothoraces. Almost any cardiothoracic surgical procedure can be complicated by the develop-

TABLE 23-5. CAUSES OF CHYLOTHORAX

- Tumors
  - Hodgkin's disease and non-Hodgkin's lymphoma
  - Burkitt's lymphoma
  - Lymphosarcoma
  - Bronchogenic carcinoma
  - Leukemia
- Trauma
  - Iatrogenic
    - Esophageal surgeries
    - Sclerosis of esophageal varices
    - Coronary artery bypass grafting
    - Heart transplants
    - Lung transplants
    - Central venous cannulation
  - Noniatrogenic
    - Penetrating chest trauma (gunshot, knife-wound)
    - Nonpenetrating chest trauma (crush injury, collision)
  - Minor injuries
    - Lifting
    - Severe cough
    - Severe emesis
    - Childbirth
- Idiopathic
  - Congenital
  - Acquired (includes minor traumas listed above)
- Other
  - Sarcoidosis
  - Tuberculosis
  - Histoplasmosis
  - Filariasis
  - Lymphangioleiomyomatosis
  - Tuberous sclerosis
  - Behçet's syndrome
  - Yellow nail syndrome
  - Thoracic radiation therapy
  - Superior vena cava thrombosis
  - HIV-associated Kaposi's sarcoma
  - Subclavian vein thrombosis
  - Chylous ascites (with transdiaphragmatic leak)

Modified from Doerr CH, Miller DL, Ryu JH. Chylothorax. *Semin Respir Crit Care Med* 2001;22(6): 617–626.

ment of a chylothorax, which may be delayed by 1–2 wks after the surgery. In addition, the traumatic event may be as benign as lifting weights, coughing, or vomiting. These less common causes are important to consider, especially when the etiology of the effusion is more obscure.

In a considerable number of cases, the cause of the chylothorax remains undiagnosed. Occasionally, chyle from a chylous ascites may leak transdiaphragmatically and fill the pleural space. Causes of **chylous ascites** include nephrotic syndrome, hypothyroidism, and cirrhosis.

The key to diagnosing a chylous effusion is to suspect its presence. As mentioned previously, chylous effusions are generally nonirritating. As such, complaints of pain (typically associated with pleurisy) are uncommon with chylothoraces. **Common complaints** usually involve shortness of breath, a feeling of restricted breathing, and occasional chest heaviness. Exam findings are typical for those of any pleural effusion. Most commonly, chylous effusions are unilateral owing to the unique anatomy of the thoracic duct, the most common source of chyle in chylous effusions. The duct runs upward along the right side of the thoracic vertebral bodies below the level of T5. Thus, injuries along this portion of the thoracic duct result in a right-sided chylothorax. At the level of T5, the duct crosses from the right to the left side of the thoracic vertebral bodies, continuing its course into the neck. Chylothoraces above the level of T5 are therefore usually left sided.

A **classic chylothorax** appears white, milky, and opalescent on removal from the affected hemithorax. However, only approximately 50% of all chylous effusions have this appearance. They may range from yellow to green and be serosanguineous or even bloody. In these cases, a chylothorax as the etiology of the pleural effusion is easily overlooked.

Chemically, a chylothorax is defined by the presence of chylomicrons in the pleural effusion in question. The diagnosis of chylothorax is therefore confirmed by high levels of pleural **triglycerides** (the most common constituent of chylomicron particles). A pleural fluid triglyceride level of **>110 mg/dL** is considered diagnostic of chylothorax.

The amount of triglyceride in a chylous effusion is variable and is dependent on the type, amount, and timing of food recently ingested. Thus, values in the range of **50–110 mg/dL** are still consistent with a diagnosis of chylothorax, especially in more **chronic cases** in which the patient already has malnutrition or is ingesting a low-fat diet. Effusions with triglyceride levels <50 mg/dL are almost never chylous. In cases in which doubt exists (pleural triglyceride level, 50–110 mg/dL), a lipoprotein electrophoresis can be carried out to confirm the presence of chylomicrons in the pleural space.

Just as a chylous effusion may be confused with other effusions, the opposite can occur, too. A **pseudochylothorax** is a cholesterol-rich effusion that may have the typical milky appearance of a chylothorax. These effusions are typically long-standing (>5 yrs old at the time of assessment) and are typical of old rheumatoid or tuberculous effusions. They characteristically contain cholesterol crystals and typically have cholesterol levels in excess of 250 mg/dL. They are chylomicron poor, with triglyceride levels of <50 mg/dL. This diagnosis can be confirmed by measuring the levels of both triglyceride and cholesterol in the effusion, or by performing a lipoprotein electrophoresis.

The optimal management of chylothorax is controversial. The approach used for **management** depends on the underlying cause of the effusion, the patient's functional status and nutritional state, comorbid illnesses, and local expertise. Despite this, the three mainstays for the management of pleural effusion are treatment of the underlying cause, specific conservative therapy, and surgical therapy.

Conservative therapy usually involves **tube thoracostomy** to achieve drainage of the effusion and expansion of the underlying lung tissue. **Repeated thoracentesis** to remove fluid has lost favor owing to the fact that complete drainage is almost never achieved and because of the risk of complications. Once the effusion is adequately drained, a **pleurodesis** (usually using talc as a sclerosing agent) can be performed if needed. Results using this approach are moderately successful with lower rates of resolution than with nonchylous effusions both with and without pleurodesis.

Irrespective of whether a chest tube is inserted, the patient's **nutritional status** must be closely monitored to prevent unnecessary malnutrition. Body weight, serum electrolytes, and albumin levels should be followed and maintained as close to normal as possible.

Medium-chain triglyceride (MCT) diets have been touted as a way of reducing chyle drainage into the pleural space and preventing malnutrition. Because chylomicrons (and hence chyle) are derived from long-chain triglycerides in the diet, a MCT diet should in theory minimize the amount of chyle formed. However, MCT diets have met with variable success because oral intake of any kind still results in chyle formation. Therefore, **total parenteral nutrition** with complete bowel rest is preferred to MCT diets and has in fact been shown to result in better outcomes.

Using this approach, most patients can be managed conservatively with a combination of chest tube thoracostomy and either MCT diet or total parenteral nutrition. Once the effusion is drained and the lung reexpanded, a regular diet can be resumed. If the effusion does not recur, the chest tube can be removed. If, however, the effusion reaccumulates or does not resolve over a 10- to 14-day period, pleurodesis or operative management needs to be considered.

Anecdotally, the **surgical management** of chylothoraces has met with greater success than conservative therapies. However, randomized, controlled studies comparing the two modalities have not been performed. The most frequent surgical intervention for chylothorax is ligation of the thoracic duct. This procedure can be performed by either open thoracotomy or video-assisted thoracoscopic surgery (VATS). In the majority of cases, a parietal pleurectomy or pleurodesis is performed in conjunction with the duct ligation to achieve pleural fusion.

Certain chylothoraces have been shown to warrant **early surgical intervention.** These include chylothorax with chest tube output >1500 mL/day, chylothorax complicated by malnutrition, chylothorax with immunologic compromise, and chylothorax complicating esophagectomy.

In patients who need surgical intervention but are poor operative candidates, **pleuroperitoneal shunting** can be performed. The procedure is safe and relatively simple, and in well-selected patients is also effective. Chylous effusions secondary to chylous ascites of any cause are an obvious contraindication to this procedure.

HEMOTHORAX

A hemothorax is the presence of blood in the pleural space. It is most commonly the result of some form of **trauma** involving the chest wall. Occasionally, a hemothorax may occur secondary to abdominal trauma, especially penetrating trauma such as knife or gunshot wounds. In these cases, the thoracic involvement may not always be obvious. In rare cases, hemothoraces may occur spontaneously (Table 23-6).

Diagnosis of hemothorax is based on a **high index of suspicion.** A hemothorax presents with clinical features similar to any other effusion, but the cause of the hemothorax (e.g., pain from a gunshot wound) may dominate the presenting complaint. Hemothoraces are visible on most chest imaging modalities but are difficult to differentiate from other causes of pleural effusion, especially on CXR. Thus, a high index of suspicion should always be maintained.

Like any acute bleeding, the presence of a hemothorax may not initially be obvious when a peripheral blood Hct is checked, because hemodilution has not yet had time to occur. A **coagulation profile** (PT, PTT) should always be checked when evaluating a patient with a possible or confirmed hemothorax.

The definitive diagnosis of hemothorax is made by sampling the effusion. Sometimes the sample may be grossly bloody. In more subtle cases, the effusion Hct may need to be evaluated. When the **hematocrit of the effusion is >50%** of the corresponding value for peripheral blood, a hemothorax is confirmed.

Delayed hemothorax may occur in up to 10% of cases of penetrating thoracic trauma. Clinically, this may manifest with any combination of worsening dyspnea, hemodynamic instability, or falling Hct. Repeating the CXR 3–6 hrs after the injury may help avoid clinical deterioration by detecting worsening effusions before they become symptomatic.

The first step in treating any hemothorax is **volume resuscitation.** Once the patient is stable, drainage of blood from the pleural space is performed. In most cases, the bleeding causing a hemothorax stops spontaneously, with or without chest tube insertion. Less commonly, patients cannot be adequately stabilized owing to ongoing bleeding. This complication occurs in approximately 30% of penetrating injuries and 15% of blunt injuries. In these cases, immediate thoracotomy is indicated.

TABLE 23-6. ETIOLOGY OF HEMOTHORAX

Penetrating trauma
- Knife wounds
- Gunshot wounds
- Other

Blunt trauma
- Motor vehicle accidents
- Falls
- Beating
- Other

Iatrogenic injury
- Central line placement
- Surgery (neck, thorax, abdomen)
- Thoracentesis
- Pleural biopsy (needle, video assisted)

Spontaneous
- Anticoagulation
- Hereditary hemorrhagic telangiectasia (and other arteriovenous malformations)
- Malignancy (usually metastatic)
- Pulmonary embolus (with complicating pulmonary infarct)
- Ruptured aortic aneurysm (thoracic or abdominal)
- Aortic dissection
- Catamenial pneumothorax
- TB

Modified from Eggerstedt JM. Hemothorax. Available at: http://www.emedicine.com/med/topic2915.htm. Accessed October 5, 2005.

Drainage of the pleural space is best achieved by tube thoracostomy. The purpose of evacuating the intrapleural blood is threefold. First, it allows apposition of the visceral and parietal pleura, which assists in hemostasis. Second, it allows for reexpansion of the pulmonary parenchyma, which helps tamponade any pulmonary parenchymal bleeding. And third, it removes clotted blood, which may lyse later, leading to further bleeding.

In general, the **largest tube possible** should be placed—usually a 36 French tube in adults. The amount of blood obtained on insertion and every hour thereafter should be accurately recorded. Once inserted, the chest tube should be placed to 20 cm H_2O suction.

If the hemothorax persists despite a functional thoracostomy tube, the blood in the pleural space may already have clotted. **Decubitus** films may help in the evaluation of a clotted hemothorax, because clotted blood in the pleural space does not layer out. A **second chest tube** may also be placed to assist with further drainage if the effusion layers on CXR. The addition of a **lytic agent** such as streptokinase can be considered if clotting is confirmed. In up to 30% of cases, these measures fail, and a VATS with removal of old blood is indicated to prevent the development of fibrothorax or empyema. The optimal timing for VATS therapy of a clotted hemothorax is usually 1–3 days after the injury has occurred.

Massive hemothorax is defined as an initial chest tube output of >1500 mL of blood, or continued chest tube output of >200 mL of blood over 2 hrs. In these cases, bleeding continues unabated and surgical intervention is necessary. The approach may be either open thoracotomy or VATS. The chest tube should never be clamped in

TABLE 23-7. CAUSES OF SECONDARY PNEUMOTHORAX

COPD	Usually related to rupture of apical blebs.
	ABG may be abnormal with hypoxemia and hypercapnia.
	Recurrence rate higher than other types.
AIDS	Pneumothorax significantly more common in AIDS patients.
	There is often a history of PJP.
	Etiology is likely due to large subpleural cysts with underlying necrosis seen in PJP.
Cystic fibrosis	Incidence is related to predisposition to severe COPD.
	Usually large apical subpleural cysts.
Tuberculosis	Usually due to a cavitary lesion that ruptures into the pleural space while communicating with a bronchus.
Sarcoidosis	Multisystemic granulomatous disease.
Pulmonary fibrosis	Fibrosis may be due to connective tissue disease, infection, occupational exposure, drugs.
	Often idiopathic.
Asthma	Related to hyperinflation and overdistention of alveoli.
	More commonly seen with positive-pressure ventilation.
Marfan's disease	Related to connective tissue abnormality.
Lung abscess	Related to cavity formation and rupture of a pus collection.
Menstruation	Catamenial pneumothorax (rare).
Acute respiratory distress syndrome	Usually related to positive-pressure ventilation.
Lymphangioleiomyomatosis	Women of childbearing age have recurrent pneumothorax.
	Pulmonary function tests reveal obstruction.
	X-ray reveals hyperinflation, reticulonodular infiltrates, and thin-walled cysts.
Pulmonary Langerhans' cell histiocytosis	Abnormal histiocyte proliferation.
	Histiocytes → nodules → irregular thin-walled cysts.
	Strong link to smoking.
Trauma	Penetrating and nonpenetrating chest trauma can cause pneumothorax.
	Iatrogenic causes include insertion of central venous catheters, thoracentesis, transbronchial biopsy, and mechanical ventilation.

PJP, *Pneumocystis jiroveci* pneumonia.

these situations because the maneuver will not arrest the bleeding and may lead to the development of a tension hemothorax and cardiopulmonary instability.

UNCLASSIFIED PLEURAL EFFUSIONS

Despite the standard evaluation, in 5–15% of pleural effusions an etiology is not found. In these cases, the following should be considered:

1. Blind needle biopsy (with an Abrams needle)
2. Thoracoscopic biopsy
3. Open pleural biopsy

PNEUMOTHORAX

Pneumothorax is defined as the presence of gas in the pleural space. It is important to note that **large subpleural blebs** and **skin folds** can mimic a pneumothorax on CXR.

Primary spontaneous pneumothorax occurs when there is no obvious underlying lung disease. The usual cause is rupture of apical subpleural blebs, which have no known etiology. They are most likely related to airway inflammation and smoking. This type of pneumothorax is more common in tall, thin individuals and recurs up to 50% of the time.

Secondary spontaneous pneumothorax is usually a complication of an underlying lung disease (Table 23-7).

Treatment is generally the same for primary and secondary pneumothoraces. The difference in recurrence rates between the different etiologies guides aggressiveness of the management. Table 23-8 shows the escalating options available for treatment of pneumothoraces.

TENSION PNEUMOTHORAX

Unlike a simple pneumothorax, with a tension pneumothorax there is a ball-valve effect whereby air enters the pleural space during inhalation but cannot exit it on exhalation. The intrapleural pressure exceeds alveolar pressure, resulting in lung collapse of the ipsilateral lung, mediastinal shift, and eventual respiratory failure from compression of the

TABLE 23-8. TREATMENT OPTIONS FOR PNEUMOTHORAX

Observation	Usually if pneumothorax is <15% of the hemithorax volume, it is safe to observe.
	Always give supplemental high-flow oxygen, which increases the rate of pleural air reabsorption (by increasing the nitrogen gradient between the air in the pneumothorax and the pleural capillaries).
Aspiration	Can be the initial treatment if pneumothorax is >15% of the hemithorax volume and the patient is clinically stable.
	Repeat chest x-ray after 4 hrs to confirm reexpansion.
Tube thoracostomy	Indicated if pneumothorax is >15% of the hemithorax volume, patient has failed aspiration, or there is recurrence.
	If the patient is clinically stable, interventional radiology can be consulted to put in a smaller chest tube.
Tube thoracostomy with pleurodesis	Pleurodesis by intrapleural injection of doxycycline or tetracycline is used for recurrent pneumothoraces. These injections are painful, and patients should be given analgesia for pain.
	Talc is also used, but complications can include ARDS, calcification, and pleural thickening.
VATS	Can be considered in patients who have failed other treatments (above), lack of lung reexpansion with tube thoracostomy, or persistent bronchopleural fistula.
	With this procedure, an endoscopic stapler is used to do a wedge resection of the bulla or fistula. This can be combined with chemical pleurodesis. With this procedure, there is usually <5% recurrence of pneumothorax.
Open thoracotomy	Has been replaced by VATS.
	Is still used if VATS has failed or is unavailable as an option. Usually is associated with longer hospitalization and more postop pain.

VATS, video-assisted thoracoscopy.

contralateral lung. **Clinical clues** include severe dyspnea, chest pain, hypotension, distended neck veins, pulsus paradoxus, no tactile fremitus on the affected side, hyperresonance on percussion of the affected side, and tracheal deviation away from the affected side representing shifting of the mediastinum. The most common etiologies are mechanical ventilation and CPR.

Never obtain a CXR to confirm the diagnosis of a tension pneumothorax. It is a medical emergency that is diagnosed clinically and needs immediate management to save the patient's life.

Immediate aspiration of the pleural space is life saving in this situation. A 20-cc syringe is obtained and the plunger removed. The syringe is filled with sterile saline and a 14- to 18-ga needle is attached to it. The needle (attached to the syringe) is inserted into the affected hemithorax in the second intercostal space in the midclavicular line after it has been cleaned. The presence of a tension pneumothorax is confirmed by a rush of bubbles through the saline. The procedure can also be performed without the syringe and saline if indicated—in this case, the tension pneumothorax is confirmed by an outward rush of air through the needle, which, again, is easily heard.

The patient is then evaluated clinically for resolution of the findings mentioned above while a chest tube is inserted in the affected hemithorax. A CXR may be obtained once the chest tube is inserted and the patient has been stabilized.

KEY POINTS TO REMEMBER

- Symptoms of pleural effusions include dyspnea and pain that may be induced by deep breathing, coughing, sneezing, or body movement. Referred pain in the abdomen is also possible due to the shared nerve supply to the abdominal wall.
- A thoracentesis should be performed after localizing the effusion to define it as transudate or exudate. This helps to evaluate the underlying etiology and facilitates the management of the effusion.
- Parapneumonic effusions and empyemas are specific types of exudative effusions related to infection in or adjacent to the pleural space and are most frequently due to extension of infection from an underlying pneumonia.
- Chylothorax, the presence of chyle within the pleural space, is nonirritating. It commonly presents with shortness of breath, a feeling of restricted breathing, and occasional chest "heaviness." Secondary infection is rare because chyle is bacteriostatic.
- A coagulation profile should always be checked when evaluating a patient with a possible or confirmed hemothorax.

REFERENCES AND SUGGESTED READINGS

Andrews CO, Gora ML. Pleural effusions: pathophysiology and management. *Ann Pharmacother* 1994;28(7–8):894–903.

Ashbaugh DG. Empyema thoracis: factors influencing morbidity and mortality. *Chest* 1991;99(5):1162–1165.

Bartter T, Santarelli R, Akers SM, Pratter MR. The evaluation of pleural effusion. *Chest* 1994;106(4):1209–1214.

Baumann MH, Strange C. The clinician's perspective on pneumothorax management. *Chest* 1997;112(3):822–828.

Blackmore CC, Black WC, Dallas RV, et al. Pleural fluid volume estimation: a chest radiograph prediction rule. *Acad Radiol* 1996;3(2):103–109.

Colice GL, Curtis A, Deslauriers J, et al. Medical and surgical treatment of parapneumonic effusions: an evidence-based guideline. *Chest* 2000;118(4):1158–1171.

Dev D, Basran GS. Pleural effusion: a clinical review. *Monaldi Arch Chest Dis* 1994; 49(1):25–35.

Doerr CH, Miller DL, Ryu JH. Chylothorax. *Semin Respir Crit Care Med* 2001;22(6):617–626.

Eggerstedt JM. Hemothorax. Available at: http://www.emedicine.com/med/topic2915.htm. Accessed October 5, 2005.

Ferrer JS, Munoz XG, Orriols RM, et al. Evolution of idiopathic pleural effusion: a prospective, long-term follow-up study. *Chest* 1996;109(6):1508–1513.

Fraser RS, Muller NL, Colman N, et al. Pneumothorax. In: Fraser RG, Paré AJ, eds. *Fraser and Paré's diagnosis of diseases of the chest*, 4th ed. Philadelphia: WB Saunders, 1999:2781–2794.

Good JT Jr, Taryle DA, Maulitz RM, et al. The diagnostic value of pleural fluid pH. *Chest* 1980;78(1):55–59.

Gustman P, Yerger L, Wanner A. Immediate cardiovascular effects of tension pneumothorax. *Am Rev Resp Dis* 1983;127:171–174.

Heffner JE, Brown LK, Barbieri CA. Diagnostic value of tests that discriminate between exudative and transudative pleural effusions. *Chest* 1997;111:970–980.

Jacoby RC, Battistella FD. Hemothorax. *Semin Respir Crit Care Med* 2001;22(6):617–626.

Jantz MA, Pierson DJ. Pneumothorax and barotrauma. *Clin Chest Med* 1994;15:75–91.

Jay SJ. Pleural effusions. 1. Preliminary evaluation—recognition of the transudate. *Postgrad Med* 1986;80(5):164–177.

Kennedy L, Sahn SA. Noninvasive evaluation of the patient with a pleural effusion. *Chest Surg Clin North Am* 1994;4(3):451–465.

Kinasewitz GT, Fishman AP, Winterbauer RH, Sahn SA. Pleural dynamics and effusions; nonneoplastic pleural effusions; malignant pleural effusions. In: Fishman AP, ed. *Pulmonary diseases and disorders*. New York: McGraw-Hill, 1988:2117–2170.

Kirby TJ, Ginsberg RJ. Management of pneumothorax and barotrauma. *Clin Chest Med* 1992;13:97–112.

Light RW. A new classification of parapneumonic effusions and empyema. *Chest* 1995;108(2):299–301.

Light RW. Clinical manifestations and useful tests. In: Light RW. *Pleural diseases*, 4th ed. Baltimore: Lippincott Williams & Wilkins, 2001:42–86.

Light RW, Broaddus VC. Pneumothorax, chylothorax, hemothorax, and fibrothorax. In: Murray RF, Nadel JA, eds. *Textbook of respiratory medicine*, 3rd ed. Philadelphia: Elsevier Science, 2000:2043–2055.

Light RW, Girard WM, Jenkinson SG. Parapneumonic effusions. *Am J Med* 1980;69(4):507–512.

Light RW, Jenkinson SG, Minh VD, George RB. Observations on pleural fluid pressures as fluid is withdrawn during thoracentesis. *Am Rev Respir Dis* 1980; 121(5):799–804.

Light RW, Macgregor MI, Luchsinger PC, et al. Pleural effusions: the diagnostic separation of transudates and exudates. *Ann Intern Med* 1972;77(4):507–513.

Ludwig J, Kienzle GD. Pneumothorax in a large autopsy population. A study of 77 cases. *Am J Clin Pathol* 1978;70(1):24–26.

Miller AC, Harvey JE. Guidelines for the management of spontaneous pneumothorax. Standards of Care Committee, British Thoracic Society. *BMJ* 1993;307(6896):114–116.

Ogata ES, Gregory GA, Kitterman JA. Pneumothorax in the respiratory distress syndrome: incidence and effect on vital signs, blood gases, and pH. *Pediatrics* 1976; 58:117–183.

Sahn SA. State of the art. The pleura. *Am Rev Respir Dis* 1988;138(1):184–234.

Sahn SA, Heffner JE. Spontaneous pneumothorax. *N Engl J Med* 2000;342(12):868–874.

Spillane RM, Shepard JO, Deluca SA. Radiographic aspects of pneumothorax. *Am Fam Physician* 1995;51:459–464.

Staton GW, Ingram RH. Disorders of the pleura, hila, and mediastinum. In: Dale DC, Federman DD, eds. ACP Medicine 2005. Available at http://online.statref.com/document.aspx?docid=2386&fxid=48&sessionid=5cee44mqdlwimnfi&scroll=1&index=0. Accessed May 3, 2005.

Urschel JD. Thoracoscopic treatment of spontaneous pneumothorax. A review. *J Cardiovasc Surg* 1993;34:535–537.

Woodring JH. Recognition of pleural effusion on supine radiographs: how much fluid is required? *AJR Am J Roentgenol* 1984;142(1):59–64.

Yeam I, Sassoon C. Hemothorax and chylothorax. *Curr Opin Pulm Med* 1997;3(4): 310–314.

Yim APC, Ho JK, Chung SS, Ng DCY. Video-assisted thoracoscopic surgery for primary spontaneous pneumothorax. *Aust N Z J Surg* 1994;64:667–670.

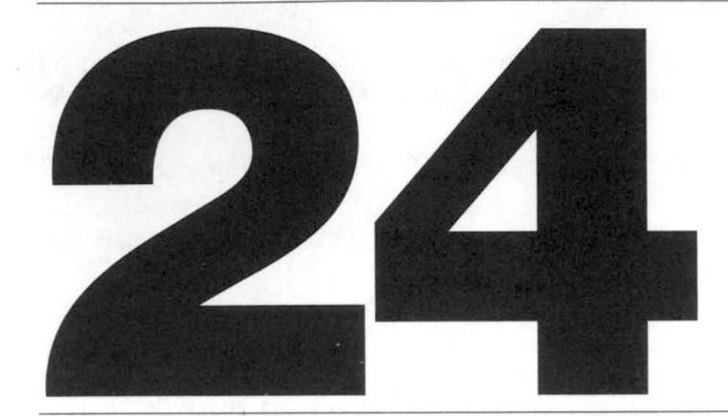

Radiographic Evaluation of Pleural Disease

Shan Cheng

INTRODUCTION

The pleural sacs encase each lung, forming a smooth surface over which the lungs expand and contract. The pleural membranes are composed of connective tissue covered with mesothelial cells, and they form two apposing layers. The parietal layer covers the thoracic wall, the diaphragm, and the mediastinum. The visceral layer adheres to the lung across its surfaces. The pleural cavity between these two layers is under negative pressure and typically contains a scant amount of fluid, estimated at <8 mL/cavity. Disease of the pleural sac may involve the pleural membranes or the potential space between them. There are a few general patterns of pleural disease generated on chest radiographs (CXRs), including effusion, thickening, plaque, calcification, mass, and pneumothorax. A particular radiograph may have one or more of these findings, and overlap exists between the various radiographic patterns. However, taken together with the clinical history, plain radiographs offer invaluable clues to making a specific diagnosis.

PLEURAL EFFUSIONS

Appearance

Fluid within the pleural space accumulates in dependent areas. On a standard upright posteroanterior (PA) and lateral chest film in a patient with a pleural effusion, the lower lung zones are **opacified** and the costophrenic angles appear **blunted.** Opacification is more prominent in the lateral portions of the lung fields owing to a meniscus effect. At least **175–200 cc of pleural fluid** is usually required to generate blunting on a standard upright film. The posterior angles are deeper and may appear blunted on upright lateral CXRs before blunting of the lateral angles on PA views. The lateral decubitus film provides an even more sensitive study for pleural effusions. It detects as few as 50–75 cc of fluid in the pleural space. In very large effusions, opacification of the hemithorax, mediastinal shift (away from the side of the effusion), and inversion of the diaphragm may occur.

Supine films are less sensitive for pleural effusions. Fluid within the pleural space layers posteriorly in the supine patient and may not be associated with the classic changes noted above. **Between 175 and 525 cc of fluid** is necessary to demonstrate costophrenic blunting on a supine film. An apical cap or density seen on supine views should raise suspicion for pooling of fluid within dependent areas.

Loculated effusions are important to identify on plain radiographs both for diagnostic and therapeutic reasons. Loculations occur when adhesions exist between the visceral and parietal pleural layers. The radiographic appearance is that of **limited free flow of fluid** within the pleural space on decubitus films. This appearance is often difficult to differentiate from masses involving the chest wall or pleura. Loculated effusions are more likely to exist in the setting of an exudative effusion and especially with an empyema or hemothorax. These effusions may ultimately require chest tube drainage for full treatment.

Etiology

In most cases, the history, physical exam, and lab evaluation of the pleural fluid serve as the primary tools guiding the differential diagnosis of a pleural effusion. The distinction between transudative and exudative effusions is not readily apparent on most plain radiographs. However, associated radiographic findings on plain films are helpful in elucidating the underlying diagnosis.

Pleural effusions associated with **cardiac enlargement** may be caused by heart failure, collagen vascular disease (lupus, rheumatoid arthritis), malignancy, or infection (myocarditis, pericarditis). Pleural effusions seen with **hilar enlargement** may indicate primary lung cancer, metastatic tumor, lymphoma, or granulomatous disease. Pleural effusions with lobar opacification may represent pneumonia, malignancy, or pulmonary embolus.

Congestive heart failure is the most common cause of pleural effusions. Associated radiographic findings include cardiomegaly, interstitial edema, and prominence of the pulmonary vasculature. Effusions in the setting of congestive heart failure are most commonly bilateral but, if unilateral, are most often right sided.

Pulmonary embolism may present with a pleural effusion and cardiac enlargement on CXR. The cardiac failure is right sided and less likely than in congestive heart failure to cause an effusion. Other radiographic features of pulmonary embolism include subsegmental atelectasis, lobar opacification, and hilar enlargement.

An **empyema** occurs when purulent fluid accumulates within the pleural space. Pneumonia is the most common cause of empyema. Empyema also may develop in the setting of a thoracic procedure, chest trauma, mediastinitis, intraabdominal infection, esophageal perforation, malignant effusion, or pharyngeal abscess. The typical radiographic appearance is that of a pleural effusion and accompanying lung consolidation. These findings are also seen in parapneumonic effusion and pulmonary abscess. In the later stages, an empyema often becomes loculated. U/S may demonstrate septations, but it cannot accurately identify the cause of an empyema in all cases.

The appearance of **malignant effusions** on plain films is variable. The spectrum includes isolated pleural effusions as well as complex, loculated effusions with associated masses. Most malignant pleural effusions are secondary to lung or breast carcinoma and may therefore have associated radiologic findings consistent with those malignancies. In general, patients with pleural metastases have large volume effusions, and approximately 10% demonstrate opacification of an entire hemithorax on CXR.

Hemothorax is most often the result of trauma, although it may occur with pulmonary embolism, metastatic disease, or aortic aneurysm. Pleural fluid identified on a chest film after acute trauma, especially in the setting of associating rib fractures, is most likely intrapleural blood. In some cases, this posttraumatic fluid may not be identified until delayed images are taken. CT is helpful in delineating the locations of active bleeding sites, which appear as high attenuation areas. Empyema and calcified fibrothorax are potential complications of hemothorax.

Chylous effusions have a nonspecific appearance on CXR. Most chylous effusions are unilateral, but they may be bilateral and of varying sizes. Chylous effusions are usually right sided, as the longest portion of the thoracic duct runs in the right hemithorax. The effusion is more likely to be left sided if associated with disease at the level of the aortic arch or above. CT scan is useful in delineating the source of a chylothorax. If a chylous effusion is associated with lymphangioleiomyomatosis, reticulonodular infiltrates and cystic changes may also be seen on the CXR.

Additional Imaging

Additional imaging with U/S or CT scan may be useful in the evaluation of a pleural effusion. **U/S** delineates the size and location of an effusion while serving as a useful guide for thoracentesis. U/S may also provide insight into the nature of an effusion; septate and echogenic effusions are more likely to be exudative. **CT imaging** of the chest, which can reveal pleural enhancement, nodules, or other disease, may aid in determining the source and composition of pleural effusions.

PLEURAL THICKENING

Pleural thickening represents a nonspecific response to injury of the pleura, and it has a broad differential diagnosis. The differential diagnosis includes exposure to asbestos and talc; infectious sources such as bacterial empyema, TB, and aspergillosis; various forms of malignancy including metastatic disease, mesothelioma, and primary lung tumors; collagen vascular diseases; sarcoidosis; and trauma. Organizing serous pleural effusions can also be a source of pleural thickening.

Appearance

Pleural thickening is diagnosed by the appearance of a thick, white line in the area between the lung fields and the body wall. It must be distinguished from a pleural effusion, which is usually evident by the shifting of fluid on lateral decubitus films. Loculated effusions are difficult to differentiate from pleural thickening, although the effusions may be identified both by serial imaging and by comparison with old films (recent appearance over a period of days to weeks favors effusion).

Patterns of Pleural Thickening

Pleural thickening may be localized or diffuse and may affect different areas of the pleural sac. Identifying a particular distribution and any associated features on plain radiograph may help to confirm a diagnosis.

Apical pleural thickening is a common finding on plain radiographs and is typically idiopathic. If apical thickening is associated with pulmonary cavities, TB or histoplasmosis should be suspected. Malignancy, such as a Pancoast tumor, may also present with apical pleural thickening. Pleural thickening owing to neoplasm is usually asymmetric, appears thicker than benign disease, and may be associated with bony changes and complaints of pain.

Basal pleural thickening is a nonspecific finding. In association with parenchymal scars and a history of pneumonia, the presence of basal thickening on radiograph suggests a previous organizing effusion or empyema. Noninfectious causes of pleural effusions, such as chronic rheumatologic disease, may also generate a fibrous pleural reaction.

A **diffuse pattern** of pleural thickening occurs in the setting of asbestos exposure, TB, prior thoracotomy, pleurodesis, and trauma. Diffuse thickening may also be due to other causes, and the pattern of diffuse nodular disease in particular should generate concern for a loculated effusion, metastatic pleural disease, or malignant mesothelioma.

PLEURAL PLAQUES

The term pleural plaque generally refers to a discrete, asymptomatic lesion involving the **parietal pleura.** Pleural plaques are flat or nodular when viewed on plain radiographs. **Calcification,** lack of spread around the lung, and noninvolvement of the apex suggest the diagnosis of pleural plaque.

Asbestos exposure is the most common benign source of pleural plaquing. These typically appear ≥ 20 yrs after asbestos exposure. Although these lesions are not premalignant, they remain important to identify because they are markers for patients at risk of future complications owing to previous asbestos exposure. The sensitivity of CXRs for plaques of all types ranges from 30% to 80% when compared with CT.

Appearance

Pleural plaques are best imaged on tangential views. They typically involve the parietal pleura with thickness ranging from 1 mm to 10 mm. Larger thickness should raise suspicion for malignancy. **Plaque thickness** is usually more pronounced overlying the ribs or other rigid structures. Plaques are not usually seen at the apex or costophrenic angles, although they have marked variability from patient to patient in number, size, and distribution. Noncalcified plaques are more difficult to visualize on plain films. Pleural plaques are unilateral in approximately 25% of cases with a predominance on the left. If the plaques are bilateral, they typically appear asymmetric. High-resolution CT further delineates pleural plaques and distinguishes them from extrapleural fat.

PLEURAL CALCIFICATION

Appearance

Pleural calcification appears as white lines at the lung periphery on tangential views, or as fields of white opacification overlying the lung when viewed *en face*. **Calcification** is often found in association with other abnormalities, such as pleural thickening or plaquing. The presence of calcification usually suggests a long-standing process.

Etiology

Although not seen with all cases of asbestos pleural plaquing, **asbestos exposure** is a common cause of pleural calcification. In pleural plaques followed up to 40 yrs after the initial exposure to asbestos, approximately 40% contain calcifications. Pleural calcification related to asbestos may be diffuse and bilateral, but it is commonly asymmetric with a nodular, linear, or sheetlike appearance. Talcosis (talc exposure) can result in a similar radiographic appearance.

Infection is a common source of pleural calcification. TB should be strongly suspected when pleural calcification is seen in older patients. These calcifications are typically apical and asymmetric and may be very extensive. TB also results in parenchymal changes with scarring, cavitation, and calcified granulomas. Some cases of nontuberculous empyema also result in pleural calcification, and a careful history should seek a previous episode of pneumonia or penetrating injury.

Hemothorax results in pleural calcification and should be suspected in cases of prior chest trauma. The calcification typically occurs in the visceral pleura and is unilateral in nature. Findings of prior rib fractures support this diagnosis.

PLEURAL MASSES

Pleural masses appear as focal or diffuse opacities on CXRs. The radiographic pattern of a pleural mass is similar to the appearance of pleural plaques and pleural thickening. However, the diagnosis of a pleural mass should be concerning for an underlying malignancy and should encourage further evaluation.

Appearance of a Solitary Pleural Mass

A solitary pleural mass may be very difficult to identify and localize. A **lateral view** is valuable in verifying the peripheral location of the mass when it is in an anterior or posterior position. Masses involving the medial pleural membranes are especially difficult to localize and differentiate from mediastinal masses. Peripheral pleural masses must be distinguished from processes involving the chest wall or subpleural lung. Typically, smooth borders represent pleural or chest wall disease, although some peripheral lung masses, such as metastatic tumor deposits, may also be smooth-walled. CT imaging is useful to reliably localize an abnormality seen on CXR.

Etiology of a Solitary Pleural Mass

Metastatic disease is the most common cause of pleural masses. In contrast, primary pleural tumors represent only 10% of cases. Lung and breast cancer are responsible for approximately 60% of solitary pleural masses owing to metastatic disease.

Mesothelioma occasionally presents as a solitary mass. The typical appearance is that of an irregular, nodular opacity in the periphery of the lung. When solitary, this represents an early stage of disease and the mass does not typically extend to the chest wall or lung parenchyma.

Localized fibrous tumor of the pleura is an uncommon neoplasm that appears as a well-circumscribed mass without invasion into the chest wall or lung. It is often rounded or oval with a homogenous appearance and may contain lobulations. Localized fibrous tumor of the pleura may be benign or malignant and accounts for approximately 10% of primary pleural tumors.

Lipoma and **liposarcoma** appear as soft tissue masses contiguous with the pleural surface. CT is useful for verifying fat attenuation within these lesions.

Nonmalignant etiologies of solitary masses include hematoma, organized empyema, mesothelial cyst, and loculated pleural effusion.

Appearance of Multiple Pleural Masses

Multiple pleural masses typically appear as separate, circumscribed opacities or as pleural thickening with inner surface lobulation. Multiple pleural masses may appear identical on CXR to loculated effusions. Lateral decubitus imaging is often not of value in differentiating these entities because pleural masses are often associated with free fluid.

Etiology of Multiple Pleural Masses

Metastatic disease is the most common cause of multiple pleural-based nodules. Pleural effusion is often the only major finding of malignant disease involving the pleura, but nodules and extensive pleural thickening occur in some cases. Adenocarcinoma, especially of the lung or breast, is prone to generate this pattern. Advanced lymphoma also metastasizes to the pleural surface, although the typical pattern is that of an effusion.

Malignant mesothelioma is the most common primary pleural neoplasm. The typical presenting appearance is that of a unilateral pleural effusion. Involvement of the pleura on CXR appears as irregular, nodular lesions at the lung periphery, which preferentially involve the parietal pleura. This diagnosis may be a difficult one to distinguish from metastatic disease based purely on CXRs. The presence of asbestos-related pleural plaques does not secure the diagnosis, and only 20% of those with malignant mesothelioma have findings of asbestos-related lung disease.

Malignant thymoma is a rare source of pleural masses, which usually appear to spread contiguously around the lung. Splenosis is the presence of ectopic splenic tissue, which can enter the left-sided pleural space, usually after splenic and diaphragmatic injury.

PNEUMOTHORAX

Pneumothorax is the presence of air within the pleural space. Air is introduced by a variety of mechanisms including trauma, ruptured lung cyst, barotrauma, diaphragmatic damage, and iatrogenic injury. Small pneumothoraces (usually <15% of the hemithorax) may be treated with observation, but larger pneumothoraces can result in life-threatening consequences even in the otherwise healthy patient. Serial imaging becomes crucial in monitoring progression of a pneumothorax as well as following resolution after intervention. See Pneumothorax section in Chap. 23, Pleural Diseases, for more information.

Appearance

An erect PA CXR taken on expiration is the ideal study if pneumothorax is suspected. When pneumothorax occurs, the lung recoils from the chest wall, generating the findings seen on CXR. Pneumothorax classically presents as radiolucency with absent lung markings and a free lung edge representing the visceral pleura. Typically, air migrates to apicolateral areas in the standing patient. At least **50 cc or more of air** is required to be visible on upright chest films.

In critically ill patients, a supine CXR is often the only available study. Unless the pneumothorax is large (approximately >500 cc air), detection of free air in the supine view is difficult. Significant free air may accumulate in the anterior chest or subpulmonic area without demonstrating a free lung edge. Air in the anterior chest sharply delineates the superior vena cava (**right-sided** pneumothorax) and the left subclavian artery (**left-sided** pneumothorax). Air in the subpulmonary spaces may present with a

deep sulcus sign. This sign results from the costophrenic angle that extends more inferiorly than expected on a supine film as air accumulates between the inferior surface of the lung and the superior surface of the diaphragm. A lateral decubitus film with the affected side placed superiorly may help to reveal a pneumothorax in a patient unable to have an upright film.

False Positives

Several findings seen on CXR may cause a **false reading** of pneumothorax. Skin folds, tubing, dressings, and IV bags may simulate a pleural edge. In these cases, careful study should reveal lung markings that extend beyond the artifact. Bowel gas may be present in the thorax as the result of a hernia or diaphragmatic rupture. In these cases, bowel folds and diaphragmatic irregularity rule out true pneumothorax. Giant emphysematous bullae at the lung periphery may also mimic pneumothoraces. An absent lung edge, the rounded shape of the lucency, and other bullae in the remaining lung fields support the diagnosis of a giant bulla.

TENSION PNEUMOTHORAX

When pressure in the pleural space is greater than atmospheric pressure, a tension pneumothorax develops. Radiographic signs include **inversion of the diaphragm, shifting of the mediastinum away from the pneumothorax,** and **flattening of the heart border** and **great vessels.** If the diagnosis of tension pneumothorax is suspected, therapeutic intervention should not be delayed for confirmation by CXR because this represents a **true medical emergency.** (See Chap. 23, Pleural Diseases, for more information on management of tension pneumothorax.)

KEY POINTS TO REMEMBER

- The general patterns of pleural disease generated on CXRs include effusion, thickening, plaque, calcification, mass, and pneumothorax.
- On a standard upright PA and lateral chest film in a patient with a pleural effusion, the lower lung zones are opacified and the costophrenic angles appear blunted.
- Loculated effusions are important to identify on plain radiographs for diagnostic and therapeutic reasons. Loculations occur when adhesions exist between the visceral and parietal pleural layers.
- Congestive heart failure is the most common cause of transudative pleural effusions.
- Lung diseases (e.g., pneumonia, cancer, TB) are the most common cause of exudative effusions.

REFERENCES AND SUGGESTED READINGS

Bonomo L, Feragalli B, Sacco R, et al. Malignant pleural disease. *Eur J Radiol* 2000;34(2):98–118.

Davies CL, Gleeson FV. Diagnostic radiology. In: Light RW, Lee YC, eds. *Textbook of pleural diseases*. London: Arnold, 2003.

Gallardo X, Castaner E, Mata JM, et al. Benign pleural diseases. *Eur J Radiol* 2000;34(2):87–97.

Henschke CI, Davis SD, Romano PM, Yankelevitz DF. Pleural effusions: pathogenesis, radiologic evaluation, and therapy. *J Thorac Imag* 1989;4(1):49–60.

Rankine JJ, Thomas AN, Fluechter D, et al. Diagnosis of pneumothorax in critically ill adults. *Postgrad Med J* 2000;76(897):399–404.

Reed J. *Chest radiology*. St Louis: Mosby, 1997.

25 Sleep-Disordered Breathing

Robin Kundra

INTRODUCTION

Sleep-disordered breathing (SDB) is a continuum of malfunctions in the control or mechanics of the respiratory system, resulting in varying degrees of arterial hypoxemia, sleep fragmentation, and cognitive dysfunction. The recognized pathologic sequelae of SDB continue to expand as this multidisciplinary field is explored.

PATHOPHYSIOLOGY OF SLEEP-DISORDERED BREATHING

SDB denotes recurrent cessations of breathing **(apnea)** or decrements in airway flow **(hypopnea),** resulting in varying degrees of hypoxemia and sleep fragmentation. Abnormalities in the activity or structure of the pharyngeal dilator muscles and/or surrounding soft tissues may cause **narrowing** and subsequent **obstruction of the airway.** In addition, abnormalities in the shape and size of the airway, as a consequence of obesity or craniofacial malformation, can contribute to airway obstruction. During sleep, the activity of these muscles is diminished. As respiratory efforts continue, negative intrathoracic pressure is generated, further collapsing the partially or completely obstructed airway. Less commonly, **central respiratory drive** is diminished as the etiology of SDB in the absence of upper airway pathology. In either setting, airflow to the lungs is compromised, and sleep is interrupted with or without the development of hypoxemia and transient hypercapnia. Frequent apnea/hypopnea causes physiologic changes that have pathologic sequelae (Table 25-1).

TYPES OF SLEEP-DISORDERED BREATHING

Obstructive Sleep Apnea

The **criteria** for diagnosing **obstructive sleep apnea (OSA)** are based on clinical experience and continued research. For reference, a standard is included (Table 25-2). Respiratory disturbance index (RDI) of >15 events/hr in the presence of both daytime and nighttime symptoms is also an accepted criterion for diagnosing OSA. However, current data indicate that an RDI >5 is abnormal. OSA may coexist with obesity hypoventilation syndrome, central sleep apnea, and **upper-airway resistance syndrome (UARS).**

Upper-Airway Resistance Syndrome

Increased upper-airway resistance leads to **crescendo snoring,** which ends abruptly in an arousal from sleep and the restoration of pharyngeal tone. In contrast to OSA, neither apnea nor significant oxygen desaturations occur. However, **sleep fragmentation** causes daytime somnolence, cognitive dysfunction, and depression, and may be associated with other comorbidities (e.g., ischemic heart disease and HTN). Diagnosis of this syndrome requires the placement of an esophageal bal-

TABLE 25-1. EFFECTS OF SLEEP-DISORDERED BREATHING

Cardiovascular
Right ventricular dysfunction
Left ventricular dysfunction
Pulmonary hypertension
Systemic hypertension
Tachyarrhythmias
Bradyarrhythmias
Ischemic heart disease
Cerebrovascular
Transient ischemic attacks
Stroke
Neuropsychiatric
Depression
Anxiety
Irritability
Hallucinations
Cognitive impairment (difficulty concentrating, poor work performance)
Excessive daytime sleepiness
Other
Impaired insulin resistance (independent of obesity)
Erythrocytosis
Impaired sexual function
Increased risk of traffic accidents
Sleep disturbances in the patient's bed partner
Increased overall mortality (when other factors are controlled for)

loon to document low intraesophageal pressure, which subsequently leads to upper-airway collapse.

Obesity Hypoventilation Syndrome

The development of hypoventilation may be associated with obesity, although obesity is not a sufficient cause. Obesity hypoventilation syndrome describes a **decrease in effective ventilation** during both sleep and wakefulness, reflecting defective central respiratory control. Decreased ventilatory responsiveness to both hypoxemia and hypercapnia is further complicated by diminished total lung capacity, increased work of breathing, and increased carbon dioxide production.

Chest Wall Deformities

Major thoracic surgery or the presence of **kyphoscoliosis** may result in decreased chest wall compliance and consequentially lower tidal volumes during both sleep and wakefulness. As a result, physiologic dead space ventilation is increased, which eventually causes hypercapnia and hypoxemia. In addition, pulmonary vascular resistance is increased. These defects are accentuated during sleep as hypoventilation decreases arterial oxygen saturation and increases end-tidal carbon dioxide.

TABLE 25-2. TERMINOLOGY

Breathing disturbances

Apnea: Cessation of airflow at the nose/mouth for at least 10 secs.

Hypopnea: Abnormal respiratory event lasting at least 10 secs with a decrement in airflow of at least 30% or a 4% fall in oxygen saturation or electroencephalographic arousal.

Respiratory disturbance index (RDI) = the number of apneas + hypopneas occurring in 1 hr. The RDI required to make the diagnosis of a sleep-related breathing disorder ranges from 5 to >15 depending on the clinical study consulted. RDI is typically determined by a full night of polysomnography.

Classes of apnea

Central: Both airflow and respiratory effort are absent.

Obstructive: Continued respiratory effort without airflow.

Mixed: Central apnea (i.e., no airflow or respiratory effort) that becomes obstructive (i.e., respiratory effort without airflow) in the same episode.

Adapted from Loredo JS. Sleep apnea, alveolar hypoventilation and obesity-hypoventilation. In: Bordow RA, Ries AL, Morris TS, eds. *Manual of clinical problems in pulmonary medicine*. Philadelphia: Lippincott Williams & Wilkins, 2001:406–412; and Schwab RJ, Goldberg AN, Pack AI. Sleep apnea syndromes. In: Fishman A, Elias JA, Fishman JA, et al., eds. *Fishman's pulmonary diseases and disorders*, 3rd ed. New York: McGraw-Hill, 1998:1617–1637.

Neuromuscular Disorders

Respiratory muscle weakness and decreased chest wall compliance in neuromuscular disease lead to rapid shallow breathing and subsequent increased dead space ventilation. This can progress to hypopnea despite an intact central respiratory drive. Patients may have significant respiratory dysfunction in the absence of reported symptoms. Indeed, **oxygen desaturations during sleep** may be early indications of respiratory dysfunction in the absence of dyspnea.

Central Sleep Apnea

Approximately 10% of SDB is due to central sleep apnea. Under normal conditions, central sleep apnea can occur at **high altitude,** as hyperventilation secondary to hypoxia drives $Paco_2$ to levels below the sleep-related apneic threshold.

Idiopathic Central Sleep Apnea

Idiopathic central sleep apnea occurs in response to a decrease in the signal that drives respiration—namely **Pco_2**. Patients with idiopathic central sleep apnea have both lower wakeful and nocturnal Pco_2, indicating chronic hyperventilation secondary to an increased central ventilatory drive. An increase in tidal volume associated with a transient arousal decreases the $Paco_2$ to below the sleeping apneic threshold, causing central apnea. Secondary pulmonary HTN with cor pulmonale and right-heart failure may be present.

Primary Alveolar Hypoventilation

Primary alveolar hypoventilation, also termed **Ondine's curse,** is a rare condition affecting mainly male patients. Hypercapnia and hypoxemia develop in the absence of underlying chest pathology.

Central Alveolar Hypoventilation

Central alveolar hypoventilation is similar to primary alveolar hypoventilation, except an **underlying neurologic disease** is responsible for the inability to integrate chemoreceptor signals (e.g., Shy-Drager syndrome, meningitis or encephalitis, multiple sclerosis, and primary brainstem lesions).

Cheyne-Stokes Respiration

Cheyne-Stokes respiration is characterized by **crescendo-decrescendo** alteration in tidal volume separated by periods of apnea or hypopnea. Cheyne-Stokes respiration may be present in the setting of cortical injury or in patients with congestive heart failure (prevalence 40% in patients with ejection fraction <40%). The mechanism for developing the periodic breathing associated with Cheyne-Stokes respiration is not defined but may stem from overcompensation of inputs from chemoreceptors.

SIGNIFICANCE OF SLEEP-DISORDERED BREATHING

Even SDB as seemingly innocuous as snoring has social and pathologic sequelae that generally go unrecognized. The prevalence of SDB has been reported to affect 2–29% of the population in various studies. SDB is a **risk factor** for HTN, myocardial infarction, nocturnal arrhythmia, and cor pulmonale. Animal studies have demonstrated a direct role of OSA in the development of HTN that is supported by clinical data. Furthermore, the fragmentation of sleep intrinsic to SDB causes significant cognitive decline and hypersomnolence, which can make patients a danger to themselves and others in the workplace and on the road. Studies have demonstrated the causal relationship between OSA and increased frequency of automobile accidents, and consequentially negligent patients driving with untreated OSA have been convicted of vehicular homicide. As such, diagnosis and successful treatment of SDB have tremendous merit.

DIAGNOSIS OF SLEEP-DISORDERED BREATHING

Screening for daytime somnolence is a sensitive although nonspecific method for identifying patients with OSA or SDB. The **Epworth Sleepiness Scale** is an example of a standard tool to determine a patients self-rated level of daytime somnolence. Input from a patient's spouse or bed partner may be invaluable, as patients may be unaware of sleep disturbances such as gasping, choking, or apnea. The presence of both daytime and nighttime symptoms is typical. A table of signs and symptoms suggesting OSA or SDB is included to facilitate clinical evaluation (Table 25-3). Risk factors for OSA include the conditions listed in Table 25-4. When a constellation of signs and symptoms suggests that SDB is present, rapid referral to a sleep specialist should be made, and the patient should not drive until the SDB is treated or excluded if the patient is somnolent.

The standard for diagnosis of SDB is **full-night attended polysomnography (PSG)** during which sleep architecture, arousals, airflow, respiratory efforts, and pulse oximetry are assessed. Further monitoring with an intraesophageal catheter may be required to confirm that arousals are due to upper airway obstruction (UARS). Although lab assessment has the advantage of allowing the attendant to optimize monitoring conditions, the patient's sleep quality may not be typical because of the unfamiliar environment. Further disadvantages of full-night attended PSG are cost and accessibility.

Devices for **in-home unattended PSG** are available, but the American Sleep Disorders Association only recommends their usage in (a) patients with severe symptoms indicative of OSA when initiation of treatment is urgent and standard PSG is not readily available, (b) follow-up studies of patients with established OSA, and (c) patients who are unable to be studied in the sleep lab, such as nonambulatory and medically unstable patients. Further study is needed to validate the sensitivity and specificity of home monitoring devices. Currently, full-night attended PSG remains the gold standard for the diagnosis of SDB and evaluation of therapeutic interventions.

TREATMENT OF OBSTRUCTIVE SLEEP APNEA AND SLEEP-DISORDERED BREATHING

The treatment modality is in part dictated by the **severity of symptoms** as perceived by the patient and the RDI (see Table 25-2) as measured by PSG. Therapy may be as

TABLE 25-3. SIGNS AND SYMPTOMS ASSOCIATED WITH SLEEP-DISORDERED BREATHING

History
Loud snoring
Witnessed episodes of apnea, choking, or gasping during sleep
Hypersomnolence
Unrefreshing sleep
Insomnia (reported in central sleep apnea)
Fatigue (particularly female patients who deny daytime sleepiness)
Nocturia
Nocturnal cardiac arrhythmias
Personality changes (depression, irritability)
Impaired intellectual performance
Morning headache
Sexual impotence
History of automobile or industrial accidents
Physical exam and lab findings
Normal
HTN
Cor pulmonale in advanced stages
Truncal obesity (may be present in 70% of patients)
Narrow, high-arching palate
Erythematous, enlarged uvula
Prominent tonsil pillars
Low-lying soft palate
Macroglossia
Retrognathia
Erythrocytosis (reflecting chronic hypoxemia)

basic as **modifying sleeping position** to the lateral decubitus or as complex as oral appliances, surgery, and/or positive pressure ventilation. **Behavioral changes** such as weight loss can improve symptoms in part by increasing the size of the airway. Other lifestyle modifications include avoidance of alcohol and sedatives, because these CNS depressants decrease pharyngeal-dilator muscle tone.

Positive pressure therapy acts as a pneumatic splint that stabilizes the collapsible upper airway. Three modes of noninvasive positive pressure therapy are currently used to treat OSA: continuous positive airway pressure (CPAP), bilevel positive airway pressure (BiPAP), and autotitrating CPAP.

CPAP by means of a nasal mask, nasal prongs, or facemask delivers a fixed pressure throughout the breathing cycle. CPAP has been documented to improve both obstructive and mixed sleep apneas. In addition, nocturnal desaturation, ventilatory-related arousals, nocturnal dysrhythmias, pulmonary HTN, and right heart failure associated with OSA are frequently improved. Both nasal CPAP and tracheostomy have been associated with improved survival compared with untreated patients. However, unlike in tracheostomy, significant complications of CPAP are rare and include case reports of pulmonary barotrauma and pneumocephalus. However, patient-reported side effects stemming from the mask–nose interface and pressurized air delivery may

TABLE 25-4. RISK FACTORS AND PATHOLOGIC CONDITIONS ASSOCIATED WITH OBSTRUCTIVE SLEEP APNEA

Gender[a] (male/female 2:1)	Lingual tonsillar hypertrophy
Obesity[a] >120% ideal body weight or elevated BMI	Macroglossia
	Acromegaly
Neck size[a] [circumference at cricothyroid membrane >17 in. (male) and >15 in. (female)]	Micrognathia
	Congenital
	Acquired
Use of CNS depressants/ethanol[a]	Retrognathia
Genetic diseases associated with craniofacial abnormalities	Lipoma of neck
	Head and neck burns
Treacher Collins syndrome	Larynx
Down syndrome (macroglossia)	Papillomatosis
Apert's syndrome	Edema of supraglottic structures
Achondroplasia	Vocal cord paralysis
Hunter syndrome	Neuromuscular
Hurler syndrome	Cerebral palsy
Nose	Myotonic dystrophy
Deviated septum	Muscular dystrophy
Polyposis	Myasthenia gravis
Septal hematoma	Multiple sclerosis
Septal dislocation	Hypothyroidism
Nasopharynx	Chiari malformation
Carcinoma	Syringomyelobulbia
Adenoidal hypertrophy	Shy-Drager syndrome
Lymphoma	Dysautonomia
Stenosis	Olivopontocerebellar degeneration
Mouth and oropharynx	Spinal cord injuries
Hypertrophic tonsils	Bulbar stroke
Lymphoma of tonsils	

[a]Major risk factor.

reduce compliance with CPAP therapy. These include skin abrasions, conjunctivitis, aerophagia, sinus discomfort, rhinorrhea, noise, and spouse intolerance, to name a few. Close follow-up and encouragement are needed to ensure the long-term compliance required for effective therapy.

To expedite care, CPAP therapy may be instituted during split-night attended PSG, meaning that the diagnosis of OSA is made during the first portion of the sleep study, and the remainder of study time is devoted to determining optimal CPAP conditions. Split-night PSG should only be used for patients with a clinical history consistent with OSA and an RDI >30 episodes/hr on the baseline portion of the study. Furthermore, 20–40% of patients may not achieve an adequate CPAP prescription during a partial-night sleep study. Thus, full-night PSG is still the standard of care.

The use of **BiPAP** therapy allows independent adjustment of inspiratory and expiratory pressures delivered by nasal or facemask. Because upper-airway instability represents the primary factor that promotes airway closure during expiration, but both airway instability and negative intraluminal pressure combine to promote airway closure during inspiration, the pressure requirement to maintain upper-airway patency is reduced during expiration compared with that during inspiration. Thus, BiPAP therapy can prevent apnea/hypopnea at lower mean mask pressures, which may increase patient comfort and compliance.

BiPAP therapy is currently more expensive than CPAP and is generally reserved for patients who fail CPAP therapy. The lower mean airway pressures of bilevel therapy may lessen symptoms of nasal congestion, rhinorrhea, chest discomfort, and difficulty exhaling against positive pressure. Compliance with BiPAP therapy appears to be equivalent to that of CPAP use.

The initiation of BiPAP therapy also requires titration of conditions in a sleep lab. Unlike in CPAP, variable inspiratory and expiratory pressures are delivered and may be adjusted independently in BiPAP. Inspiratory positive airway pressure is initiated in response to low-level patient-generated inspiratory airflow and cycles to the set expiratory positive airway pressure when inspiratory airflow declines below a threshold. If the upper airway closes during expiration, such as in the setting of insufficient expiratory positive airway pressure, inspiratory positive airway pressure cannot be triggered, and apnea occurs.

Autotitrating CPAP has recently been developed, and these systems are designed to respond dynamically to changes in upper airway resistance. Positive airway pressure is variably increased or decreased in response to changes in pressure, flow, or reflections of snoring sounds. Autotitrating CPAP has been studied almost exclusively in the monitored setting of a sleep lab to determine a fixed CPAP prescription.

Oral appliances of two basic types have been developed for treatment of OSA, but no specific custom device has been shown to be more effective than the others. The common effect of these dental devices is to produce changes in the shape and function of the upper airway during sleep, particularly by increasing the posterior airway space between the base of the tongue and the posterior pharyngeal wall, thereby opening the velopharynx. Devices that advance the tongue, such as the tongue-retaining device, are designed to hold the tongue forward via a suction bulb held in place by a flange between the lips and teeth. Another class of devices advances the mandible and is also typically custom made. Evaluation of the airway using radiographic studies and a comprehensive oral/dental exam may help determine if a patient's symptoms will be responsive to an oral appliance.

An American Sleep Disorders Association–commissioned review reported that 51% of study participants achieved normal breathing with a variety of oral appliance therapies when normal breathing was defined by an RDI of <10 episodes/hr. However, patients with initial RDIs >20 episodes/hr were less likely to improve with oral appliance therapy (39% vs 51% improved). Studies comparing mandibular advancement and CPAP have shown the efficacy of both therapies in mild to moderate disease but an increased efficacy of CPAP in more severe cases. After therapy is instituted, follow-up of symptoms in cases of mild severity can be adequate. However, moderate to severe disease should be reevaluated using PSG with the device in place. Patients may more readily accept oral appliance therapy, perhaps reflecting its simplicity of use.

Successful **surgical therapy** of UARS and OSA has the appeal of providing a permanent solution to the disorder without the need for further therapy. The first surgical therapy for OSA was tracheostomy. However, adverse psychological and cosmetic effects along with significant morbidity in comparison to nonsurgical therapy have made tracheostomy nearly a last resort. **Uvulopalatopharyngoplasty (UPPP)** involves the removal of soft tissue from the palate in conjunction with a tonsillectomy if indicated. Improvement of OSA after surgery depends in part on appropriate patient selection (e.g., retropalatal collapse may respond to this procedure, whereas hypopharynx obstruction is not corrected). Laser-assisted uvulopalatoplasty has been used to trim the soft tissues of the palate and uvula but is ineffective for OSA.

Obstruction of the hypopharynx (base of tongue) with or without an obstruction at the palate is more effectively treated by maxillofacial surgery, often in combination with soft tissue surgery such as UPPP. One surgical approach, mandibular osteotomy with genioglossus advancement, expands the airway by placing the pharyngeal muscles and base of tongue on tension by means of anterior repositioning of the genioglossus muscle through a mandibular osteotomy and advancement of the hyoid bone. Success rates of approximately 60% have been reported, with greater improvement in patients with initial RDIs <60 episodes/hr, without oxygen desaturations <70%, and with lower BMIs. The second surgical approach, bimaxillary advancement, is reserved for patients who do not respond to UPPP, mandibular osteotomy with genioglossus advancement, or other surgeries in conjunction with CPAP. The goal of the surgery is to enlarge the posterior airway space by moving the mandible and maxilla as far forward as possible. In general, PSG should be performed several months postop to document improvement.

KEY POINTS TO REMEMBER

- SDB denotes cessations of breathing (apnea) or decrements in airway flow (hypopnea), resulting in varying degrees of hypoxemia and sleep fragmentation.
- The standard for diagnosis of SDB is full-night attended PSG, during which sleep architecture, arousals, airflow, respiratory efforts, and pulse oximetry are assessed.
- CPAP by means of a nasal mask, nasal prongs, or facemask delivers a fixed pressure throughout the breathing cycle; it has been documented to improve both obstructive and mixed sleep apneas.
- The three modes of noninvasive positive pressure therapy that are currently used to treat OSA are CPAP, BiPAP, and autotitrating CPAP.
- Surgery and oral appliances have more limited roles in the management of OSA and are usually secondary lines of therapy.

REFERENCES AND SUGGESTED READINGS

Badr SM. Pathophysiology of upper airway obstruction during sleep. *Clin Chest Med* 1998;19:21–31.

Bahammam A, Kryger M. Decision making in obstructive sleep-disordered breathing. *Clin Chest Med* 1998;19:87–97.

D'Alessandro R, Magelli C, Gamberini G. Snoring every night as a risk factor for myocardial infarction: a case-control study. *BMJ* 1990;300:1557–1558.

Debacker WA, Verbraecken J, Willemen M, et al. Central apnea index decreases after prolonged treatment with acetazolamide. *Am J Respir Crit Care Med* 1995;151: 87.

Ellis PDM, Harries ML, Fowcs-Williams JE, Shneerson JM. The relief of snoring by nasal surgery. *Clin Otolaryngol* 1992;17:525–527.

Fairbanks DNF. Snoring: surgical vs. nonsurgical management. *Laryngoscope* 1983;94:1188–1192.

Fairbanks DNF, Fujita S, eds. *Snoring and obstructive sleep apnea,* 2nd ed. New York: Raven, 1994:1–16.

Feinsilver SH. Current and future methodology for monitoring sleep. *Clin Chest Med* 1998;19:213–218.

He J, Kryger MH, Zorick FJ, et al. Mortality and apnea index in obstructive sleep apnea: experience in 385 male patients. *Chest* 1988;94:9–14.

Javaheri S, Parker TJ, Wexler L, et al. Effect of theophylline on sleep disordered breathing in heart failure. *N Engl J Med* 1996;335:562.

Johns MW. A new method for measuring daytime sleepiness. *Sleep* 1991;14:540–545.

Koskenvuo M, Kaprio J, Telakivi T, et al. Snoring as a risk factor for ischemic heart disease and stroke in men. *BMJ* 1987;294:16–19.

Krachman S, Criner GJ. Hypoventilation syndromes. *Clin Chest Med* 1998;19:139–155.

Kump K, Whalen C, Tishler PV, et al. Assessment of the validity and utility of a sleep-symptom questionnaire. *Am J Respir Crit Care Med* 1994;150:735–741.

Lawrence KS. *The international classification of sleep disorders: diagnostic and coding manual*, 2nd ed. Rochester, MN: American Sleep Disorders Association, 1997.

Loredo JS. Sleep apnea, alveolar hypoventilation and obesity-hypoventilation. In: Bordow RA, Ries AL, Morris TS, eds. *Manual of clinical problems in pulmonary medicine*. Philadelphia: Lippincott Williams & Wilkins, 2001:406–412.

Meoli AL, Casey KR, Clark RW, et al. Hypopnea in sleep-disordered breathing in adults. *Sleep* 2001;24:469–472.

Mickelson SA. Laser-assisted uvulopalatoplasty for obstructive sleep apnea. *Laryngoscope* 1996;106:10–13.

Millman RP, Rosenberg CL, Kramer NR. Oral appliances in the treatment of snoring and sleep apnea. *Clin Chest Med* 1998;19:69–75.

Naughton MT, Bradley TD. Sleep apnea in congestive heart failure. *Clin Chest Med* 1998:19:99–113.

Peppard PE, Young T, Palta M, Skatrud J. Prospective study of the association between sleep-disordered breathing and hypertension. *N Engl J Med* 2000;342:1378–1384.

Phillips B, Anstead M, Gottlieb D. Monitoring sleep and breathing: methodology. *Clin Chest Med* 1998;19:203–211.

Piccirillo J, Duntley S, Schotland H. Obstructive sleep apnea. *JAMA* 2000;284:1492–1494.

Powell NB, Riley RW, Robinson A. Surgical management of obstructive sleep apnea syndrome. *Clin Chest Med* 1998;19:77–85.

Rapoport DM, Sorkin D, Garay SM, Goldring RM. Reversal of the "pickwickian syndrome" by long-term use of nocturnal nasal-airway pressure for obstructive sleep apnea. *N Engl J Med* 1982;807:931–933.

Redline S, Strohl K. Recognition and consequences of obstructive sleep apnea hypopnea syndrome. *Clin Chest Med* 1998;19:1–19.

Sanders MH. Nasal CPAP effects on patterns of sleep apnea. *Chest* 1984;68:830–844.

Schellenberg JB, Maislin G, Schwab RJ. Physical findings and the risk for obstructive sleep apnea. *Am J Respir Crit Care Med* 2000;162:740–748.

Schmidt-Nowara WW, Coultas D, Wiggins C, et al. Snoring in a Hispanic-American population. Risk factors and association with hypertension and other morbidity. *Arch Intern Med* 1990;150:597–601.

Schwab RJ. Upper airway imaging. *Clin Chest Med* 1998;19:33–53.

Schwab RJ, Goldberg AN, Pack AI. Sleep apnea syndromes. In: Fishman A, Elias JA, Fishman JA, et al., eds. Fishman's pulmonary diseases and disorders, 3rd ed. New York: McGraw-Hill, 1998:1617–1637.

Sher AE. The upper airway in obstructive sleep apnea syndrome: pathology and surgical management. In: Thorpy MJ, ed. *Handbook of sleep disorders*. New York: Marcel Dekker Inc, 1990:311–335.

Skatrud JB, Dempsy JA, Iber C, Berssenbrugge A. Correction of CO_2 retention during sleep in patients with chronic obstructive pulmonary disease. *Am Rev Respir Dis* 1981;124:260.

Strollo OJ, Sanders MH, Atwood CW. Positive pressure therapy. *Clin Chest Med* 1998;19:55–67.

Sutton FD, Zwillich CW, Creagh CE, et al. Progesterone for outpatient treatment of the pickwickian syndrome. *Ann Intern Med* 1975;63:476.

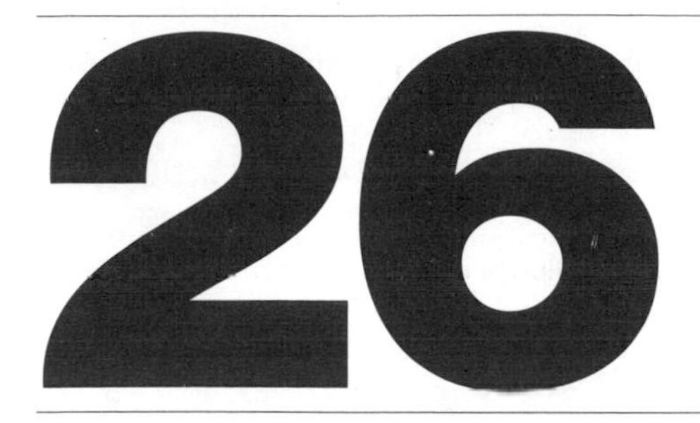

Interstitial Lung Diseases

Adrian Shifren and
Lee E. Morrow

INTRODUCTION

The term **interstitial lung disease (ILD)** refers to a wide spectrum of pulmonary disorders that are grouped together on the basis of similar clinical, radiologic, and physiologic findings. The term is a misnomer because it comprises a diverse range of pulmonary pathologies that may in fact involve the lung parenchyma, airways, blood vessels, and pleura. They have widely discrepant courses, responses to therapy, and prognoses. As a group, they are very important, accounting for approximately 15% of pulmonary practice. To evaluate and treat these diseases, a thoughtful and concise approach is needed, one that maximizes diagnostic efficiency while minimizing inconvenience to the patient. Owing to the broad range of diseases covered, this text concentrates on evaluation only, and treatment is not discussed specifically.

PATHOGENESIS

Very little is known about the pathogenesis of the ILDs. They are generally thought to result from an **initial insult** to the alveolar epithelium. The agent of injury may be delivered via the **airways** [occupational lung diseases, **hypersensitivity pneumonitis (HP)**] or the **circulation** (drug-induced lung disease, collagen vascular disease). The resulting repair response spills over to the lung interstitium, which is comprised of the alveolar basement membrane, loose connective tissue, macrophages, fibroblasts, and occasionally other cell types.

With limited injury and an intact repair response, the insult is reversed, and normal physiology is restored. However, if the injurious agent persists or the repair responses are abnormal, unrestrained injury and/or pathologic "repair" continue (analogous to keloid formation seen in skin wounds). The end result is an alteration in the alveolar–capillary interface and a distorted lung architecture, which results in the clinical, radiologic, and physiologic picture characteristic of the ILDs.

CLASSIFICATION

There is no universal system for classifying the ILDs. Classification systems based on clinical features, lung histology, disease chronicity, radiographic appearance, and pos-

---

Abbreviations used in this chapter: ACE, angiotensin-converting enzyme; Ag, antigen; ANA, antinuclear antibody; ANCA, antineutrophil cytoplasmic antibody; BAL, bronchoalveolar lavage; BUN, blood urea nitrogen; CBC, complete blood count; CF, cystic fibrosis; COP, cryptogenic organizing pneumonia; COPD, chronic obstructive pulmonary disease; CT, computed tomography; CXR, chest x-ray; DIP, desquamative interstitial pneumonia; DLCO, diffusing capacity of lung for CO; FOB, fiber-optic bronchoscopy; HP, hypersensitivity pneumonitis; HRCT, high-resolution CT; HTN, hypertension; ILD, interstitial lung disease; IPF, idiopathic pulmonary fibrosis; LAM, lymphangioleiomyomatosis; LCH, Langerhans' cell histiocytosis; NSAIDs, nonsteroidal antiinflammatory drugs; NSIP, nonspecific interstitial pneumonia; PAP, pulmonary alveolar proteinosis; PFT, pulmonary function test; RB-ILD, respiratory bronchiolitis–interstitial lung disease; RV, right ventricle; SLB, surgical lung biopsy; SLE, systemic lupus erythematosus; TBBx, transbronchial biopsy; VATS, video-assisted thoracoscopy; V/Q, ventilation/perfusion.

sible etiology all exist. None of these is all encompassing or intuitive. For the purposes of simplicity, a system based loosely on etiology and/or disease association is presented in Table 26-1. Note that it is far from extensive.

EVALUATION

The text on patient evaluation is laid out to follow a dedicated algorithm (Fig. 26-1) for the evaluation of ILD.

HISTORY

The history is an extremely important part of the patient evaluation. It can help direct the physical exam and reduce the need for extensive testing by considerably narrowing down the differential diagnosis.

The most common presenting symptom is **dyspnea.** The dyspnea is characteristically progressive, occurring initially with exertion but later needing less and less effort to produce symptoms. Eventually, the patient becomes dyspneic at rest. Typically, the dyspnea runs a chronic course over months to years. However, presentation may be much more acute over a course of days (acute eosinophilic pneumonia) to weeks (acute interstitial pneumonia). **Episodic dyspnea** may also occur with intermittent exposure to environments that precipitate symptoms [hypersensitivity pneumonitis (HP)]. It is therefore important to quantify the duration of the patient's dyspnea and the amount of effort necessary to elicit it (effort tolerance). The effort tolerance can be used as a clinical measure of disease progression over time.

Cough is a very frequent complaint. Dry cough is most common and may become particularly irritating (sarcoidosis, lymphangitic carcinomatosis). **Chest pain** is unusual but when it occurs can be pleuritic (SLE, rheumatoid arthritis) or atypical (sarcoidosis). **Wheezing** is very infrequent and occurs in diseases that involve the airways [HP, **respiratory bronchiolitis–interstitial lung disease (RB-ILD)**]. **Hemoptysis** is also infrequent and is more common with diseases that result in diffuse alveolar hemorrhage (Wegener's granulomatosis, microscopic polyangiitis, Goodpasture's syndrome). **Constitutional symptoms** occur with variable frequency and include fevers, chills, weight loss, fatigue, and night sweats. Significant weight loss should raise the possibility of cancer-related ILD.

Past and current medical histories are important. Multiple systemic diseases are associated with ILD (see Table 26-1). In most cases, the systemic disease concerned is present at the time of the diagnosis of the ILD. However, in certain cases the ILD predates the systemic disease by up to a number of years (collagen vascular diseases). In these cases, a high index of suspicion needs to be maintained.

A **social history** needs to be obtained, too. **Smoking** has an integral relationship with certain ILDs [Langerhans' cell histiocytosis (LCH), desquamative interstitial pneumonia (DIP), and RB-ILD are seen almost exclusively in smokers, whereas diffuse alveolar hemorrhage occurs in almost 100% of patients with Goodpasture's syndrome who smoke and only 20% of those who do not]. Some diseases, however, have the opposite relationship and are less common in smokers (sarcoidosis, chronic eosinophilic pneumonia, HP). **Recreational drug abuse** is being increasingly recognized as a cause of ILD (see Table 26-1).

Therapeutic drug history is invaluable. Although obtaining a current medication list is easy enough, it is very common for patients to forget drugs that they have taken in the past, even when having taken them for prolonged periods of time. Ask about these drugs carefully and note them. Whereas most cases of drug-induced lung disease have a close temporal relationship to use of the drug concerned, the latency period for drug-induced lung disease after drug discontinuation spans weeks to years **(cyclophosphamide, amiodarone).** Another oft-forgotten category of drugs is the **over-the-counter medications** that can also lead to ILD (lipoid pneumonia with mineral oil drops or laxatives).

A **detailed occupational history** is paramount in the evaluation of ILDs. An extremely large number of exposures may lead to ILD (see Table 26-1). The occupa-

TABLE 26-1. CLASSIFICATION OF INTERSTITIAL LUNG DISEASE

- Occupation/environmental exposure
  - Inorganic
    - Asbestosis
    - Coal miner's pneumoconiosis
    - Silicosis
    - Berylliosis
    - Hard metal pneumoconiosis (cobalt)
    - Talc pneumoconiosis
    - Siderosis (iron)
    - Stannosis (tin)
  - Organic[a]
    - Bird fancier's lung (pigeons, parakeets, other)
    - Farmer's lung (moldy hay)
    - Humidifier lung
    - Machine operator's lung
    - Bagassosis (sugar cane)
    - Cheese-worker's lung
    - Suberosis (cork)
- Collagen vascular disease
  - Scleroderma
  - Systemic lupus erythematosus
  - Rheumatoid arthritis (RA)
  - Polymyositis/dermatomyositis
  - Mixed connective tissue disease
  - Sjögren's syndrome (primary/secondary)
  - Ankylosing spondylitis
- Autoimmune disease
  - Inflammatory bowel disease
  - Cryoglobulinemia
  - Celiac disease
  - Chronic hepatitis C
  - Primary biliary cirrhosis
  - Autoimmune hemolytic anemia
- Drug related
  - Antibiotics
    - Cephalosporins
    - Nitrofurantoin
    - Sulfasalazine
  - Antiarrhythmic
    - Amiodarone
    - Beta-blockers
  - Antiinflammatory
    - NSAIDs
    - Gold
    - Penicillamine
  - Neuropsychiatric
    - Phenytoin
    - Carbamazepine
    - Fluoxetine
  - Chemotherapy
    - Bleomycin
    - Methotrexate
    - Azathioprine
    - Cyclophosphamide
    - Busulfan
    - Chlorambucil
    - Paclitaxel
  - Recreational
    - Heroin
    - Cocaine
    - Methadone
  - Others
    - Oxygen
    - Radiation therapy
    - Bacille Calmette-Guérin vaccination
- Idiopathic interstitial pneumonias
  - Usual interstitial pneumonia[b]
  - Nonspecific interstitial pneumonia
  - Desquamative interstitial pneumonia
  - Respiratory bronchiolitis–interstitial lung disease
  - Acute interstitial pneumonia[c]
  - Cryptogenic organizing pneumonia[d]
  - Lymphocytic interstitial pneumonia
- Cancer related
  - Amyloidosis (primary/secondary)
  - Lymphoma
  - Lymphangitic carcinomatosis
  - Micrometastases
  - Bone marrow transplant
  - Treatment (see drug related above)

(continued)

TABLE 26-1. (*continued*)

Inherited disease	Nonclassified
Cystic fibrosis	Sarcoidosis
Tuberous sclerosis	Lymphangioleiomyomatosis
Neurofibromatosis	Langerhans' cell histiocytosis (eosinophilic granuloma)
Hermansky-Pudlak syndrome	Alveolar proteinosis
Gaucher's disease	Eosinophilic pneumonia (acute and chronic)
Niemann-Pick disease	Lipoid pneumonia
Vasculitis	Alveolar microlithiasis
Wegener's granulomatosis	Diffuse pulmonary ossification
Microscopic polyangiitis	Hereditary hemorrhagic telangiectasia
Goodpasture's syndrome	
Churg-Strauss syndrome	
Giant cell arteritis	

[a]Also known as hypersensitivity pneumonitis.
[b]Also known as idiopathic pulmonary fibrosis.
[c]Also known as Hamman-Rich syndrome.
[d]Also known as bronchiolitis obliterans organizing pneumonia.
Adapted from British Thoracic Society and Standards of Care Committee. The diagnosis, assessment and treatment of diffuse parenchymal lung disease in adults. *Thorax* 1999;54[Suppl 1]:S1–S28; and Schwarz M, King TE, Raghu G. Approach to the evaluation and diagnosis of interstitial lung disease. In: Schwarz M, King T Jr., eds. *Interstitial lung disease*. Hamilton, Ontario: BC Decker, 1998.

tional history needs to span the patient's **entire life** because the time between exposure and disease onset may be many years. Also, **details of the exposure** including length of exposure, level of exposure, and the presence/absence of respiratory protection need to be recorded. Patients should also be questioned about the occupations of close contacts, because ILD may be related to exposure to agents with which the contacts work (e.g., asbestos-related lung disease in the wives of miners). Nonoccupational exposures also need to be recorded. These include pets (bird-fancier's lung), hobbies, and travel history (eosinophilic pneumonia from parasites).

Family histories should be taken, as certain ILDs have familial forms [**idiopathic pulmonary fibrosis (IPF),** sarcoidosis]. **Gender** is also important because some ILDs occur more frequently (collagen vascular disease in women, pneumoconiosis in men) or even almost exclusively **[lymphangioleiomyomatosis (LAM) in women]** in one gender. Noting the patient's age also helps, because some diseases preferentially affect younger patients (e.g., sarcoidosis, collagen vascular disease) and some older patients (e.g., IPF).

PHYSICAL EXAM

Because the pulmonary exam in patients with ILDs is nonspecific, the goal of the physical exam is to search for any evidence of systemic disease that may help narrow the differential diagnosis.

Examination of the **head and neck** should exclude enlarged lachrymal, parotid, and salivary glands (sarcoidosis, systemic sclerosis), conjunctivitis and episcleritis (collagen vascular diseases, sarcoidosis), dry mouth or eyes (primary or secondary Sjögren's syndrome), lymphadenopathy (sarcoidosis, lymphoma), and alopecia (SLE, sarcoidosis).

Respiratory exam is most commonly characterized by fine inspiratory crackles, which in IPF and other fibrotic ILDs are typically noted to be Velcro in nature. However, many diseases can present without crackles depending on where in the airways

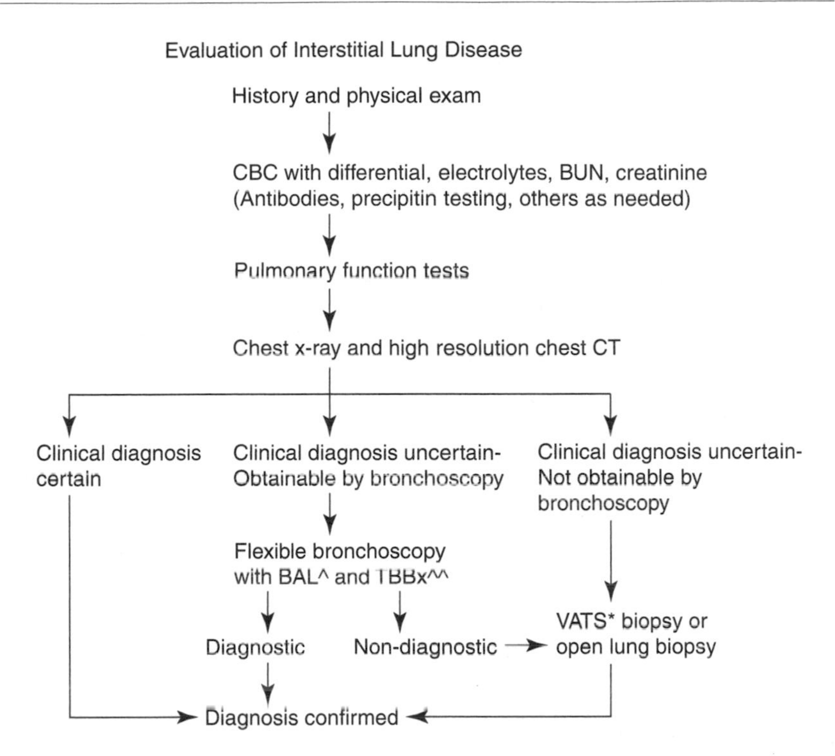

FIG. 26-1. Evaluation of interstitial lung disease. Adapted from American Thoracic Society/European Respiratory Society International Multidisciplinary Consensus Classification of the Idiopathic Interstitial Pneumonias. *Am J Respir Crit Care Med* 2002;165:277–304; and British Thoracic Society and Standards of Care Committee. The diagnosis, assessment and treatment of diffuse parenchymal lung disease in adults. *Thorax* 1999;54[Suppl 1]:S1–S28.

or parenchyma the disease manifests. Other respiratory findings include coarse crackles [cystic fibrosis (CF)], wheezing [sarcoidosis, HP, LCH, cryptogenic organizing pneumonia (COP)], and normal vesicular sounds (many diseases).

Cardiac exam should focus on eliciting evidence of pulmonary HTN, which may complicate almost any ILD. An elevated jugular venous pressure may be present due to elevated right-sided cardiac pressures. A displaced apex beat and right parasternal heave owing to RV enlargement, a palpable S_2, and loud pulmonic component of S_2 owing to closure of the pulmonic valve under higher pressures may also be present. Tricuspid and possibly pulmonic regurgitation secondary to RV enlargement and an altered RV geometry may be heard, as may a right-sided S_3 owing to RV volume overload. Pulsatile hepatomegaly and peripheral edema may also be present.

Multiple ILDs can be associated with **hepatomegaly** (sarcoidosis, collagen vascular diseases, cancers) or **splenomegaly** (sarcoidosis, lymphoma, lymphocytic interstitial pneumonia, collagen vascular diseases, amyloidosis), for which one should carefully examine when palpating the abdomen.

The **skin** is involved in numerous systemic diseases that may also affect the lungs. Involvement includes (but is certainly not limited to) malar rash (SLE), heliotrope rash (dermatomyositis), telangiectasias (hereditary hemorrhagic telangiectasia, scleroderma), palpable purpura (vasculitides), erythema nodosum (sarcoidosis, collagen vascular diseases), plaques (collagen vascular diseases, sarcoidosis), and café au lait spots and neurofibromas.

The **joints and muscles** may also be involved. Arthritis is a common manifestation of many systemic diseases (collagen vascular diseases, vasculitides, sarcoidosis), whereas muscle involvement is less so (collagen vascular diseases, sarcoidosis). Neurologic defects can also occur, including cerebral lesions (collagen vascular diseases, sarcoidosis) that may be as subtle as a personality change or as obvious as a dense hemiparesis; spinal cord lesions (collagen vascular diseases, vasculitides); peripheral nerve lesions (sarcoidosis, vasculitides, amyloidosis); and cranial nerve lesions (sarcoidosis, amyloidosis).

LAB TESTING

Lab testing in the ILDs needs to be directed by findings on the history and physical exam. Many of the tests used for diagnosing ILDs share a common feature—a positive test is helpful, but a negative test is not.

General testing should include a CBC with a full differential and an electrolyte panel with BUN and creatinine. Where indicated, the following tests may be helpful: urine sediment examination (collagen vascular diseases, vasculitides, all acutely presenting ILDs), ANA, double-stranded DNA, and rheumatoid factor (collagen vascular diseases, all acutely presenting ILDs), ANCA, and possibly anti–glomerular basement membrane antibodies (vasculitides and all cases of diffuse alveolar hemorrhage).

The routine use of serum **ACE levels** in sarcoidosis is not recommended because ACE levels have a poor sensitivity and specificity for diagnosis, do not correlate with chest x-ray (CXR) findings, and have no prognostic utility.

Serum precipitin testing in HP can be used to confirm the presence of precipitating serum antibodies against an Ag, which may be responsible for the lung disease. However, routine test panels for serum precipitins contain a limited number of Ags, which may not include the suspected agent. Thus, the suspected agent must be made known to the lab so that it can be included in the test panel. Also, a positive test is indicative only of exposure to the suspected agent and does not confirm that the agent is responsible for the disease. To complicate this test further, patients with positive serum precipitins may not have lung disease at all. Hence, the use of serum precipitins should be limited to cases in which the offending agent is very strongly suspected to maximize the utility of the results.

Pulmonary Function Tests

Spirometry and Lung Volumes

Pulmonary function tests (PFTs) in ILD are classically described as having a **restrictive pattern.** There are **two problems** with this description: (a) Owing to the large number of diseases classified as ILDs, many diseases show a mixed or even obstructive pattern on PFTs; and (b) the finding of restriction on PFTs is nonspecific and may be due to a number of causes, including chest wall disease, obesity, neuromuscular disease, previous lung surgery, and others.

The finding of **obstruction** in a patient with ILD can be helpful, however. The ILDs with an obstructive pattern on PFTs are limited and include sarcoid, LCH, LAM, eosinophilic pneumonia, HP, and CF. The presence of obstruction usually implies involvement by the disease of the bronchioles, with resulting obstruction of airflow during the expiratory phase of the respiratory cycle.

It is very important to know the smoking status of the patient, because **superimposed COPD** may result in a mixed or obstructive pattern on PFTs and needs to be recognized and taken into account when interpreting the PFT data.

Diffusion Capacity

The **DLCO** in patients with ILDs is almost invariably **reduced.** This reduction may be due to a number of factors depending on the etiology of the ILD, including abnormal V/Q, decreased surface area for gaseous diffusion, and in extreme cases, a thickened alveolar–capillary interface.

6-Min Walk Test

The 6-min walk test is an extremely useful tool in the evaluation of ILD. It provides a measurement of a patient's **exercise capacity,** it can be used to follow a patient's progression and/or response to therapy, it has prognostic value, and it allows for the assessment of a patient's oxygen needs both at rest and with exertion. A 6-min walk in which the patient does not drop his or her oxygen saturation into the hypoxemic range almost always rules out the diagnosis of IPF.

Radiologic Testing

Chest X-Ray

Despite the advent of CT, plain film CXR is still a very useful modality for the evaluation of ILD. It is common for findings on CXR to predate the clinical presentation, sometimes by 5–10 yrs. In some cases, asymptomatic patients have disease detected on CXR obtained for incidental reasons. Thus, looking at **old studies** is invaluable when seeing the patient for the first time and should be considered a routine part of the ILD workup. Old studies may also give an idea of how rapidly or slowly a disease is progressing.

Markings that indicate ILD include lines, nodules, opacities, and honeycombing. Honeycombing suggests an end-stage fibrotic process, which may be the result of progression of any number of diseases (IPF, HP, sarcoidosis, scleroderma). Ground-glass opacity, an increased attenuation of lung parenchyma that does not obscure pulmonary vessels, can be found in both interstitial (DIP, sarcoidosis) and alveolar diseases. Linear (or reticular) markings [sarcoid, pneumoconiosis, nonspecific interstitial pneumonia (NSIP)] are almost always associated with interstitial processes, as are nodular markings (pneumoconiosis, sarcoidosis, LCH, Wegener's granulomatosis).

That being said, CXR yields the **correct diagnosis** in only **approximately 50%** of all cases. Certain diseases, however, do have characteristic appearances on CXR that may allow a diagnosis. These include LCH, LAM, chronic eosinophilic pneumonia (radiographic negative of pulmonary edema), silicosis, asbestosis, and sarcoidosis (particularly stage I). Also, approximately 10% of patients with proven ILD have a normal CXR (most commonly those with DIP, sarcoidosis, and HP).

The **clinical severity** of ILDs can often be difficult to predict from radiographic findings. In IPF, for example, the clinical severity of disease is often greater than would be predicted by the CXR. The converse is often true in the case of nodular diseases such as sarcoidosis, LCH, and pneumoconiosis, in which patients can be asymptomatic despite extensive radiographic abnormalities.

As mentioned with PFTs, **most ILDs** produce lung **restriction** with a resulting **decrease in lung volume** that can be seen on CXR. Thus, the presence of **normal** or **even increased lung volume** on CXR is very **useful** (and corresponds to the presence of mixed or obstructive physiology on PFTs). Again, the number of diseases that can produce this is limited (sarcoid, LCH, LAM, eosinophilic pneumonia, HP, CF). It is important to be wary of the presence of superimposed obstructive lung disease (e.g., COPD) that may complicate the restrictive picture.

The presence of **pleural involvement** on a CXR may be helpful in narrowing down the differential diagnosis because involvement of the pleura in ILD is generally uncommon. Diseases that affect the pleura include collagen vascular diseases (pleural effusion, pleural thickening), asbestosis (pleural plaquing, pleural calcification), LAM and LCH (pneumothorax), and *Pneumocystis jiroveci* pneumonia (pneumothorax).

Finally, the **distribution of interstitial markings** on CXR can be useful because certain diseases have a predilection for affecting certain areas of the lung. In general, diseases can be grouped into those affecting predominantly the **upper lobes** and those affecting predominantly the lower. Diseases affecting the upper lobes include CF, ankylosing spondylitis, sarcoidosis, silicosis, eosinophilic granuloma (the former name for LCH), tuberculosis, *P. jiroveci* pneumonia, Crohn's disease–associated ILD, ulcerative colitis–associated ILD, and ILD secondary to bischloroethylnitrosourea chemotherapy. (These can be remembered with the mnemonic **CASSET-P-CUB.**) Diseases affecting the **lower lobes** include bronchiectasis, asbestosis, lymphangitic carcinomatosis, DIP/usual interstitial pneumonia/NSIP, aspiration, sarcoidosis (note, also included under upper lobe diseases), and scleroderma-associated ILD. (These can be remembered with the mnemonic **BALDASS.**)

Computed Tomography

High-resolution CT **(HRCT)** has revolutionized the evaluation of ILDs, as it offers much improved spatial resolution when compared with routine CXR. The diagnostic power of HRCT scanning has increased substantially in diffuse lung diseases as a result of the radiologic experience accumulated over the last 10 yrs. As such, HRCT may be diagnostic in certain diseases and is useful in evaluating patients in whom CXR is unrevealing (up to 10% of ILD cases).

One disease in which the role of HRCT has proved useful is **idiopathic pulmonary fibrosis (IPF),** a disease of unknown etiology characterized by **relentless pulmonary fibrosis and death.** Pathologically, it is characterized by the finding of usual interstitial pneumonia on biopsy. Much study has been dedicated to the diagnosis of IPF using HRCT in an effort to spare patients from high-risk biopsies. In one study in a group of patients with ILD (including a subgroup with biopsy-proven IPF as controls), HRCT findings considered typical of IPF had a sensitivity of 88%, a specificity of 93%, and an accuracy of 91%. The series was compiled when open-lung biopsy was routinely performed in patients with suspected IPF. Other studies have yielded similar results. However, the results at referral centers in these studies tend to overstate the accuracy of HRCT in suspected IPF when compared to routine clinical practice in which the level of expertise may not be as high. It is important to note that the accuracy of making an HRCT diagnosis of IPF is improved when the pretest probability of the disease is high—in other words, HRCT adds to a good history and physical exam but does not replace them.

There is good circumstantial evidence that HRCT diagnosis is similarly accurate in other ILDs. HRCT appearance is highly suggestive of, or sometimes pathognomic for, **LAM, LCH, pulmonary alveolar proteinosis (PAP), HP,** and **lymphangitic carcinomatosis.** In one study of patients with ILD in which the majority had a preexisting histologic diagnosis, the correct first choice HRCT diagnosis was made in 87% of cases, with a remarkable level of agreement between the radiologic observers.

One of the great advantages of HRCT is the **ability to detect coexisting pathology** at the time of scanning. One example is the coexistence of lung cancers and COPD in smoking patients with ILD. IPF is more common in patients who smoke. Therefore, both COPD and lung cancer can be predicted to occur with greater frequency in these patients. HRCT allows for the evaluation of IPF, emphysema, and lung masses on the same scan. Similarly, LCH occurs almost exclusively in smokers, as do RB-ILD and DIP. Therefore, all these patients are at higher risk of developing emphysema and lung cancers, which can be detected at the time of scanning. Once all coexisting conditions are diagnosed, management of these patients can be optimized.

Finally, although a number of clinicians believe that serial CT evaluation is a valuable adjunct for monitoring disease progression in selected ILD cases, the clinical usefulness of HRCT scanning in this capacity is overwhelmingly anecdotal and is in desperate need of formal evaluation. As such, no firm recommendations can be made at the present time.

Lung Biopsy

Bronchoalveolar Lavage

Bronchoalveolar lavage (BAL) is the process of instilling sterile saline into the distal lung units and then aspirating the fluid back for microscopic analysis. It is performed during

fiber-optic bronchoscopy (FOB) and is a relatively innocuous procedure. The fluid may contain, depending on the disease process, particles, cells, and/or pathogens, and can be used for culture, cytology, and histology. BAL is always performed at the time of FOB and can be **diagnostic** of certain diseases, including **PAP** (the aspirated fluid is milky white and periodic acid–Schiff–positive on microscopy), **eosinophilic pneumonia** (BAL cell differential contains >25% eosinophils), **diffuse alveolar hemorrhage** (increasingly bloody aliquots of aspirated fluid), **malignancy** (positive cytology), **infection** (positive bacterial, fungal, or viral cultures), **pneumoconiosis** (fluid contains asbestos bodies or silica), and **LCH** (BAL cell differential contains >3% Langerhans' cells).

In addition, BAL may be useful for excluding the above diagnoses, although the lack of diagnostic findings is not as significant as their presence. IPF is one condition in which the absence of any of the above findings is useful in aiding the diagnosis by excluding known causes of ILD. In addition, in cases in which the diagnosis of IPF is established, patients with predominantly lymphocytic BAL differentials are believed to have a more favorable prognosis than those with neutrophilic differentials. However, this theory may have been based on errors in the diagnosis of IPF rather than different responses to treatment.

Transbronchial Biopsy

There is some controversy about the ideal biopsy technique for patients with ILD. Essentially, two forms of biopsy exist: **transbronchial biopsy (TBBx)** performed via FOB, and **surgical lung biopsy (SLB)** performed via video-assisted thoracoscopy (VATS) or open thoracotomy. When deciding on a biopsy, a number of factors need to be taken into consideration. These factors include the condition of the patients, the skill of the surgeons or bronchoscopists, the facilities available at the medical center concerned (fewer small centers offer VATS), and the disease process itself.

The overall yield for TBBx in all forms of ILD is approximately 50% (the equivalent of a coin toss). However, certain diseases are very amenable to diagnosis by TBBx. These diseases are predominantly bronchocentric (centered around the bronchus) because the biopsy forceps must bite through the small peripheral bronchi to obtain lung tissue. Diseases with a **high diagnostic yield** on TBBx include sarcoidosis (>95% in experienced hands), berylliosis, HP (subacute form), PAP, lymphangitic carcinomatosis, and bronchoalveolar carcinoma.

Conversely, some diseases **cannot be diagnosed** using TBBx owing to the small size of transbronchial biopsies. Examples include **IPF** and **COP** (also known as **bronchiolitis obliterans organizing pneumonia**). IPF has a diffuse and heterogeneous pathology, and the findings of parenchymal fibrosis on a TBBx are nonspecific for IPF. COP is characterized by the plugging of bronchioles by ingrowths of myxoid connective tissue, which occurs diffusely throughout the lower zones of the lungs. However, localized injury can result in the formation of identical lesions as part of a reparative response. In these cases, TBBx can lead to the incorrect diagnosis.

In addition to errors resulting from biopsy size, TBBx can yield poor results from **sampling error** (biopsying unaffected areas of lung), and **crush artifact** (crushing of the tissue by the biopsy forceps). To overcome these errors and increase the TBBx yield, the lung is sampled multiple (10–20) times in different lobes. Yields are further increased by the use of HRCT to localize affected areas that are then targeted for biopsy.

Surgical Lung Biopsy

As mentioned, certain diseases are not amenable to BAL or TBBx for diagnosis. The **indications for SLB** therefore include these diseases (IPF, NSIP, vasculitis, COP) and cases in which BAL and TBBx have been attempted but have not yielded a diagnosis. As with all biopsies, decision on SLB should not be made without a full history, physical exam, and radiographic investigation. Again, the role of HRCT is stressed because HRCT may make or suggest a diagnosis, allow for TBBx (instead of a surgical procedure), and assist in planning SLB to increase the diagnostic yield.

VATS biopsy is less invasive than open-lung biopsy obtained through an open thoracotomy. It results in similar diagnostic yields with less morbidity and shorter hospital stays. It is, however, unavailable in some centers and depends on the skill of the surgeon performing the procedure. As with TBBx, **multiple HRCT-targeted samples** improve the yield. Where available, it is the procedure of choice for SLB.

CONCLUSION

ILD comprises a wide spectrum of diseases accounting for a considerable portion of everyday pulmonary practice. Evaluation and treatment of these diseases require a thoughtful approach to optimize the benefits for the patient. By following a dedicated diagnostic algorithm and building on information garnered at each step of the process, these ideals can be easily achieved.

KEY POINTS TO REMEMBER

- The most common presenting symptom of ILDs is dyspnea. The dyspnea is characteristically progressive, initially being exertional, but later needing less and less effort to produce symptoms.
- Occupational and therapeutic drug histories are very important. A careful examination of all work performed during the patient's lifetime is essential. Information on current medications as well as drugs taken in the past is necessary. Over-the-counter medications should always be included.
- Lab testing should be directed by clinical findings.
- Looking at old CXR studies is invaluable when seeing a patient for the first time and should be considered a routine part of the ILD workup.

REFERENCES AND SUGGESTED READINGS

American Thoracic Society. Idiopathic pulmonary fibrosis: diagnosis and treatment. International consensus statement. American Thoracic Society (ATS), and the European Respiratory Society (ERS). *Am J Respir Crit Care Med* 2000;161:646–664.

American Thoracic Society/European Respiratory Society International Multidisciplinary Consensus Classification of the Idiopathic Interstitial Pneumonias. *Am J Respir Crit Care Med* 2002;165:277–304.

Andersen SJ, Arvidsson U, Fransson L, et al. The relationship between the transfer factor obtained at rest, and arterial oxygen tension during exercise, in patients with miscellaneous pulmonary diseases. *J Intern Med* 1992;232:415–419.

Bettencourt PE , Del Bono EA, Spiegelman D, et al. Clinical utility of chest auscultation in common pulmonary diseases. *AJR Crit Care Med* 1994;150:1291–1297.

Bonelli FS, Hartman TE, Swensen SJ, et al. Accuracy of high resolution CT in diagnosing lung diseases. *AJR Am J Roentgenol* 1998;170:1507–1512.

British Thoracic Society and Standards of Care Committee. The diagnosis, assessment and treatment of diffuse parenchymal lung disease in adults. *Thorax* 1999;54[Suppl 1]:S1–S28.

du Bois RM. The genetic predisposition to interstitial lung disease: functional relevance. *Chest* 2002;121:14S–20S.

Fulmer JD, Roberts WD, Crystal RG. Diffuse fibrotic lung disease: a correlative study. *Chest* 1976;69:263–265.

Johnston IDA, Gomm SA, Kalra S, et al. The management of cryptogenic fibrosing alveolitis in three regions of the United Kingdom. *Eur Respir J* 1993;6:891–893.

Kim EA, Lee KS, Johkoh T, et al. Interstitial lung diseases associated with collagen vascular diseases: radiologic and histopathologic findings. *Radiographics* 2002;22:S151–165.

Lama VN, Flaherty KR, Toews GB, et al. Prognostic value of desaturation during a 6-minute walk test in idiopathic interstitial pneumonia. *Am J Respir Crit Care Med* 2003;168:1084–1090.

Michaelson JE, Aguayo SM, Roman J. Idiopathic pulmonary fibrosis: a practical approach for diagnosis and management. *Chest* 2000;118:788–794.

Monaghan H, Wells AU, Colby TV, et al. Prognostic implications of histologic patterns in multiple surgical lung biopsies from patients with idiopathic interstitial pneumonias. *Chest* 2004;125:522–526.

National Heart and Lung Institute. Task force on research in respiratory diseases. Report on problems, research approaches, needs. DHEW No: 73-432. Washington: The Lung Program, NHLI; 1972 October. Washington: 1973.

O'Donnell DE. Physiology of interstitial lung disease. In: Schwarz M, King T Jr, eds. *Interstitial lung disease*. Hamilton, Ontario: B. C. Decker, 1998:51–70.

Primack SL, Hartman TE, Hansell DM, et al. End-stage lung disease: CT findings in 61 patients. *Radiology* 1993;189:681–686.

Raghu G, Mageto YN, Lockhart D, et al. The accuracy of the clinical diagnosis of new-onset idiopathic pulmonary fibrosis and other interstitial lung disease: a prospective study. *Chest* 1999;116:1168–1174.

Schwarz MI, King TE, Raghu G. Approach to the evaluation and diagnosis of interstitial lung disease. In: Schwarz M, King T Jr, eds. *Interstitial lung disease*. Hamilton, Ontario: B.C. Decker, 1998.

Selman M. The spectrum of smoking-related interstitial lung disorders: the never-ending story of smoke and disease. *Chest* 2003;124:1185–1187.

Studdy PR. Sarcoidosis. In: Brewis RAL, Gibson GJ, Geddes DM, eds. *Respiratory medicine*. London: Bailliere Tindall, 1990:1133–1139.

Sundar KM, Gosselin MV, Chung HL, et al. Pulmonary Langerhans cell histiocytosis: emerging concepts in pathobiology, radiology, and clinical evolution of disease. *Chest* 2003;123:1673–1683.

Tozman ECS. Sarcoidosis: clinical manifestations, epidemiology, therapy, and pathophysiology. *Curr Opin Rheumatol* 1991;3:155–159.

Tung KT, Wells AU, Rubens MB, et al. The accuracy of the typical CT appearances of fibrosing alveolitis. *Thorax* 1993;48:334–338.

Watters LC, Schwarz MI, Cherniack RM, et al. Idiopathic pulmonary fibrosis: pretreatment bronchoalveolar lavage cellular constituents and their relationships with lung histopathology and clinical response to therapy. *Am Rev Respir Dis* 1987;135:696–704.

Wells A. Clinical usefulness of high resolution computed tomography in cryptogenic fibrosing alveolitis. *Thorax* 1998;53:1080–1087.

Xaubet A, Agusti C, Luburich P, et al. Pulmonary function tests and CT scan in the management of idiopathic pulmonary fibrosis. *Am J Respir Crit Care Med* 1998;158:431–436.

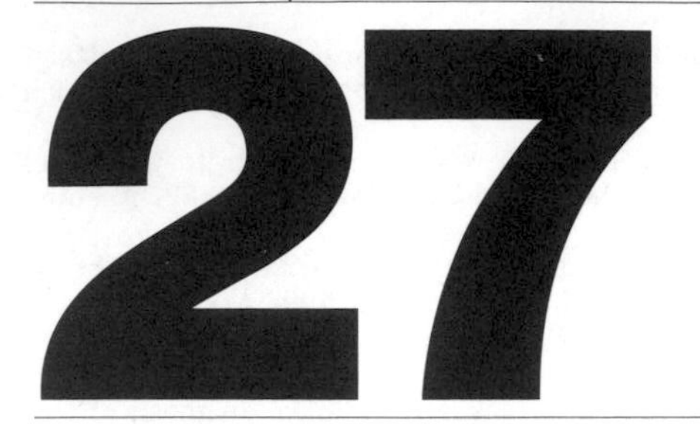

Occupational Lung Disease

Barbara A. Lutey and
Peter G. Tuteur

INTRODUCTION

The workplace contains a wide range of materials that can cause pulmonary disease in susceptible hosts or aggravate preexisting conditions. Virtually every occupation has some potential for hazardous exposure. Table 27-1 lists a number of potentially hazardous agents, many of which are relatively common. Safety must be evaluated continually as new technology is introduced into traditional workplaces or used to develop new industries.

At times, there is an obvious exposure/disease relationship because of temporal proximity. In contrast, clinically symptomatic disease may not develop until many years after the initial insult and may even progress in severity despite avoidance of the provocative agent. Signs and symptoms and radiographic findings are often nonspecific and fleeting. Thus, in many cases, there is no clear temporal relationship between an exposure and the development of symptoms that lead the patient to consult a physician. Consequently, a **high index of suspicion** and a **detailed occupational history** are essential when evaluating a patient for a possible workplace-related pulmonary disease.

With a diagnosis of workplace-related pulmonary disease, issues of impairment, disability, and workers' compensation frequently arise. It is important for the physician to realize that the terms *impairment* and *disability* have very specialized definitions in this context. Generally, **impairment** means objectively determined abnormality of functional assessment. **Disability** implies inability to perform specific tasks owing to impairment. The disability certification process often involves multiple agencies and procedures that vary from state to state. For assistance with definitions and criteria, the American Medical Association *Guides to the Evaluation of Permanent Impairment* is a valuable resource.

OCCUPATIONAL HISTORY

The object of an occupational history is to obtain a detailed, comprehensive, and chronologic list of the **nature** and **duration** of all remunerative work the patient has ever done, as well as unpaid chores, short-term/temporary employment, summer jobs, internships, volunteer work, and military service. To make this history meaningful, the physician must not only rely upon job titles such as "machinist" but also must make systematic inquiries about the **activities** and **environment** of each job to obtain all the information necessary to clearly define the nature of the patient's responsibilities, activities, and associated exposures. A detailed **description of the workplace** is also important (Table 27-2).

ASBESTOS-ASSOCIATED LUNG DISEASE

Asbestos is composed of hydrated silicates with varying combinations of other elements such as sodium, magnesium, and iron. It occurs in many forms and can be primarily classified according to the shape of its fibers. Amphibolites have straight fibers and serpentines have curly fibers. All asbestos-containing materials, whether made

TABLE 27-1. POTENTIALLY HAZARDOUS AGENTS IN THE WORKPLACE

Gases/vapors	Solvents
Carbon monoxide	Benzene
Formaldehyde	Carbon tetrachloride
Hydrogen sulfide	Methanol
Ethylene oxide	Chloroform
Nitrogen dioxide	Trichloroethylene
Ozone	Xylene
Phosgene	Metals
Smoke	Aluminum
Sulfur dioxide	Arsenic
Fumes from welding and metal processing	Cadmium
Acids/alkalis	Cobalt
Ammonia	Iron
Chlorine	Lead
Biological agents	Mercury
Bacteria	Chromium
Fungi	Other
Molds	Plastics
Rickettsia	Vinyl chloride
Spores	Acrylonitrile
Dusts—inorganic	Styrene
Asbestos	Dyes
Silica	Petrochemicals
Coal mine dust	Creosote
Fiberglass	Asphalt and tar
Nickel	Poisons
Talc	Insecticides
Beryllium	Herbicides
Dusts—organic	
Cotton dust	
Wood dust	

from amosite, crocidolite, tremolite, or chrysotile, can cause fibrosis, lung cancer, and diffuse malignant mesothelioma. Chrysotile and vermiculite are often contaminated with tremolite.

Exposure

Asbestos was widely used in construction and manufactured products until 1975. It remains in place in such materials as **floor tiles, insulated pipes, roofing materials,** and **brake linings.** Workers at risk for exposure include those in construction, maintenance, textile, or roofing industries, as well as those who are required to disturb or remove asbestos-containing materials currently in place and those who are involved in the manufacturing of asbestos-containing products. Workers, once exposed, remain

TABLE 27-2. SAMPLE OCCUPATIONAL HISTORY

1. List all jobs you have ever held and the dates of employment beginning with the very first one
2. For each job identify:
   (a) Chemicals/dusts or other substances you may have been exposed to
      (i) Nature of exposure risk: contact/inhalation/ingestion
   (b) Protective equipment
      (i) Was equipment available? Did you use it? Describe
      (ii) Was the equipment fit tested?
      (iii) Did you use the equipment as instructed? When? What percentage of the time? Under what circumstances did you not use it?
   (c) Air quality
      (i) What kind of active ventilation was provided? What was the maintenance schedule?
      (ii) Were there strong odors/taste in the air?
      (iii) Could you see haze/dust in the air?
      (iv) Did your eyes burn/water?
   (d) Facilities for washing/showering present?
   (e) Were uniforms provided? Did you wear them? Were they washed at home? By whom?
   (f) Did you eat, drink, or smoke in the workplace?
   (g) Procedures for accidental exposure?
   (h) Your symptoms
      (i) Date of onset
      (ii) Relationship to exposure: Worse at beginning/end of shift/week? Better after weekend off/vacation?
      (iii) Do you blow dust from your nose or cough it up?
   (i) Coworkers
      (i) Coworkers with similar symptoms? Other problems?
   (j) Were there animals/insects in the workplace?
   (k) Is the workplace damp? Is there standing water?
   (l) Any usual event such as spills, excessive exposure, or fires?
3. Other exposures
   (a) Smoking history
   (b) Alcohol history
   (c) Chemicals used at home in housekeeping/hobbies/lawn care/automobile maintenance
   (d) Animals at home: pets, livestock, birds

at risk for developing asbestos-related disease in the future because clinical and radiographic manifestation may be **delayed for decades.**

Asbestos fibers have several characteristics that contribute to their **toxicity:**

- Fibers can be suspended in air and inhaled
- Inhaled fibers penetrate deeply into the lungs and cellular structures
- Fibers are incompletely cleared

Both the lung parenchyma and the pleura can be damaged by asbestos fibers; the processes by which asbestos fibers cause asbestosis and pleural disease are complex and incompletely understood.

General Diagnostic Principles

It is important to note that the **exposure history** may be essential to making the diagnosis because the presentation, exam, pulmonary function tests (PFTs), and some radiologic findings are nonspecific. It is also important to eliminate other potentially treatable causes for the patient's symptoms.

Benign pleural disease (plaques) invariably is asymptomatic. With **asbestosis,** patients describe dry cough, persistent progressive dyspnea, and sometimes chest discomfort. Chest pain is commonly associated with diffuse malignant mesothelioma. Findings are nonspecific. Patients appear dyspneic, dry inspiratory crackles may be heard on auscultation, and clubbing may be seen in some cases.

CT is more sensitive than chest x-ray (CXR) for detecting subtle findings, as well as for characterizing pleural disease. **PFTs** show decreased lung volumes, especially total lung capacity (TLC), and **decreased forced vital capacity** with **decreased DLCO** is most common. Impairment of gas exchange is most sensitively determined by **ABG** analysis conducted at rest and during exercise. **Special studies** such as bronchoalveolar lavage, tissue biopsy, and sputum evaluations may be necessary to find asbestos fibers if exposure cannot be documented.

The patient should have a **history of exposure** to asbestos fibers and a suitable **latency period** before developing symptoms or radiographic findings. (Pleural effusions >1 yr; pleural plaques >10 yrs; asbestosis, lung cancer, diffuse malignant mesothelioma >20 yrs.)

Asbestosis

The presence of asbestos fibers results in a persistent inflammatory process culminating in diffuse interstitial fibrosis, with distortion of the lung parenchyma. **Diffuse interstitial fibrosis** usually develops 20 yrs after first and heavy exposure. CXR shows irregular linear opacities. On CT scan, multiple abnormalities may be seen, such as curving subpleural lines, parenchymal banding, short peripheral lines, and honeycombing in advanced disease. To make the diagnosis, **both bilateral plaques** and **intraparenchymal processes** must be present.

Pleural Disease

Pleural disease may result from translocation of fibers into the pleural space to stimulate an inflammatory and fibrotic response.

Pleural Effusion

Pleural effusion is the earliest clinical phenomenon after initiation of asbestos exposure, but it is relatively infrequent. Typically, it occurs **approximately 10 yrs** after first exposure, but it may occur as early as 1 yr after exposure commencement. CXR usually shows a unilateral effusion. Thoracentesis yields an exudative bloody effusion. Fibers are not often found in pleural fluid.

Pleural Thickening

Fibrosis of the visceral pleura with adhesions to the parietal pleura occurs. These obliterate the pleural space and extend into lung parenchyma, making surgical resection difficult to impossible. On CXR, plaques are widely distributed and do not spare the apices or costophrenic angles, which may be blunted.

Rounded Atelectasis

Pleural thickening may trap a section of lung, causing atelectasis. CXR shows a thickened pleura surrounding a section of atelectatic lung with a "comet tail" extending in the direction of the hilum. There may be associated volume loss of affected lung.

Diffuse Malignant Mesothelioma

Diffuse malignant mesothelioma (DMM) is a malignant process of the parietal surface of thoracic and/or abdominal cavities with invasion of heart and lung by direct extension. Exposure may have been apparently minimal, indirect, and not occupational but almost always **>20 yrs earlier.** Almost all DMM in the United States is due to asbestos exposure. Although dose related, the relationship is rather flat. Persons may present rather subtle exposures (aiding a parent to clean work clothes as a child or being present during ship refitting). Radiographic findings include lobulated growth over the parietal pleural surface. The diagnosis usually requires tumor biopsy. There is no significantly effective treatment. The prognosis for this malignancy is very grim, but new surgical and chemotherapeutic regimens may show some therapeutic promise.

Management

No specific treatment is available for asbestosis or asbestos-related pleural diseases. The most important intervention is to **avoid further exposure.** This intervention may involve a change in job responsibilities, and patients should be made aware of this fact.

Other **supportive care** measures depend on individual patient requirements. These include supplemental oxygen if needed, pulmonary rehabilitation, smoking cessation, bronchodilators, and influenza/pneumonia vaccinations.

Because the disease can progress even after exposure has ended, the patient should be **followed with CXR and PFTs.**

Association with Lung Cancer

Asbestos has been classified by the International Agency for Research on Cancer as Group I, Carcinogenic to Humans. Exposure to asbestos, both in serpentine or amphibole forms, clearly is associated with increased risk of lung cancer.

Tobacco smoking increases the risk of lung cancer in persons who have even short-term exposure to asbestos. This risk is at least additive and possibly synergistic. Therefore, it is imperative that asbestos-exposed persons stop smoking immediately and permanently.

Because asbestos exposure has been associated with a substantial increased risk of developing lung cancer, many believe that patients should have regular CXRs with CT correlation and tissue diagnosis as needed. The outcome of such active surveillance in changing outcome is unclear.

COAL DUST–ASSOCIATED PULMONARY DISEASE

Coal is ranked according to its carbon content, and anthracite coal contains the highest percentage. The rank of coal mined locally depends on the geologic setting in which it was formed—for example, anthracite coal is chiefly found in northeast Pennsylvania.

Exposure

The amount and nature of exposure during coal mining depend on the rank of coal and the individual worker's responsibilities. Coal dust is primarily carbon but may be contaminated by other potentially harmful substances such as silica, kaolin, mica, and metal dusts. The **greatest exposure occurs underground,** working at the coal face; however, workers above ground, who operate drills or who handle coal, also have sufficient exposure to produce disease in a susceptible host.

Spectrum of Disease

The spectrum of disease is wide. Not all coal workers develop **coal workers' pneumoconiosis.** Coal workers may develop measurable **decreases in pulmonary function** (TLC, forced vital capacity, impairment of gas exchange) owing to coal mine dust inhalation without noticeable changes on CXR. Rarely, an isolated obstructive abnormality may develop. However, pathologic findings of disease may be found on biopsy or at autopsy even in those with normal CXR and/or no pulmonary functional impairment. Similarly, radiographic abnormalities may precede impairment. Miners also develop lung disease unrelated to coal dust—most notably **cigarette-induced COPD.**

Coal Workers' Pneumoconiosis

The hallmark symptom of coal workers' pneumoconiosis is **shortness of breath.** Crackles are heard on exam. On CXR, small nodular opacities found in the upper lobes in early stages become more numerous and confluent as disease progresses. **PFTs** most frequently show a **restrictive ventilatory defect,** with impaired gas exchange seen first during exercise. Obstructive ventilatory defects are rare and difficult to distinguish from tobacco-related disease in a smoking miner.

Progressive Massive Fibrosis

Patients complain of shortness of breath and cough. CXR shows coalescence of nodules >20 mm. PFTs can show both obstructive and restrictive ventilatory defects.

Chronic Obstructive Pulmonary Disease Phenotype

Rarely, never-smoking miners present with cough, expectoration, and/or wheezing with manifestations of airflow obstruction on physical exam and function studies associated with a CXR free of interstitial changes. If no other cause for this clinical presentation is present (bronchiectasis, asthma, cystic fibrosis, alpha-1 antitrypsin deficiency), it should be attributed to coal dust.

Industrial Bronchitis

Industrial bronchitis is associated with a clinical picture of coughing during times of exposure that resolves with cessation of coal mine dust exposure. Regularly, no associated impairment is seen.

Management

No specific treatment is available for simple coal workers' pneumoconiosis or progressive massive fibrosis. The most important intervention is to **avoid further exposure.** This intervention may involve a change in job responsibilities, and patients should be made aware of this fact.

Other **supportive care measures** depend on individual patient requirements. These may include supplemental oxygen if needed, pulmonary rehabilitation, smoking cessation, bronchodilators, and influenza/pneumonia vaccinations.

Because the disease can progress even after exposure has ended, the patient should be **followed with CXRs and PFTs,** especially during the first years after retirement.

Association with Lung Cancer

There is no association between coal mining and lung cancer. Miners may be exposed to multiple carcinogens, including radon gas and cigarette smoke. Those miners are at increased risk for lung cancer.

SILICA-ASSOCIATED LUNG DISEASE

Silica (SiO_2), in its amorphous form, is noncrystalline and relatively nontoxic if inhaled. In its crystalline form, most commonly occurring as quartz, it can clearly cause pulmonary toxicity if inhaled.

Exposure

Silica is found in soil and rock. In the workplace, it is a hazard for tunnelers, sandblasters, and foundry workers. Silica is also found in materials as diverse as plaster and toothpaste, and a detailed occupational history may be needed to identify sources of exposure. It is important to note that even workers who believe they worked under safe conditions may still have a significant potential risk of developing disease regardless of the chronology of exposure.

Acute Silicosis

Acute silicosis may develop within weeks to months after exposure to very high concentrations of silica in small particles of airborne dust, such as may occur when sandblasting, rock drilling, tunneling, or quartz milling. Patients develop dyspnea, hypoxemia, and possible respiratory failure. Radiographic findings including abundant **ground-glass infiltrates** are seen on CXR and CT. On PFTs, restrictive and or obstructive ventilatory defects may develop, usually with **impaired gas exchange.** A subset of acute silicosis patients develop silicoproteinosis, which mimics pulmonary alveolar proteinosis radiographically and pathologically.

Accelerated Silicosis

Accelerated silicosis develops **2–10 yrs after exposure.** Patients complain of progressive exertional dyspnea and cough. CXR and CT show multiple small nodules in the upper lungs and midzone of the lungs. Patients may have restrictive and/or obstructive ventilatory defects.

Chronic Silicosis

Develops after ≥**10 yrs of exposure** to relatively low concentrations of silica. Patients report progressive exertional dyspnea and cough. CXR and CT show **multiple small nodules** in the upper lungs and midzone of the lungs, becoming larger and more diffusely distributed with disease progression. **Progressive massive fibrosis** results from enlargement and confluence of nodules. Progression may occur after cessation of exposure. Patients may have restrictive and/or obstructive ventilatory defects.

Management

No specific treatment is available for silicosis. The most important intervention is to **avoid further exposure.** This intervention may involve a change in job responsibilities, and patients should be made aware of this fact. Other **supportive care measures** depend on individual patient requirements. These measures could include supplemental oxygen if needed, pulmonary rehabilitation, smoking cessation, bronchodilators, and influenza/pneumonia vaccinations. Because silicosis can progress even after exposure has ended, disease progression should be **monitored with CXRs and PFTs.**

Patients with silicosis are prone to infection with both TB and nontuberculous mycobacteria. Patients who are **PPD positive** should be given **lifelong TB prophylaxis.**

Association with Lung Cancer

The International Agency for Research on Cancer has classified silica as Group I, Carcinogenic to Humans. This classification has been a somewhat controversial decision because not all studies have shown a clear relationship between exposure to silica and the development of cancer. Further complicating the matter in many studies is smoking history and other confounding factors that must also be taken into account. In other studies, data were used directly from notoriously unreliable death certificates. It should be stated, however, that silica exposure, especially with silicosis, may cause a slight increase in risk for malignancy. An official statement of the American Thoracic Society published in 1997 noted that, “the balance of evidence indicates that silicotic patients have increased risk for lung cancer. It is less clear whether silica exposure in the absence of silicosis carries increased risk for lung cancer.”

Until the relationship among silica exposure, silicosis, and the development of lung cancer can be clarified, it seems prudent to recommend that **abnormalities seen on CXR** should be **followed closely,** and any findings **concerning for malignancy** should be evaluated with **chest CT** and **tissue diagnosis** as appropriate.

WORKPLACE-ASSOCIATED BRONCHIAL REACTIVITY

A clinical phenotype based on bronchial reactivity can result when some workers interact with some workplace environments. It is the genetic makeup of the worker and the variability of apparently similar workplaces that produce great diversification of the clinical picture and the response to therapy. Thus, the etiology and pathophysiology of this syndrome are not unique. An oft-used generic term applied to this condition is **occupational asthma.**

Bernstein and colleagues developed a set of applicable consensus definitions. Occupational asthma is characterized by **variable airflow limitation and/or airway hyperresponsiveness attributable uniquely to the workplace environment.** This same syndrome can occur outside the workplace, too. These criteria can be met when the etiology is either immunologic or nonimmunologic. Typically, workplace-associated bronchial reactivity is a result of exposure to high-molecular-weight substances, resulting in an immunologic mechanism that is either IgE mediated or non–IgE mediated.

In contrast, exposure to low-molecular-weight chemicals (inorganic acids, alkalis, and other irritants) may induce this syndrome either immediately after a single massive exposure or not so suddenly after multiple, less intense ones. For this reaction, there is no apparent immunologic mechanism.

Exposure

When evaluating a person who develops symptoms of bronchial reactivity, whether in response to antigenic stimuli or to irritants, evaluation of a broad differential diagnosis may lead to concern about a workplace etiology.

Immunologic

A careful history may suggest a relationship to cotton or other textile dust exposures; animal, insect, or shellfish allergies; employment in the lumber industry with particular exposures to western red cedar dust; work in the baking industry with exposure to wheat or rye dusts; or other food industry exposures to garlic dust, cinnamon, and mushrooms. Interaction with isocyanates (toluene diisocyanate, methylene diphenyl isocyanate, hexamethylene diisocyanate) may produce an asthmalike clinical picture, but an IgE-based immunologic mechanism for this has not been established robustly.

Nonimmunologic

Exposure to a variety of low-molecular-weight irritant and nonantigenic chemicals produces the phenotype. Chronic formaldehyde exposure occurring both in the industrial setting as well as from the use of products, particularly particleboard often used in mobile home construction, has resulted in clinical bronchial reactivity. Furthermore, exposures to significant and clinically meaningful concentrations of low-molecular-weight irritant chemicals such as hydrochloric acid, sulfuric acid, sodium hydroxide, and chlorine have resulted in syndromes in which bronchial hyperreactivity either develops immediately or is delayed following repeated and less intense exposures.

Susceptibility

In almost all settings, there is substantial individual variation of the dose–response curve and the type of symptoms that result. Often, several workers may experience what appears to be a similar exposure in an industrial spill, but not all are adversely affected.

One must also be aware that it appears that persons with either retrospectively identified or extremely quiescent atopy may have a greater susceptibility to develop latency-associated occupational asthma of any sort (immunologic and nonimmunologic), especially with repeated exposures. The clinician may be required to opine if such a worker has occupational asthma or a preexisting asthma phenotype aggravated by the workplace.

Presentation

The patient complains of breathlessness, cough, expectoration, wheezing, and chest tightness. Over time, persistent bronchial reactivity is manifested by different symptom patterns triggered by irritants differing from the initial etiologic agent, but the specific trigger(s) varies among the affected. In general, irritant triggers include extremes of temperature and humidity, ambient tobacco smoke, perfumes, colognes, hairspray, cooking fumes, products of combustion, and cleaning materials. The physical exam may be normal; intermittently, wheezing may be heard on auscultation.

CXRs are typically normal. Pulmonary function studies often are normal at baseline but may demonstrate airflow obstruction with or without improvement after bronchodilators are administered. A positive methacholine challenge test is considered diagnostic for the presence of bronchial reactivity.

Management

Environmental

Irrespective of the specific etiology of environmental/occupational-induced bronchial reactivity, treatment principles are similar. Foremost is **environmental control.** Specifically, persons should not return to the workplace without proper respiratory protection, which can be difficult to achieve. Also, persons must be fastidious in their avoidance of other non–workplace-associated triggers, both allergic and irritant.

Pharmacologic

Pharmacologic intervention with **beta-2 agonists** and **inhaled corticosteroids** should be the first-order approach to blunt the effect of inadvertent breaches in environmental control.

Special Problems

Reports to Patients and Third Parties

Because of the nature of reversible or partially reversible airflow obstruction, and because appropriate treatment may preclude an individual's return to the workplace, the physician may be faced with difficulty in explaining the apparent inconsistency between no measurable impairment on routine pulmonary function studies and the presence of disability owing to dysfunction that develops when returning to the workplace. Although this is well understood by the worker, others may be less accepting.

Family and Social Problems

Because regularly occurring irritants in the household initiate bronchial narrowing, not only may a former wage earner be unable to return to work, but he or she may also be limited in ability to perform routine household chores (cleaning, cooking, transport, shopping). This limitation may result in unsuccessful role reversal and substantial family stress and may require appropriate counseling.

HYPERSENSITIVITY PNEUMONITIS

Hypersensitivity pneumonitis is an immunologically mediated lung disease that occurs in susceptible hosts who become **sensitized** and then are **repeatedly exposed** to one of an enormous number of offending antigens (Table 27-3). Persons who work in virtually any environment may be affected, resulting in such colorfully named disorders as *cheese washer's disease* and *paprika splitter's lung*.

TABLE 27-3. HYPERSENSITIVITY PNEUMONITIS—CAUSATIVE AGENTS

- Organisms
  - Bacteria
    - Thermophilic actinomycetes
      - Various sources:
        - Moldy hay, grain, compost
        - Air conditioners, humidifiers
    - *Mycobacterium avium-intracellulare*–contaminated water
    - Mixed bacteria/fungi–contaminated metal-working fluids
  - Fungi
    - *Aspergillus* species—moldy malt dust
    - *Alternaria* species—moldy wood dust
    - *Cryptostroma corticale*—wet maple bark
    - *Pullularia* species—moldy redwood dust
    - *Trichosporum cutaneum*—Japanese house mold
  - Amoebae
    - *Naegleria gruberi*–contaminated ventilation system
    - *Acanthamoeba castellani*–contaminated ventilation system
- Animal proteins
  - Bovine/porcine protein
  - Rat urinary protein—rat urine
  - Oyster/mollusk shell protein—shell dust
  - Animal fur protein
  - Fish meal dust
  - Pigeons/doves
- Plants
  - Soybean hulls
  - Coffee bean dust
  - *Lycoperdon* species
- Chemicals and manufactured products
  - Amiodarone
  - Procarbazine
  - Toluene diisocyanate—paints, plastics
  - Diphenylmethane diisocyanate—paints, plastics
  - Phthalic anhydride—plastics
  - Trimellitic anhydride—plastics
  - Nylon flock

Exposure

Although many persons may be exposed to a particular antigen, relatively few develop hypersensitivity pneumonitis. Smokers may be less prone to develop the disease. Multiple exposures may be necessary to become sensitized. Ultimately, disease may progress to diffuse fibrosis.

With time, industries, work conditions, and products change; these changes can create new venues for this disease. A high level of suspicion is needed to make the diagnosis.

One of the most commonly mentioned hypersensitivity pneumonitides develops in agricultural workers and is known as **farmer's lung.** It is the result of exposure to the fungi *Micropolyspora faeni* and *Thermoactinomyces vulgaris*. Exposure occurs when moldy hay is disturbed and spores are distributed into the air and inhaled by susceptible persons. The risk of developing disease is increased by weather conditions predisposing to the growth of mold, frequent and heavy exposure to hay, and poor-quality ventilation in the workplace.

General Diagnostic Considerations

A high level of clinical suspicion is necessary. Because the patient presentation and radiographic studies can vary according to the stage of disease, and findings are not pathognomonic, hypersensitivity pneumonitis should be considered when symptoms improve with avoidance of the suspected agent and recur or worsen with reexposure. Some attempts have been made to formalize the diagnostic process with major and minor criteria, but these criteria have not been universally accepted.

Presentation

Acute

The acute phase usually develops between **4 and 12 hrs after exposure** to the antigen and **resembles an infectious process.** The patient complains of cough, dyspnea, fever, chills, myalgias, and malaise. Exam shows elevated temperature, tachypnea, significant hypoxemia, and inspiratory crackles.

CXR shows diffuse ground-glass opacification, but a nodular or reticulonodular pattern may be seen. **Chest CT** also shows diffuse ground glass that is patchy or diffuse; small centrilobular nodules of ground-glass attenuation can also be seen. **PFTs** show restriction confirmed by a decreased TLC and associated with decreased DLCO and oxygen desaturation with exercise.

Subacute/Chronic

This phase develops after **continued, prolonged, low-level exposure.** Signs and symptoms are more subtle. The patient reports progressive dyspnea, cough, fatigue, anorexia, and weight loss. The exam may be normal or may reveal such findings as basilar crackles.

On **CXR,** the subacute phase typically presents with a prominent reticulonodular pattern. Chronic phase CXR may show irregular linear densities with upper lobe retraction, volume loss, honeycombing, and traction emphysema.

CT shows irregular linear opacities, traction bronchiectasis, lobar volume loss, honeycombing, and emphysema.

PFTs in either phase may demonstrate any combination of restrictive and obstructive ventilatory defects. Desaturation with exercise is commonly seen.

Evaluation

Lab evaluation usually is not helpful because elevations in ESR, CRP, and Igs are nondiagnostic.

Bronchoalveolar lavage may show increased cellularity, usually lymphocyte predominant, with variable proportions of CD8 and CD4 cells.

Precipitin tests are of limited usefulness. Specific tests do not exist for all potential antigens. A positive result may mean only that the patient has had sufficient exposure to develop an immunologic response, but the particular antigen is not actually responsible for the disease. Thus, positive tests may not be diagnostic. Test reagents and testing processes vary widely in quality.

Inhalation challenge, in which the expected offending agent is inhaled in a similar fashion to that used in a methacholine challenge, is usually unnecessary for diagnosis.

Such a challenge is most useful if symptoms occur promptly after exposure and improve after removal from offending agents. Suitable agents and standardized testing methods may be unavailable for the suspected antigen.

Management

Acute hypersensitivity pneumonitis usually **resolves without specific intervention** within 1–3 days if the patient is removed from exposure.

Removal/avoidance of antigen exposure is most important to prevent progression to fibrosis, reactive airway disease, and obstruction. Protective equipment includes masks and filters. Decrease exposure to the antigen in the workplace.

Corticosteroids [initially, 1 mg/kg (maximum, 60 mg) PO qd until clinical and lab improvements are noted, then tapered over 3–6 mos, monitoring symptoms and labs] may help to resolve the acute/subacute phase. **Supportive measures** include smoking cessation, bronchodilators if PFTs show a reactive airways component to the disease, supplemental oxygen if needed, and pulmonary rehabilitation.

Prognosis

Acute disease has a good prognosis if further exposure is avoided. Subacute/chronic disease is unpredictable, and some patients progress despite antigen avoidance.

KEY POINTS TO REMEMBER

- A high index of suspicion and a detailed occupational history are essential when evaluating a patient for a possible workplace-related pulmonary disease.
- The disability certification process often involves multiple agencies and procedures that vary from state to state. For assistance with definitions and criteria, the AMA *Guides to the Evaluation of Permanent Impairment* is a valuable resource.
- Tobacco smoking increases the risk of lung cancer in persons who have even short-term exposure to asbestos. The risk is at least additive and possibly synergistic. Therefore, it is imperative that asbestos-exposed persons stop smoking immediately and permanently.
- A high level of clinical suspicion is necessary when diagnosing hypersensitivity pneumonitis since patient presentation and radiographic studies can vary according to the stage of the disease. Also, findings are not pathognomonic, so this diagnosis should be considered when symptoms improve with avoidance of the suspected agent and recur or worsen with reexposure.

REFERENCES AND SUGGESTED READINGS

Akira M. High-resolution CT in the evaluation of occupational and environmental disease. *Radiol Clin North Am* 2002;40(1):43–59.

American Thoracic Society. Adverse effects of crystalline silica exposure. American Thoracic Society Committee of the Scientific Assembly on Environmental and Occupational Health. *Am J Respir Crit Care Med* 1997;155:761–768.

Ando M, Suga M, Kohrogi H. A new look at hypersensitivity pneumonitis. *Curr Opin Pulm Med* 1999;5(5):299–304.

Barron BA. Disability certifications in adult workers: a practical approach. *Am Fam Physician* 2001;64(9):1579–1586.

Beeckman LA, Wang ML, Petsonk EL, Wagner GR. Rapid declines in FEV_1 and subsequent respiratory symptoms, illnesses, and mortality in coal miners in the United States. *Am J Respir Crit Care Med* 2001;163:633–639.

Bernstein IL, Chan-yeung M, Malo L-L, Bernstein DI. *Asthma in the workplace*. New York: Marcel Dekker Inc, 1999.

Bierman CW, Pearlman DS, Shapiro GS, et al. *Allergy, asthma, and immunology from infancy to adulthood,* 3rd ed. Philadelphia: WB Saunders, 1996:560.

Brooks SM, Hammad Y, Richards I, et al. The spectrum of irritant-induced asthma: sudden and not-so-sudden onset and the role of allergy. *Chest* 1998; 113:42–49.
Brooks S, Weiss MA, Bernstein IL. Reactive airways dysfunction syndrome: persistent asthma syndrome after high-level irritant exposure. *Chest* 1985;88:376–384.
Castranova V, Vallyathan V. Silicosis and coal workers' pneumoconiosis. *Environ Health Perspect* 2000;108[Suppl 4]:675–684.
Chapman SJ, Cookson WOC, Musk AW, Lee YCG. Benign asbestos pleural diseases. *Curr Opin Pulm Med* 2003;9:266–271.
Checkoway H, Franzblau A. Is silicosis required for silica-associated lung cancer? *Am J Ind Med* 2000;37:252–259.
Cocchiarella L, Andersson GBJ, eds. *Guides to the evaluation of permanent impairment,* 5th edition. Chicago: AMA Press, 2001.
De Vuyst P, Camus P. The past and present of pneumoconioses. *Curr Opin Pulm Med* 2000;6:151–156.
Erdogdu G, Hasirci V. An overview of the role of mineral solubility in silicosis and asbestosis. *Environ Res* 1998;78:38–42.
Fink JN. Immunologic orchestration of hypersensitivity pneumonitis. *J Clin Lab Med* 2000;136(1):5–6.
Finkelstein MM. Silica, silicosis, and lung cancer: a risk assessment. *Am J Ind Med* 2000;38:8–18.
Fujimura N. Pathology and pathophysiology of pneumoconiosis. *Curr Opin Pulm Med* 2000;6:140–144.
Glazer CS, Rose CS, Lynch DA. Clinical and radiologic manifestations of hypersensitivity pneumonitis. *J Thorac Imaging* 2002;17:261–272.
Goldman RH, Peters JM. The occupational and environmental health history. *JAMA* 1981;246(24):2831–2836.
Gottschall EB. Occupational and environmental thoracic malignancies. *J Thorac Imaging* 2002;17:189–197.
Greaves IA. Not-so-simple silicosis: a case for public health action. *Am J Ind Med* 2000;37:245–251.
Hathaway GJ, Proctor NH, Hughes JP. *Proctor and Hughes' chemical hazards of the workplace,* 4th ed. New York: Van Nostrand Reinhold, 1996.
Hessel P, Gamble JF, Gee JB, et al. Silica, silicosis, and lung cancer: a response to a recent working group report. *J Occup Health Med* 2000;42(7):704–720.
Hillerdal G, Henderson DW. Asbestos, asbestosis, pleural plaques and lung cancer. *Scand J Work Environ Health* 1997;23:93–103.
Kim JS, Lynch DA. Imaging of nonmalignant occupational lung disease. *J Thorac Imaging* 2002;17(4):238–259.
Kuschner WG, Stark P. Occupational lung disease. Part 1. Identifying work-related asthma and other disorders. *Postgrad Med* 2003;113(4):70–78.
Kuschner WG, Stark P. Occupational lung disease. Part 2. Discovering the cause of diffuse parenchymal lung disease. *Postgrad Med* 2003;113(4):81–88.
Lapp NL, Morgan WKC, Zoldivar G. Airways obstruction, coal mining, and disability. *Occup Environ Med* 1994;51:234–238.
Levin SM, Kann PE, Lax MB. Medical examination for asbestos-related disease. *Am J Ind Med* 2000;37:6–22.
McSharry C, Anderson K, Bourke SJ, Boyd G. Takes your breath away—the immunology of allergic alveolitis. *Clin Exp Immunol* 2002;128:3–9.
Merrill W. Hypersensitivity pneumonitis: just think of it! *Chest* 2001;120(4):1055–1057.
Morgan WKC, Seaton A. *Occupational lung diseases.* Philadelphia: WB Saunders, 1995:548–562.
Mossman BT, Churg A. Mechanisms in the pathogenesis of asbestosis and silicosis. *Am J Respir Crit Care Med* 1998;157:1666–1680.
Murray JF, Nadel JA. *Textbook of respiratory medicine,* 3rd ed. Philadelphia: WB Saunders, 2000:1806–1807.

National Institute for Occupational Safety and Health. NIOSH Hazard Review—Health Effects of Occupational Exposure to Respirable Crystalline Silica. DHHS (NIOSH) Publication No 2002-129. Cincinnati, OH: U.S. Department of Health and Human Services, Centers for Disease Control and Prevention, National Institute for Occupational Safety and Health, 2002.

Nishimura SL, Broaddus C. Asbestos-induced pleural disease. *Clin Chest Med* 1998;19(2):311–329.

The Occupational and Environmental Health Committee of the American Lung Association of San Diego and Imperial Counties of San Diego, California. Taking the occupational history. *Ann Intern Med* 1983;99(5):641–650.

Patel A, Ryu JH, Reed CE. Hypersensitivity pneumonitis: current concepts and future questions. *J Allergy Clin Immunol* 2001;108(5):661–672.

Roach HD, Davies GJ, Attanoos R, et al. Asbestos: when the dust settles—an imaging review of asbestos-related disease. *Radiographics* 2002;22:S167–S182.

Ross RM. The clinical diagnosis of asbestosis in this century requires more than a chest radiograph. *Chest* 2003;124:1120–1128.

Salvaggio JE. Extrinsic allergic alveolitis (hypersensitivity pneumonitis): past, present, and future. *Clin Exp Allergy* 1997;27[Suppl 1]:18–25.

Schins RPF, Borm PJA. Mechanisms and mediators in coal dust induced toxicity: a review. *Ann Ind Hygiene* 1999;43(1):7–33.

Schuyler M, Cormier Y. The diagnosis of hypersensitivity pneumonitis [editorial]. *Chest* 1997;111(3):534–536.

Schwarz MI, King TE Jr. *Interstitial lung disease*, 4th ed. London: BC Decker, 2003.

Singh N, Davis GS. Review: occupational and environmental lung disease. *Curr Opin Pulm Med* 2002;8:117–125.

Sood A, Beckett WS. Determination of disability for patients with advanced lung disease. *Clin Chest Med* 1997;18(3):471–482.

Steenland K, Mannetje A, Boffetta P, et al. Pooled exposure-response analyses and risk assessment for lung cancer in 10 cohorts of silica-exposed workers: an IARC multicentre study. *Cancer Causes Control* 2001;12:773–784.

Wagner GR. Asbestosis and silicosis. *Lancet* 1997;349:1311–1315.

Weiss W. Asbestosis: a marker for the increased risk of lung cancer among workers exposed to asbestos. *Chest* 1999;115:536–549.

Weitberg AB, Klastersky J, eds. *Cancer of the lung—from molecular biology to treatment guidelines.* Totowa, NJ: Human Press, 2002.

28 Solitary Pulmonary Nodule

Sanjay Sharma

INTRODUCTION

The evaluation of a solitary pulmonary nodule found on chest x-ray (CXR) is a common clinical question encountered by pulmonary consult services. The primary goal is to determine whether the nodule is malignant or benign. Identifying an early stage of lung cancer is of great benefit, given survival rates of 40–80% after removal of malignant solitary pulmonary nodules.

The evaluation consists of a thorough history, physical exam, and evaluation of available imaging before deciding whether to recommend surgical removal of the nodule or careful watching and waiting.

DEFINITION

A solitary pulmonary nodule is defined as an **opacity <3 cm** in its greatest dimension, completely surrounded by lung parenchyma, and without evidence of atelectasis or hilar enlargement. Lesions **>3 cm** have a **high likelihood of being malignant** and should be treated as such.

DIFFERENTIAL DIAGNOSIS

The differential diagnosis of a solitary pulmonary nodule can be divided into malignant and nonmalignant causes (Table 28-1). Among the **malignant causes** are primary lung cancers (adenocarcinoma, small cell carcinoma, large cell carcinoma, squamous cell carcinoma), metastatic cancers, and carcinoid tumors. The **nonmalignant processes** include infections (granulomatous and nongranulomatous), benign neoplasms, vascular malformations, inflammatory masses, developmental abnormalities, and others. In studies, the **rate of malignancy** of solitary pulmonary nodules has varied (depending on the definition and selection criteria for the nodule) from 10% to 68%. Of the benign nodules, >80% are infectious granulomas.

EVALUATION

History

Although a pulmonary nodule is a radiographic finding, the clinician's evaluation starts with a **history and physical exam.** The emphasis should be on the **risk factors for malignancy**—in particular, **smoking history.** Tobacco smoking is the leading risk factor for primary lung cancer, with a relative risk 10- to 30-fold greater than that of a nonsmoker. The risk of cancer decreases after 5 yrs of smoking cessation but most likely does not ever fall to that of the nonsmoker. Marijuana smoking is commonly included as a risk factor under smoking history, but direct evidence of its association with lung cancer is currently controversial.

Age is another important factor. The older the patient is, the greater the likelihood of malignancy. Among patients aged >50 yrs, a solitary pulmonary nodule has a 65% chance of being cancer, whereas in patients aged <50 yrs, the chance is 33%.

TABLE 28-1. DIFFERENTIAL DIAGNOSIS OF SOLITARY PULMONARY NODULE

Malignant
- Primary lung cancer
- Lymphoma
- Carcinoid
- Metastasis (breast, kidney, thyroid, lung, melanoma, sarcoma, bladder, colon, kidney, testicle)

Benign
- Tumors
  - Fibroma
  - Lipoma
  - Leiomyoma
  - Hemangioma
- Infectious
  - TB
  - Histoplasmosis
  - Coccidioidomycosis
  - Blastomycosis
  - *Nocardia*
  - Pneumonia (round)
  - Abscess
- Autoimmune
  - Rheumatoid arthritis
  - Wegener's granulomatosis
- Vascular
  - Arteriovenous malformation
  - Infarct
  - Hematoma
- Congenital
  - Bronchial atresia
  - Pulmonary sequestration
  - Hamartoma
  - Chondroma
- Other
  - Foreign body
  - Posttransplant lymphoproliferative disorder
  - Pleural plaque

Adapted with permission from Erasmus JJ, Connolly JE, McAdams HP, Roggli VL. Solitary pulmonary nodules: part I. Morphologic evaluation for differentiation of benign and malignant lesions. *Radiographics* 2000;20(1):43–58.

Other risk factors include exposures to asbestos, secondhand smoke, radon, arsenic, ionizing radiation, haloethers, nickel, and polycyclic aromatic hydrocarbons. Environmental exposures can also alert the clinician to other possible diseases (e.g., TB).

Symptoms related to potential cancer or inflammatory or infectious disease should be sought. **Weight loss** is a poor prognostic sign in cancer but may occur with benign diseases, such as TB and pyogenic abcesses, too. **Cough** is a nonspecific symptom, and change in cough may be a more relevant symptom. **Hemoptysis** can suggest malignancy, usually squamous cell carcinoma, but with the increasing occurrence of adenocarcinomas, which are peripherally located, hemoptysis is a less common finding. **Hoarseness** can occur with compression or invasion of the left recurrent laryngeal nerve as it passes over the aortic notch. **Severe chest pain** can sometimes signify chest wall or mediastinal involvement. Symptoms of pericardial or pleural effusions should be discussed as should neurologic symptoms and joint pains.

Past Medical History

Previous nonpulmonary cancer history raises the suspicion of **metastatic lung disease.** Cancers that tend to metastasize to lung include prior lung cancers (both ipsilateral and contralateral); malignant melanomas; sarcomas; and bladder, colon, breast, testicle, and kidney cancers. A history of **COPD** alerts the clinician to a likely smoking history. **Immunosuppressed states,** including HIV, chronic steroid therapy, and posttransplant status, broaden the differential diagnosis of the nodule considerably.

Physical Exam

The physical exam should concentrate on the direct involvement of the nodule and possible metastatic or paraneoplastic disease. A thorough physical exam with a detailed respiratory exam is mandatory. **Signs** to look for include clubbing and distal long bone swelling (hypertrophic osteoarthropathy); hepatomegaly; bone tenderness (metastases); plethoric face, engorged neck, and superficial veins (superior vena cava syndrome); wasting; lymphadenopathy; and focal neurologic deficits. Wheezing limited to one area is evidence of major airway obstruction, which may be due to an intraluminal tumor. Inspiratory stridor can lend evidence for upper-airway involvement by the nodule or associated disease.

Lab Evaluation

Lab evaluation should include **complete electrolyte panel (including calcium), liver panel,** and **CBC.** Hyponatremia may be due to SIADH, which is seen in small cell carcinoma. Hypercalcemia may be due to bony metastases or release of PTH-related peptide from squamous cell carcinoma. Liver abnormalities, particularly elevated alkaline phosphatase, may suggest liver metastases.

Radiologic Evaluation

Comparison of the current film (demonstrating the solitary pulmonary nodule) with **old CXRs** is of paramount importance. An **opacity** that has been **present and stable for >2 yrs** greatly reduces the likelihood of cancer and is generally considered to be **benign.** Any other opacities need further evaluation.

Another way to evaluate a pulmonary nodule is to study its **doubling time.** Tumor doubling time refers to the volume of a mass rather than the two-dimensional characteristics seen on an imaging study. One doubling time corresponds to a 28% increase in diameter on CXR. The doubling time of malignant tumors ranges from 20 to 400 days. Benign lesions usually have shorter or longer doubling times. A chest CT exam can better identify the size and characteristics of the nodule and better evaluate the doubling time than can CXRs. However, large overlaps in doubling times make this a less than perfect method of judging malignancy.

A particular characteristic that lends evidence to the etiology of a nodule is **calcification.** The benign patterns include popcorn calcification (as occurs with hamartomas) and central calcification (which may indicate an infectious granuloma). Stippled or eccentric calcifications are indeterminate as they can be seen in both malignant and benign diseases. Any other patterns of calcification are suggestive of malignant disease.

The nodule should also be described by its **edge** and **shape.** Scalloped, spiculated, and *corona radiata* (perpendicular lines extending outwards from the nodule) patterns are worrisome for a malignancy, whereas a smooth or lobulated edge suggests benign disease. The incidence of malignancy has been reported to be as high as 90% for corona radiata patterns. Other characteristic signs include so-called tail extensions toward the hilum found in atelectasis, arteriovenous malformation, and cysts. Peripheral nodules with extensions into the pleura may be significant for carcinoma. Single lesions connected with blood vessels may be seen with arteriovenous malformations and pulmonary sequestration, whereas multiple lesions connected with pulmonary arteries may be seen with septic emboli.

Chest CT exams are almost always needed for further evaluation of a solitary pulmonary nodule. Calcification patterns and shapes are more clearly visible on CT scans. Multiple nodules and mediastinal lymphadenopathy may also be found that were not apparent on the CXR. In addition, densitometry (measured in Hounsfield units) can identify fat, blood, and bone.

Positron Emission Tomography

The use of PET is beneficial for **evaluating the malignant potential of indeterminate nodules.** F-18 fluorodeoxyglucose–labeled PET identifies metabolically active lesions. In clinical trials, PET scans have been able to discriminate favorably between malignant and nonmalignant tissue with a sensitivity of 95% and specificity of 70%. The obvious benefit arises for the patient with the indeterminate nodule who could be risk stratified based on PET scan. However, even a negative PET scan still necessitates close follow-up and routine chest imaging to monitor for growth of the solitary pulmonary nodule.

Based on the probability of malignancy of a solitary pulmonary nodule, the clinician must recommend surgical removal or observation. Judgment errors (with or without all the pertinent clinical information) can lead to nontreatment of malignant nodules. Mathematical models have been derived, based on patient risk factors and the likelihood ratios of those risks leading to cancer, to evaluate the malignant potential of solitary pulmonary nodules. Using Bayes theorem, one can calculate the probability of malignancy mathematically. Mathematical models are more reliable than interclinician judgment but are cumbersome and still far from perfect. The hope of PET scan is to eliminate the need for such calculations and provide an answer about the malignant potential of an indeterminate nodule.

MANAGEMENT

Patients with a **high risk** of cancer should be **referred for thoracotomy** to remove the nodule. This procedure is both diagnostic and (in most cases) curative. A **low risk** of cancer should prompt a vigilant **watch and wait strategy** involving serial chest CT exams q3mos over a 12-mo period, followed by serial chest CT exams q6mos over a 12-mo period. Nodules that are stable over this time should be considered benign. Any enlargement of the mass should prompt a thoracotomy as for high-risk nodules.

The **indeterminate nodule** is more problematic. Patients' influence (i.e., the need to know) or comorbidities may dictate the management strategy pursued. PET scanning can be used or tissues can be procured. The available tissue sampling methods include fiber-optic bronchoscopy, CT- or fluoroscopic-guided needle biopsy, video-assisted thoracoscopic surgery, or thoracotomy. Bronchoscopy allows the pulmonologist to obtain washings, lavages, and biopsy samples. The yield of bronchoscopy depends strongly on the location of the nodule in relation to the bronchi. In addition, a limited amount of sample may preclude extensive testing, such as special staining or immunochemistry. Percutaneous needle aspiration with CT or fluoroscopic guidance can yield good sample sizes; however, there are risks associated with the procedure, including pneumothorax. Video-assisted thoracoscopic surgery is rapidly developing as a valuable and safe method of obtaining tissue samples but is still only available in specialized centers.

CONCLUSION

There is no general consensus on the optimal management of the solitary pulmonary nodule. The approach presented here is a good one based on current evidence and allows the timely detection of malignant nodules, thus ensuring patient safety.

KEY POINTS TO REMEMBER

- A solitary pulmonary nodule is defined as an opacity <3 cm in its greatest dimension, completely surrounded by lung parenchyma, and without evidence of atelectasis or hilar enlargement.
- In the radiologic evaluation, it is of paramount importance to compare the current film to old x-rays.
- A pulmonary nodule can also be evaluated by studying its doubling time, which refers to the change in volume of a mass.
- Chest CT exams are commonly needed for further evaluation of a solitary pulmonary nodule.

REFERENCES AND SUGGESTED READINGS

Erasmus JJ, Connolly JE, McAdams HP, Roggli VL. Solitary pulmonary nodules: part I. Morphologic evaluation for differentiation of benign and malignant lesions. *Radiographics* 2000;20(1):43–58.

Erasmus JJ, McAdams HP, Connolly JE. Solitary pulmonary nodules: part II. Evaluation of the indeterminate nodule. *Radiographics* 2000;20(1):59–66.

Gurney JW, Lyddon DM, McKay JA. Determining the likelihood of malignancy in solitary pulmonary nodules: a Bayesian approach: part I: theory. *Radiology* 1993;186:405.

Gurney JW, Lyddon DM, McKay JA. Determining the likelihood of malignancy in solitary pulmonary nodules: a Bayesian approach: part II: application. *Radiology* 1993;186:415.

Ost D, Fein A. Evaluation and management of the solitary pulmonary nodule. *Am J Respir Crit Care Med* 2000;162:782–787.

Shaffer K. Role of radiology for imaging and biopsy of solitary pulmonary nodules. *Chest* 1999;116(6):519S–522S.

Strauss GM. Overview and clinical manifestations of lung cancer, UpToDate Online 9.3. August 2, 2000. Available at: www.uptodate.com. Accessed October 10, 2005.

Strauss GM. Cigarette smoking and other risk factors for lung cancer. UpToDate Online 9.3. March 13, 2001. Available at: www.uptodate.com. Accessed October 10, 2005.

Weinberger SE. Differential diagnosis and evaluation of the solitary pulmonary nodule. UpToDate Online 9.3. February 9, 2001. Available at: www.uptodate.com. Accessed October 10, 2005.

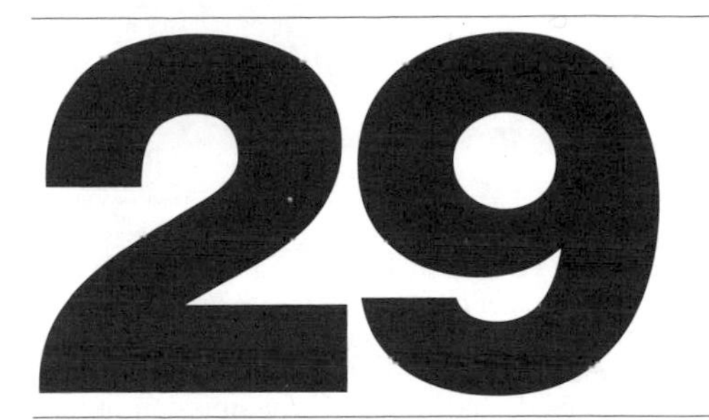

Cavitary Lung Disease

Daniel H. Cooper

INTRODUCTION

The finding of a cavitary lung lesion on chest radiograph (CXR) presents a unique and challenging clinical scenario. It requires the integration of clinical context with appropriate imaging to narrow what is a relatively broad differential diagnosis that may be readily apparent or remain elusive.

DEFINITION AND PATHOGENESIS

The regularity with which these lesions are found has not been widely reported, most likely owing to the relative disagreement of what one considers a **cavity.** Cavities are formally defined as lucent areas within the lung that may or may not contain an air–fluid level that is surrounded by a wall, usually of varied thickness. Essentially, cavities are holes in the lung with various, characteristic changes in the surrounding parenchyma. It is these surrounding changes that help elucidate the etiology of the lesions. It is also useful to distinguish between cavities and other causes of lucent radiographic defects such as cysts, bullae, and pneumatoceles. Many of these terms are used interchangeably and at times inappropriately.

The formation of a cavity is, in general, the result of either the necrosis of lung parenchyma after an insult of some form to that tissue or the central necrosis of an existing lung nodule. When the necrotic components of these processes are drained via communication with the tracheobronchial tree, air is allowed to enter the excavated space, producing the characteristic air-filled lesion. The lucency is surrounded by tissue of certain density, contour, and thickness, all of which are variable and depend on the insulting process that created the lesion.

ETIOLOGY

Pyogenic Infections

The finding of cavitation in the setting of (or after) an acute febrile illness with productive cough is often the result of **necrotizing pneumonia.** Pyogenic abscesses develop as the ongoing infection destroys the surrounding lung parenchyma. Liquefaction necrosis ensues, giving the lesion water density characteristics until communication with the airways is achieved and the material can be expectorated, thereby producing the typical clinical scenario of an air-filled lung cavity (with or without an air–fluid level, depending on degree of drainage). The organisms common in this setting include *Staphylococcus aureus, Klebsiella, Legionella,* and other gram-negative bacteria (*Pseudomonas, Escherichia coli, Proteus,* and *Serratia*). If the cavity is located in dependent portions of the lung and comorbid risk factors such as alcoholism, poor dentition, and ENT pathology exist, aspiration pneumonia with mixed gram-negative and anaerobic organisms should be suspected. Often, the finding of a cavity is in the postpneumonic period and, if the consolidation has cleared around it, a distinct hyperlucent cavity with a wall of variable thickness (usually >4 mm) and of shaggy outline is characteristic. It is rare for pneumonias caused by *Streptococcus* *pneumoniae, Haemophilus influenzae, Mycoplasma, Chlamydia psittaci,* or viruses to produce cavitary lesions.

Mycobacteria

Worldwide, the infection that is most synonymous with a finding of cavities is TB. **Cavitation** is found in most cases of **reactivation TB** and in approximately **10% of primary cases.** These patients present with symptoms of chronic respiratory illness with productive cough and often hemoptysis. **Primary TB** can present with disease in any lobe with a slight predilection for the middle and lower lung fields, given their relatively greater degree of ventilation and the inhalational route of transmission of disease. Primary TB tends to present more often with findings of hilar and paratracheal lymphadenopathy and areas of consolidation rather than nodular or cavitary lesions. During **reactivation** of the disease, there is less lymphadenopathy and consolidation, with focal nodular disease and cavitation predominating. These lesions are characteristically located in the apical and posterior portions of the upper lung fields. It is rare for a case of TB to present with cavitary lesions solely in the lower lung fields; however, it is not uncommon to find disease in both upper and lower lung fields. Therefore, although other bacterial and fungal lesions should ascend the differential with multilobar disease, TB should not be excluded. A positive tuberculin skin test and the presence of AFB on smear and correlating cultures help confirm the diagnosis.

Atypical (nontuberculous) mycobacterial infections can produce cavities as well. The most common organisms are *Mycobacterium avium-intracellulare* complex and *M. kansasii*. These lesions can appear very similar to those produced by *M. tuberculosis,* and in the setting of TB-like radiographic findings and a negative PPD, these atypical mycobacteria (and fungal disease) should be considered. Microbiological identification of the organisms is required for diagnosis and treatment.

Fungal

The various pulmonary mycoses commonly result in cavity formation. They can be found in the immunocompetent host but have an expectantly higher incidence in those who are immunocompromised. They often mimic TB in radiographic appearance and should, therefore, also be considered in a patient with apical/posterior lung cavities and a negative PPD. Most of these patients present with symptoms that are difficult to distinguish initially from those of a typical upper or lower respiratory infection (i.e., cough with sputum, myalgias, fatigue, fever, anorexia). The patient's region of origin or recent travel to areas endemic for certain fungal infections is always a vital **historical detail** to obtain.

Coccidioidomycosis, for example, is endemic to the southwestern United States, Mexico, and Central and South America. This fungus lives in the soil, and its infectious airborne spores are transmitted via inhalation when the soil is disturbed in some fashion. The location of cavitary coccidioidomycosis is more variable than that of TB and histoplasmosis, although it is still most commonly found in the upper lobes. The cavity may be either thick or thin walled. Histoplasmosis may present similarly and can often only be differentiated from TB or other fungal infections by culture. Cavitation tends to occur more often in the chronic fibrocavitary form rather than in the acute forms. It tends to be found most commonly in the southeastern, mid-Atlantic, and central United States. Another endemic mycosis is blastomycosis, which aggregates in the Missouri and Ohio River valley states (southeastern and south central United States), the Canadian provinces bordering the Great Lakes, and the area adjacent to the St. Lawrence River in New York and Canada. Serologic testing, appropriate fungal cultures, and, on occasion, skin testing help delineate between these aforementioned causes.

Aspergillus fumigatus, a ubiquitous soil fungus, presents in several different fashions with regard to pulmonary infections, all associated with cavitation. Mycetoma, or **aspergilloma,** is the formation of a fungus ball within a preexisting cavitary or cystic lesion. An air crescent is often seen between the fungus ball and cavity wall on CXR.

Aspergillomas are usually solitary findings and occur in immunocompetent patients. Invasive pulmonary aspergillosis is most commonly seen in immunocompromised patients, especially leukemia patients undergoing treatment. Multiple cavitary nodules are commonly seen. Often, these lesions have nodules suspended within the cavity (*mural nodules*) that can be differentiated from a mycetoma by their fixed rather than mobile central mass.

Opportunistic fungal infections are common in HIV/AIDS or otherwise immunocompromised patients. ***Cryptococcus neoformans*** is a common offender with regard to cavity formers. It is commonly and usually incidentally found in the immunocompetent during workups of lung nodules on CXR. If left undiscovered, the indolent infection may reactivate in patients who become immunosuppressed. The relative lack of symptoms in healthy subjects leads to the common association of pulmonary cryptococcosis with HIV/AIDS or patients who are otherwise immunocompromised. There are no particularly distinguishing features of this infection, and therefore we rely heavily on culture results to determine the pathogen.

Other Infections

***Pneumocystis jiroveci* pneumonia** (formerly *Pneumocystis carinii* pneumonia) is commonly seen in HIV-infected patients with CD4 counts <200. It is also seen increasingly in patients with posttransplant status or who are being treated with chemotherapy for malignancy. The radiologic manifestations in *P. jiroveci* pneumonia range from normal to bilateral, multifocal, "patchwork," or "mosaic" infiltrates that, on occasion, cavitate.

Parasites are another category of organisms to consider. Hydatid cysts, amebic lung abscess, and pulmonary paragonimiasis have all been described in association with cavitation. **Nocardiosis** is a well-described cause of pulmonary infection, consolidation, and cavitation in those who are immunosuppressed or in those with alveolar proteinosis. Actinomycosis, sporotrichosis, mucormycosis, and invasive candidiasis have also been known to cause cavities.

Neoplasm

Perhaps the most important consideration in the evaluation of a cavitary lung lesion is distinguishing between the benign and the malignant. With increasing age, significant tobacco use, and history of prior malignancy, suspicions for malignancy naturally grow larger. **Bronchogenic carcinoma** may lead to cavitation in two separate ways: The tumor itself may undergo central necrosis as it outgrows or thromboses off its blood supply, or a cavity may appear distal to the neoplasm as a result of obstructive pneumonitis and/or abscess formation. It has been estimated that 10–16% of primary bronchogenic carcinomas lead to cavitation. Squamous cell carcinoma is the most common variant, cavitating >30% of the time.

Metastatic disease is most often multifocal but can present as a solitary lesion as well. Only 5% of metastatic lung disease cavitates. In addition, the metastatic lesions that cavitate are most likely of **squamous cell** origin and can therefore create difficulty in differentiating between primary lung tumor and metastases. In general, it is worthwhile to search for head and neck primary disease and gynecologic disease (i.e., cervical cancer) in the setting of cavitary metastases with unknown primary origin. Metastatic malignant **sarcomas** actually cavitate more frequently than do lung carcinomas but are relatively less common. They are often associated with complicating pneumothorax (especially osteosarcoma).

Metastatic lymphoma also cavitates. However, if the patient has a known diagnosis of lymphoma and is currently or recently treated, opportunistic infection must be ruled out in the setting of multiple cavitary lesions. **Hodgkin's lymphoma** commonly cavitates, whereas non-Hodgkin's lymphoma does so less commonly. With Hodgkin's lymphoma, concomitant hilar and mediastinal lymphadenopathy and other clinical findings aid the relatively nonspecific routine plain film findings. Tissue is required to confirm these diagnoses.

Vascular

Wegener's granulomatosis and **rheumatoid arthritis** are the most common pulmonary vasculitides that cavitate. Perivascular inflammation within the granulomas and rheumatoid nodules leads to tissue necrosis and cavity formation. Both tend to present with multiple lesions. Classically, the combination of pulmonary, renal, and sinus granulomatous disease insinuates Wegener's granulomatosis, with a positive c-ANCA helping confirm the diagnosis. Cavitation in Wegener's granulomatosis occurs in approximately 50% of cases on CT scanning, typically with a thick wall and irregular inner lining. Cavitary rheumatoid nodules are usually preceded by signs and symptoms of extrapulmonary rheumatoid disease. Caplan's syndrome is the occurrence of pulmonary masses in coal miners with comorbid rheumatoid arthritis, essentially representing a pneumoconiosis that is accelerated by the patient's preexisting autoimmune disease.

Thromboembolic disease is an important consideration in the appropriate patient. Septic emboli are highly suspicious in patients demonstrating multifocal cavitary lesions, especially in concert with signs of sepsis, a history of IV drug use, history of congenital valvular disease, or an indwelling catheter. The origins of these emboli are infected thrombi or right-sided bacterial endocarditis. These lesions tend to be at the periphery of the lungs and, when cavitated, have thick walls. It is rare to see cavitation in the setting of a sterile pulmonary embolism and pulmonary infarction without superimposed infection.

Congenital

Congenital lesions are generally grouped under cystic lung abnormalities but may have characteristics similar to cavitary lesions, which prompts their inclusion in this discussion. Developmental abnormalities in the primitive foregut or lung bud may produce various cystic lesions. **Congenital adenomatoid malformation** is an entity marked by multiple circumscribed radiographic lung lucencies; it is usually discovered in childhood. **Pulmonary sequestration** refers to the congenital anomaly that leads to an isolated portion of the lung possessing an independent blood supply without communication with a normal bronchus. The intralobar variant is particularly susceptible to recurrent infections and cystic or cavitary formation. It should be considered in patients with recurrent pneumonia of the left lower lobe. Diagnosis is confirmed by angiographic evidence of an anomalous pulmonary vessel.

Other Causes

Pneumoconioses, such as coal workers' pneumoconiosis and silicosis, have been associated with cavities as well. They produce discrete masses secondary to progressive massive fibrosis that become centrally necrotic and cavitate. Cavitation is rare, however, and its presence should always prompt one to rule out TB superinfection. Pulmonary **Langerhans' cell histiocytosis** is also seen in young adults, almost always associated with a significant smoking history. Interstitial lung parenchymal changes are seen that produce reticulonodular infiltrates capable of cavitation. Diaphragmatic hernia may be mistaken for a cavitary lung lesion on routine CXR. Lucite plombage, a formerly used surgical practice of placing inert substances in the extrapleural space to induce collapse of adjacent lung for treatment of TB, produces a very characteristic appearance of multiple, tightly packed, spherical, cavitary-appearing lesions over an upper lung field. Pulmonary sarcoid, bronchiectasis, and amyloidosis rarely cause cavitation.

ROENTGENOLOGIC CHARACTERISTICS

In general, cavitation alone offers very little with regard to definitive differentiation between the benign and the malignant. Therefore, the same principles that are used to work up solitary and multiple lung nodules or masses apply to these lesions as well. Perhaps the most important aspect of this approach is the ever-present realization that disease carries an inevitable **ability to present in atypical fashion;** therefore, what is described below as typical is far from absolute and should be viewed only as guiding evidence for or against a particular diagnosis.

The approach to the cavitary lung lesion begins at its discovery with intense scrutiny of its radiographic appearance, which often begins with the analysis of routine posteroanterior and lateral CXRs.

Air–Fluid Levels

Air–fluid levels in a cavity indicate communication with airways allowing partial drainage and the entrance of air into the space. Upright or decubitus films are required to reveal the air–fluid level. They are often associated with pyogenic abscesses/infection. However, any cavity of any etiology is capable of having an air–fluid level. Therefore, **never exclude malignancy** in this instance because a malignancy may become secondarily infected, potentially masking itself as a more benign process. In addition, sterile fluid may come to occupy the space created by a cavitated neoplasm, or an obstructed neoplasm may result in distal pyogenic abscesses.

Wall Thickness

As mentioned above, the differentiation of malignant and benign is of the utmost concern. The measurement of the wall at its greatest thickness can help in this manner. Woodring et al. looked both prospectively and retrospectively at the diagnostic implications of **cavity wall thickness** and concluded that all lesions with area of greatest wall thickness of ≤ 1 mm were ultimately proven benign; of lesions with wall thickness of ≤ 4 mm, 92% were benign; of lesions with wall thickness between 5 and 15 mm, 51% were benign and 49% malignant, and of lesions with >15 mm wall thickness, 95% were malignant. Therefore, it is reasonable to conclude that lesions with walls that are **1 mm thick** can be followed without invasive intervention. Those between **1 and 4 mm thick** may only require more aggressive workup if appropriate bacterial, fungal, and mycobacterial causes are ruled out. And those that are **>15 mm** should be considered malignant, and prompt, directed attempts to obtain a tissue diagnosis via bronchoscopy or percutaneous biopsy should be undertaken without delay if no contraindications exist. Approximately 50% of lesions fall into the indeterminate range and further workup is required, guided by the clinical picture. Most thin-walled cavities **<4 mm** are more appropriately termed **cystic masses** and, in adults, are usually blebs, bullae, or pneumatoceles. Classically, coccidioidomycosis is described as producing thin-walled cysts, but on further study, appears to produce thick-walled cysts as well 50% of the time. Note that rare, thin-walled neoplastic lesions have been reported and should, therefore, always be considered in the differential diagnosis.

Outer/Inner Wall Characteristics

The various etiologies of these lesions impart wall appearances that allow for some inferences to be made. In general, an inner or outer contour that is **irregular** or **nodular** is more consistent with malignancy; if shaggy, consider acute lung abscess; if smooth, consider other causes. An irregular inner lining is also often described in cavitated Wegener's granulomas or lymphomatoid granulomatosis. TB cavities' linings can be either irregular or smooth. Eccentric cavitation with a septate, nodular inner cavity is highly suspicious for malignancy. Metastatic neoplasms are often **well circumscribed** and outwardly sharply defined, in contrast to primary neoplasm. **Cavitation** within surrounding consolidation is consistent with necrotizing pneumonia. Consider *S. aureus, Klebsiella, Legionella,* and other gram-negative bacilli. TB is also a possibility; however, the reactivation form when one sees the most cavitation presents less commonly with consolidation than the primary form does. **Granulomatous infections** (TB, coccidioidomycosis, histoplasmosis, blastomycosis), in general, produce a distinctive parenchymal reaction that is described as more reticular or reticulonodular. The radiologic course is also typically different. Benign cysts (congenital cysts, pneumatoceles, blebs, bullae) tend to have smooth, thin walls.

Focal vs Multifocal

The majority of single, focal, isolated cavitary lung lesions are bronchogenic carcinomas. Metastatic disease (usually squamous cell in origin) can present with a single lesion but more commonly presents with peripherally located multifocal metastases at different stages of growth and cavitation. Septic emboli appear similarly but often with the addition of a small area of pneumonitis or infiltrate surrounding the lesions. Wegener's granulomatosis and rheumatoid lesions are more often multifocal than solitary. Diffuse bronchiectasis, pulmonary sarcoidosis, idiopathic pulmonary fibrosis, and metastatic disease are rare causes of diffuse cavitary disease.

Location

Reactivation TB classically can be found in the **apical** or **posterior** portions of the upper lobes. It is rare for disease to be localized strictly to the lower lobe, but **multilobar** disease is not uncommon. Apical cavities in patients with a negative PPD should prompt consideration of atypical mycobacteria and fungal disease. Cavitated abscesses found in multiple lobes are usually not associated with a malignancy unless it is obstructing the mainstem bronchus. Pneumoconiosis tends to present with irregularly shaped fibrotic masses that are capable of cavitation in the upper lung fields. Cavities located in the **dependent portions of the lung** should trigger thoughts of aspiration, especially in the setting of other risk factors for aspiration. Intralobar sequestrations are typically located in the posterobasal portion of the left lower lobe.

Other

Radiologic course is important and is addressed within the clinical context discussion. Cavitation is relatively rare in primary TB and relatively common in reactivation. The **meniscus sign** or **air crescent sign** refers to the characteristic appearance of a mass within a cavitated lesion that may be produced commonly by a fungus ball or a hydatid cyst (which are usually mobile within the lesion) and less commonly by pulmonary gangrene, cavitating neoplasm, or abscesses. Cavitation in the setting of pulmonary embolism indicates the likely presence of parenchymal infarction and necrosis. Fibrocalcific findings are often indicative of old granulomatous disease. However, active TB should be investigated.

HISTORY

Age

Essentially, the older the patient, the greater risk for malignancy, especially in the setting of solitary lung lesions. Toomes et al. found that 65% of solitary lung lesions in patients aged >50 yrs were malignant, whereas 33% of those lesions were malignant in patients aged <50 yrs.

Symptoms

Most symptoms associated with cavitary lung lesions are relatively nonspecific for any one etiology. Hemoptysis, for example, indicates the invasion of pulmonary vessels, which can be seen with malignancy, invasive aspergillosis, TB, pyogenic infections, and vasculitides. Fever, malaise, productive cough, and pleuritic chest pain are common with pyogenic infections but are also seen with granulomatous infections even though the course is typically more indolent and protracted. Also, superinfection of a cavitated neoplasm or postobstructive pyogenic lung abscesses from an upstream malignancy must be considered in the febrile patient with a cavitary lung lesion. Weight loss is seen in both chronic granulomatous disease and malignancy. Low-grade fevers, progressively worsening cough, weight loss, and night sweats are often described in the context of TB but are, again, nonspecific.

Time Course

An attempt to establish the acuity of both the clinical and radiographic findings is of the utmost importance. In general, both the very acute and the extremely protracted clinical course can indicate a nonmalignant underlying etiology. A process that presents symptomatically and radiographically in a matter of days to a few weeks is more likely infectious, thromboembolic, traumatic, or perhaps immunologic (e.g., Wegener's). Chronic processes point toward neoplastic, congenital, or chronic inflammatory conditions. Specifically, lesions that demonstrate a **volume** (not diameter) **doubling** time (based on CT) of **<1 mo** or **>16 mos** suggest **a benign process.** A lesion that remains **stable >2 yrs** can be reasonably considered benign. Therefore, it is important to **review all prior radiologic studies.**

Known Malignancy

Known primary lung cancer can cavitate, especially if it is the squamous cell variant. It can also lead to obstructive pneumonia that can cause postobstructive lung abscesses that can also cavitate. Metastatic disease cavitates less commonly, with the exception of sarcomas. Lymphoma, especially Hodgkin's lymphoma, may cavitate, but one must rule out opportunistic infections if the patient is undergoing or has recently completed treatment that has caused immunocompromise. Treatment itself may accelerate cavitation.

Immune Status

One must make inquiries regarding HIV/AIDS, stem cell or solid organ transplantation, and recent radio- or chemotherapy for malignancy. In addition, any condition that may lead to some degree of immunosuppression as a result of the disease itself or its treatment must be considered. Therefore, chronic lung disease, diabetes, Cushing's syndrome, sarcoidosis, liver or renal failure, and other chronic medical conditions are all pertinent historical findings. Cavitary findings in the setting of immunosuppression or compromise are most often infectious in nature.

Exposure

One should inquire about exposure to sick contacts, with particular interest given to those with known active TB. Also, industrial exposure to the known causes of pneumoconiosis should be explored.

Travel History

Recent travel or residence in the aforementioned regions of endemic mycoses, mycobacterial, and parasitic infections should be inquired about: coccidioidomycosis (southwestern United States, Central and South America, Mexico), histoplasmosis (southeastern, mid-Atlantic, and central United States), blastomycosis (Missouri and Ohio River valley, Canadian provinces bordering the Great Lakes, and St. Lawrence River region in New York and Canada), TB (particularly prevalent in China, India, the southeastern islands of Asia, and sub-Saharan Africa; also showing increasing incidence in the United States, particularly in those with HIV/AIDS), amebiasis (developing countries, particularly those with conditions of poor sanitation), hydatid cysts (rural South and Central America, China, Russia, Middle East, sub-Saharan Africa), and paragonimiasis (Central and South America, West Africa, Far East).

Social History

Alcohol users are at greater risk for aspiration pneumonia with abscess and cavity formation. Individuals with significant long-term tobacco use make bronchogenic carcinoma more likely. **Pulmonary Langerhans' cell histiocytosis** is found almost exclusively in smokers. A careful sexual history and IV drug use history can shed light on the possibility of HIV infection. Also, IV drug use places patients at greater risk for right-sided endocarditis and septic emboli.

Other Relevant History

Patients with rheumatoid arthritis may have pulmonary manifestations (rheumatoid nodules). Recent chest trauma heightens the possibility of traumatic pneumatocele and bullae. Any patients with conditions that impair their ability to swallow are at greater risk for aspiration. Known comorbid renal and/or sinus disease may indicate Wegener's granulomatosis. Recurrent pneumonia, especially of the left lower lobe, is common in an area of pulmonary sequestration.

PHYSICAL EXAM

A thorough physical exam may yield some helpful findings. The cavitary lung lesions themselves produce relatively nonspecific respiratory exam findings or no findings at all. Hard cervical lymphadenopathy suggests metastatic cancer, especially if tobacco and age risk factors are present. Matted or fixed lymphadenopathy is consistent with malignancy. Lymphadenopathy in the presence of splenomegaly is concerning for lymphoma. Surgical scars from prior lucite plombage may be present. Malignant disease may produce superior vena cava obstruction, which would typically produce neck and chest vein distention and, potentially, facial edema. Skin findings may be useful and include all of the typical cutaneous manifestations of the diseases mentioned above (sarcoid, rheumatoid arthritis, fungal disease, others). Track marks from IV drug use should raise concern for right-sided endocarditis. Septic phlebitis or infected thrombi may produce palpable, tender cords. Right-sided endocarditis may produce an audible, new heart murmur. Peripheral findings of septic emboli such as splinter hemorrhages, Osler's nodes, and Janeway lesions could be present in patients with right-sided endocarditis and a patent foramen ovale. Physical findings consistent with consolidation on respiratory exam suggest a parapneumonic process but may be found in several other conditions.

LAB TESTS

Routine Lab Results

Routine lab results do not typically provide conclusive evidence for one etiology over another. Leukocytosis is suggestive of an ongoing, infective process but may also be seen in any secondarily infected cavity or in distal infective processes secondary to neoplastic obstruction. Leukopenia or pancytopenia may be seen in the immunocompromised state. Eosinophilia can be seen most commonly in parasitic infections. It has also been associated less commonly with lymphoma, coccidioidomycosis, and HIV. Blood cultures may reveal the offending organism if the lesion is associated with a bacteremia or fungemia.

Additional Lab Work

Serologic testing for many of the diseases mentioned above may aid in making a diagnosis. ANCA against proteinase-3 **(c-ANCA)** are present in approximately 80% of cases of Wegener's granulomatosis. An elevated **rheumatoid factor level** may suggest cavitated rheumatoid nodules. If a complicating pleural effusion is present and accessible, **pleural fluid analysis** with appropriate cell counts, chemistries, cytology, and cultures can help distinguish between infectious and malignant processes. If adequate **sputum samples** are obtained, cytologic studies, smears, and cultures may reveal the pyogenic, fungal, or mycobacterial organisms or malignancy responsible for a cavitary lesion. **Skin testing** is available for TB, coccidioidomycosis, aspergillosis, and histoplasmosis; however, positive tests do not distinguish between previous and current exposure. In addition, results may be misleading in those with compromised immune responses who may have a falsely negative dermatologic test.

ADDITIONAL IMAGING STUDIES

CT is a more sensitive and specific way to evaluate the characteristics of cavitary lesions. In modern medical practice, it is usually obtained as part of the routine workup. **High-resolution CT** allows for greater detail, with thinner slices providing more accurate depictions of the cavity, the cavity wall, and the surrounding lung parenchyma. Angiography or magnetic resonance angiography may be required if intralobar sequestration is suspected. Barium swallow readily differentiates between a diaphragmatic hernia and a true lung cavity.

INVASIVE WORKUP

Noninvasive workup is on occasion insufficient for definitive diagnosis. Tissue sampling from the cavitary pulmonary lesion is required when the diagnosis is not readily apparent or when the possibility of malignancy requires confirmation. **Bronchoscopy** is often the modality of choice. It offers several advantages, including (a) obtaining bronchial washings and secretions from the upper airways, (b) allowing bronchoalveolar lavage for representative sampling of the lower respiratory tract, and (c) allowing for brushing or biopsy of lesions within the bronchoscopist's reach. The diagnostic success of bronchoscopy is influenced greatly by the size and positioning of the lesion.

A **percutaneous approach** with needle aspiration under **fluoroscopic or CT guidance** is another option. Needle aspiration is diagnostic in most cases of metastatic and bronchogenic carcinoma. The sample aspirate is adequate for cytologic exam and the discovery of malignant appearing cells, but it does not provide a tissue core that may give further architectural detail. Therefore, it is not always diagnostic in the setting of lymphoma, infection, or immunologic causes. It also carries with it the risk of pneumothorax. Biopsies are also complicated by the fact that many lesions have necrotic components to them. If the necrotic portions are sampled, the results often prove to be nondiagnostic.

Thoracoscopy and **video-assisted thoracoscopy** have become more commonly used modalities for the diagnosis and, if necessary, excision of cavitary lung lesions. They have largely replaced traditional open thoracotomy. They are useful when all other investigative modalities have proved unsuccessful and the clinical situation warrants definitive diagnosis. The location and accessibility of the lesion via the various options often determine the initial procedure of choice.

CONCLUSION

The approach to cavitary lung lesions is one that is initiated by the thorough analysis of the available CXRs with careful consideration of the clinical context within which they were obtained. The differential diagnosis for these lesions is broad and includes infectious, neoplastic, immunologic, congenital, and iatrogenic etiologies. Wall thickness, lesion location, and the distinction between focal and diffuse disease are particularly important radiographic characteristics. The acuity or chronicity of the illness in question is vitally important to the distinction between the benign and the malignant. The presence of a comorbid disease or therapeutic intervention that may cause immunocompromise is an essential historic detail to obtain. The classic presentations of the diseases above may be mimicked by other disease processes presenting in atypical fashion. There are several potential complications inherent to the presence of a cavitary lung lesion, including superinfection, fungus balls, hemoptysis/bleeding, and pneumothorax. If diagnosis is not apparent after routine and specialized radiologic and lab workup, there are several invasive modalities that may provide definitive etiologic confirmation.

KEY POINTS TO REMEMBER

- Cavities are essentially "holes in the lung" with various characteristic changes in the surrounding parenchyma. These surrounding changes are what help elucidate the etiology of the lesions.
- Bronchogenic carcinoma may lead to cavitation in two separate ways: The tumor itself may undergo central necrosis as it outgrows or thromboses off its blood supply, or a cavity my appear distal to the neoplasm as a result of obstructive pneumonitis and/or abscess formation.
- It is worthwhile to search for head and neck primary disease in men and gynecological (i.e., cervical) disease in women in the setting of cavitary metastasis with unknown primary.
- The appearance of the wall of pulmonary cavities is helpful in deciding whether they are malignant. Features to note are the wall thickness and contour.

REFERENCES AND SUGGESTED READINGS

Bragg DG, Freundlich IM. Cysts and cavities of the lung. In: *A radiographic approach to diseases of the chest,* 2nd ed. Baltimore: Williams & Wilkins, 1997.

Chaudhuri MR. Cavitary pulmonary metastases. *Thorax* 1970;25:375–381.

Chaudhuri MR. Primary pulmonary cavitating carcinomas. *Thorax* 1973;28:354–366.

Freundlich IM. *Pulmonary masses, cysts and cavities: a radiologic approach.* Chicago: Year Book, 1981.

Goo JM, Im JG. CT of tuberculosis and nontuberculous mycobacterial infections. *Radiol Clin North Am* 2002;40(1):73–81.

Gurney JW. Determining the likelihood of malignancy in solitary pulmonary nodules with Bayesian analysis. *Radiology* 1993;186:405.

Kazerooni EA, Gross BH. Infections in the immunocompromised host. In: *Cardiopulmonary imaging.* Philadelphia: Lippincott Williams & Wilkins, 2004.

Lillington GA. Cavitary and cystic lesions. In: *A diagnostic approach to chest diseases: differential diagnoses based on roentgenographic patterns,* 3rd ed. Baltimore: Williams & Wilkins, 1987.

Nishimura K, Oguri S, Itoh H. Cystic and cavitary lung disorders. In: Sperber M, ed. *Radiologic diagnosis of chest disease,* 2nd ed. London: Springer, 2001.

Reed JC. Multiple lucent lesions. In: *Chest radiology: plain film patterns and differential diagnoses,* 3rd ed. St. Louis: Mosby-Year Book, 1991.

Reed JC. Solitary localized lucent defect. In: *Chest radiology: plain film patterns and differential diagnoses,* 3rd ed. St. Louis: Mosby–Year Book, 1991.

Ryu JH, Swenson SJ. Cystic and cavitary lung diseases: focal and diffuse. *Mayo Clin Proc* 2003;78:744–752.

Stevens DA. Coccidioidomycosis. *N Engl J Med* 1995;332(16):1077–1082.

Sundar KM, Gosselin MV, Chung HL, Cahill BC. Pulmonary Langerhans cell histiocytosis: emerging concepts in pathobiology, radiology, and clinical evolution of disease. *Chest* 2003;123(5):1673–1683.

Tan BB, Flaherty KR, Kazerooni EA, Iannettoni MD. The solitary pulmonary nodule. *Chest* 2003;123:89S–96S.

Toomes H, Delpendahl A, Manke HG, et al. The coin lesion of the lung: a review of 955 resected coin lesions. *Cancer* 1983;51:534.

Tuddenheim WJ. Glossary of terms for thoracic radiology: recommendations of the nomenclature committee of the Fleischner Society. *AJR Am J Roentgenol* 1984;143:509–517.

Vourtsi A, Gouliamos A, Moulopoulos L, et al. CT appearance of solitary and multiple cystic and cavitary lung lesions. *Eur Radiol* 2001;11:612–622.

Woodring JH, Fried AM. Significance of wall thickness in solitary cavities of the lung: a follow-up study. *AJR Am J Roentgenol* 1983;140:473–474.

Woodring JH, Fried AM, Chuang VP. Solitary cavities of the lung: diagnostic implications of cavity wall thickness. *AJR Am J Roentgenol* 1980;135:1269–1271.

Wright FW. Cavitation. In: *Radiology of the chest and related conditions.* New York: Taylor and Francis, 2002.

Diseases of the Mediastinum

Audreesh Banerjee and
Raghu Tadikamalla

INTRODUCTION

The mediastinum is located at the center of the thoracic cavity. The thoracic inlet, a bony rim created by the first ribs and clavicles that protects the vessels, airway, and esophagus, forms its superior border. Inferiorly, the mediastinum is bordered by the diaphragm, and laterally by the pleural cavities. The structures within the mediastinum give rise to multiple pathologies, which are more easily assessed based on their location within the mediastinum.

The mediastinum can be divided into anterior, posterior, and middle portions based on anatomic structures in the thorax. The **anterior** mediastinum is the area between the sternum anteriorly and the heart and brachiocephalic vessels posteriorly. It contains the thymus gland, fat, and lymph nodes. The **middle** mediastinum is bordered by the pericardial sac and extends superiorly to the fourth thoracic vertebra. The middle mediastinum contains the heart, pericardium, ascending and transverse aorta, brachiocephalic vessels, superior vena cava (SVC), main pulmonary arteries and veins, trachea, bronchi, and lymph nodes. The **posterior** mediastinum is bordered anteriorly by the heart and posteriorly by the thoracic vertebra. It contains the descending thoracic aorta, the esophagus, the azygous vein, autonomic ganglia and nerves, inferior vena cava, lymph nodes, and fat.

PNEUMOMEDIASTINUM

Pneumomediastinum is defined as the presence of air in the mediastinum, outside of the normal confines of the respiratory tract. A pneumomediastinum is never ignored and always needs to be explained.

Spontaneous pneumomediastinum occurs most often in young men. It may be the result of straining against a closed glottis or a sudden increase in lung volume causing elevated alveolar pressures with subsequent alveolar rupture. Alveolar rupture leads to the accumulation of air in the interstitial space (also known as pulmonary interstitial emphysema), which tracks back along the bronchial tree to the hilum of the lung. The air then accumulates in the mediastinum.

Causes of pneumomediastinum include vigorous coughing, vomiting, or exercising; localized airway obstruction with a ball-valve effect leading to localized hyperinflation; and mechanical ventilation in patients with high alveolar pressures. Mechanically ventilated patients at risk for pneumomediastinum are those with abnormal airway parenchyma, high tidal volumes, high levels of positive end-expiratory pressure, and who are synchronizing poorly with the ventilator.

Patients with spontaneous pneumomediastinum usually **present with substernal pain** that is often pleuritic in nature and radiates to the neck or back. Patients may also experience dyspnea, dysphagia, odynophagia, and dysphonia. Air in the subcutaneous tissues of the neck can cause a high-pitched and nasal voice. Patients with pneumomediastinum may also present with **Hamman's sign,** a crunching or clicking sound heard over the precordium that is synchronous with the heartbeat. On chest x-ray (CXR), a thin radiolucent stripe is seen along a mediastinal focal plane, commonly at the left heart border.

Most patients with pneumomediastinum are not acutely ill and need only **supportive care,** although decompensation can occur very rapidly. Patients with pneumomediastinum **associated with mechanical ventilation** are at risk for life-threatening tension pneumomediastinum, or related tension pneumothorax, and must be managed aggressively. CXRs should be checked frequently and pneumothoraces managed in a timely fashion with chest tube insertion.

MEDIASTINITIS

Mediastinitis refers to infection in the mediastinum and has multiple causes, including extension of infection from the sternum, lungs, retroperitoneum, or oropharynx. **Hemorrhagic mediastinitis** is a complication of inhalational anthrax.

Descending necrotizing mediastinitis is the result of oropharyngeal infections that infiltrate the cervical lymph nodes and extend down the prevertebral or visceral space into the mediastinum. These infections tend to be mixed aerobic and anaerobic infections. CT scans should be obtained for any severe neck infections, as descending necrotizing mediastinitis requires rapid diagnosis and treatment, with aggressive surgical drainage and prolonged antibiotic therapy.

Mediastinitis may occur by **direct extension** of necrotizing pneumonias, or from extension of pancreatitis into the mediastinum from the retroperitoneum. These patients require surgical drainage and debridement along with appropriate antibiotic therapy.

Granulomatous mediastinitis results from infection with *Histoplasma capsulatum, Mycobacterium tuberculosis,* and other fungi or mycobacteria. Necrotic lymph nodes coalesce and create a single large mass that incites a fibrotic response. This process causes encapsulation and a mediastinal granuloma. The most common area for this mass to develop is the right paratracheal area.

Broncholithiasis is the presence of calcified lymph nodes within the bronchi. Granulomatous involvement of mediastinal lymph nodes may result in calcified lymph nodes, which then erode into the tracheobronchial tree, forming broncholiths. The condition is often asymptomatic but can present as bronchial obstruction or hemoptysis owing to bleeding within the bronchi. Occasionally, patients expectorate the broncholiths. Broncholiths often have to be removed surgically if they result in symptoms.

Fibrosing mediastinitis may be thought of as the most severe end of a spectrum of involvement of the mediastinum by granulomatous diseases. It is caused by the proliferation of collagen and fibrous tissue within the mediastinum and is commonly believed to be the result of an abnormal immunologic response to infection with *H. capsulatum* or *M. tuberculosis*. It can be a benign condition, but symptoms occur when mediastinal structures are compressed. Patients can develop SVC syndrome from compression in the right peritracheal area, esophageal obstruction, pulmonary venous congestion, or tracheobronchial occlusion.

Patients are usually managed symptomatically (stenting open of vessels and airways), but the disease is often relentlessly progressive, and outcomes are usually poor.

MEDIASTINAL MASSES

Mediastinal pathology presenting as a mass is the most common form of mediastinal disease seen in clinical practice. **Mediastinal masses** may be benign or malignant. They can occur in all compartments of the mediastinum, but certain masses tend to occur in specific mediastinal compartments, making the differential diagnosis of mediastinal masses important (Table 30-1). Masses can be asymptomatic or cause **local symptoms** due to compression of or impingement on thoracic structures. These include (but are not limited to) dyspnea, dysphagia, odynophagia and dysphonia, hoarseness, neurologic fallout secondary to spinal cord compression, diaphragmatic paralysis, Horner's syndrome, and SVC syndrome. **Systemic symptoms** (e.g., fever, chills, anorexia, weight loss, and malaise) may also occur.

Anterior Mediastinal Masses

The anterior mediastinum contains the thymus gland, fat, and lymph nodes. Half of all mediastinal tumors are found in the anterior mediastinum, and anterior mediasti-

TABLE 30-1. DIFFERENTIAL DIAGNOSIS OF MEDIASTINAL MASSES

Locations of mediastinal masses		
Anterior	**Middle**	**Posterior**
Thymoma	Pericardial cyst	Neuroenteric cyst
Thymolipoma	Cardiac tumor	Nerve sheath tumor
Thymic carcinoma	Bronchogenic cyst	Neurilemmoma
Thymic carcinoid	Enterogenic cyst	Neurofibroma
Thymic cyst	Lymphoma	Neurogenic fibrosarcoma
Germ cell tumor	Cardiac aneurysm	Ganglioneuroma
Teratoma		Ganglioneuroblastoma
Seminoma		Neuroblastoma
Goiter		Preganglionic tumor
Thyroid carcinoma		
Parathyroid adenoma		
Lymphoma		
Castleman's disease		

Adapted with permission from Kaiser LR, Putnam JB. The mediastinum: overview, anatomy, and diagnostic approach. In: Fishman AP, Elias JA, Fishman JA, et al., eds. *Fishman's manual of pulmonary diseases and disorders*, 3rd ed. New York: McGraw-Hill, 2002:521–534.

nal tumors are most likely to be malignant. The so-called **terrible Ts** are used as a mnemonic (of sorts) to remember the most common anterior mediastinal masses. They include thymic tumors, thyroid masses, teratomas (and other germ cell tumors), and T-cell lymphomas.

Thymic Masses

Thymomas are a common tumor in the anterior mediastinum. They are classified as lymphocytic, epithelial, or spindle cell depending on the predominant cell type. Thymomas look like solid encapsulated lesions on CT scanning but can have cystic, necrotic, or hemorrhagic areas. Approximately one-third of thymomas invade the pleura, pericardium, or lung. Thymomas are usually discovered incidentally, although one-third of patients have symptoms, predominantly cough and dyspnea. Patients with thymomas also present with or develop myasthenia gravis in 30–50% of cases. These patients also can have pure red cell aplasia and hypogammaglobulinemia. Diagnosis is usually made by CT scanning, although MRI can be used if vascular invasion by a thymoma is suspected. Therapy is usually complete surgical resection. If resection is not possible or the disease is metastatic, patients are treated with a combination of chemotherapy and radiation.

Thymic carcinomas are aggressive epithelial malignancies found in the anterior mediastinum. They are classified into low- and high-grade histologic types, with squamous cell carcinoma and lymphoepitheliomalike variants being the most common. Thymic carcinomas typically appear in middle-aged men. These carcinomas present with pain and cough and occasionally constitutional symptoms such as fatigue, anorexia, and weight loss. Patients do not typically develop myasthenia gravis or the other paraneoplastic syndromes seen with thymomas. Some patients develop SVC syndrome. On CT scans, thymic carcinomas appear as a larger, firm, infiltrating mass, with multiple areas of cystic change and necrosis. Few of these tumors are encapsulated, and pleural or pericardial effusions are common. Complete surgical resection is the preferred treatment if infiltration or metastases have not occurred. If thymic carcinomas have infiltrated, combination chemotherapy and radiation are used with some success.

Thymic carcinoid tumors are similar to carcinoid tumors at other sites. They are commonly seen in middle age and are associated with Cushing's syndrome or the multiple endocrine neoplasia syndrome. Thymic carcinoid tumors metastasize frequently. These tumors appear as large, lobulated, invasive masses in the anterior mediastinum and can have areas of hemorrhage and necrosis. They are highly resistant to chemotherapy and radiation, and surgical resection is the treatment of choice.

Thymolipomas are rare benign tumors of the thymus gland. They grow slowly and are commonly seen in young adults. They appear as large fatty tumors in the mediastinum. They are treated with surgical resection.

Thymic cysts are also rare benign tumors that can be congenital or acquired. The congenital forms are usually remnants of the thymopharyngeal duct, whereas the acquired tumors are often associated with inflammation. They are usually surgically resected.

Thymic hyperplasia is a benign condition and results from massive thymic enlargement. It is a large bulky tumor and is commonly seen in young boys. It can occur after treatment of other malignancies and after recovery from systemic disease.

Germ Cell Tumors

Germ cell tumors are responsible for **15% of all anterior mediastinal masses** in adults. They are thought to originate from primitive germ cells that fail to migrate properly during embryonic development. They can be benign or malignant and are usually diagnosed in young adults. Malignant germ cell tumors are more common in men and can be associated with production of AFP and beta-hCG. Germ cell tumors are classified by cell type.

Benign teratomas are the most common mediastinal germ cell tumors. They contain tissue from the primitive germ layers (ectoderm, mesoderm, and endoderm). Tissue from at least two of these layers must be present in a teratoma. The ectodermal tissues usually predominate and can include skin, hair, sweat glands, sebaceous material, and toothlike structures. Mesodermal tissues include fat, cartilage, smooth muscle, and bone, whereas endodermal tissues may contain respiratory and intestinal epithelium. Mature teratomas are benign and histologically well differentiated. Immature teratomas contain fetal tissue and can become malignant, metastasize, and recur. Teratomas usually do not cause symptoms but can cause dyspnea and cough by compressing surrounding organs. Occasionally, a teratoma can rupture into the airway and cause expectoration of hair. These tumors are diagnosed by CXR and CT, where they appear as well-defined round and lobulated masses in the anterior mediastinum. Approximately one-fourth of teratomas have bone or teeth in them, which are easily seen on CXR. Teratomas are usually surgically resected.

Mediastinal seminomas represent 25–50% of malignant mediastinal germ cell tumors. They occur predominantly in young men between the ages of 20 and 40 yrs and present with symptoms such as substernal pain, dysphagia, weakness, cough, fever, gynecomastia (the result of beta-hCG secretion), and weight loss. These tumors are rare in women with normal ovaries. These tumors appear as bulky, lobulated heterogeneous masses in the anterior mediastinum. Patients with a mediastinal seminoma need a testicular exam to exclude a primary genitourinary seminoma that has metastasized to the mediastinum. Localized tumors are treated with resection followed by chemotherapy, whereas tumors that spread beyond the mediastinum require chemotherapy.

Nonseminomatous germ cell tumors are a diverse group of tumors that include embryonal cell carcinomas, endodermal sinus tumors, choriocarcinomas, and mixed germ cell tumors with heterogeneous cellular components. They commonly affect young men and present with chest pain, cough, hemoptysis, fever, and weight loss. Patients can also develop gynecomastia. AFP and beta-hCG levels are elevated in these patients. High AFP levels suggest an endodermal sinus tumor or embryonal carcinoma. On CT, these tumors usually appear as large irregular masses in the anterior mediastinum with central necrosis, cyst formation, and hemorrhage. They can invade adjacent structures and metastasize. They are treated with chemotherapy and surgical resection. Nonseminomatous germ cell tumors carry a poor prognosis.

Thyroid Masses

Mediastinal goiters can extend into all compartments of the mediastinum but are seen most commonly in the anterior mediastinum. They are usually benign and found incidentally. Patients are usually euthyroid and present with symptoms such as local neck fullness, choking, stridor, and dysphagia. Mediastinal goiters appear as encapsulated heterogeneous lobulated tumors that connect to the cervical thyroid. Surgical resection is the treatment of choice.

Parathyroid adenomas are discussed here owing to their intimate relationship to the thyroid gland. They occur in the mediastinum in 20% of cases and can cause hypercalcemia (with or without related symptoms). They appear as small, encapsulated round structures and can occasionally be confused with lymph nodes on CT scan. In these cases, MRI is helpful in making the diagnosis.

Mediastinal Lymphomas

Primary mediastinal lymphomas are the most common mediastinal neoplasms and can be found in any mediastinal compartment but are most common in the anterior mediastinum. Approximately 10% of all lymphomas in adults originate in the mediastinum and can be of both the Hodgkin's and non-Hodgkin's types. Treatment for lymphomas depends on the stage, histologic subtype, and extent of disease.

Hodgkin's disease is the most common form of mediastinal lymphoma. The nodular sclerosing subtype most commonly affects the anterior mediastinum. Lymphoma is seen most often in young women and presents with fever, pruritus, night sweats, and weight loss. Patients can also develop symptoms of local compression such as pain, stridor, and SVC syndrome. Enlarged thoracic lymph nodes are seen on CT.

Non-Hodgkin's lymphoma also frequently affects the mediastinum. It is more common in males and whites and affects all age groups. Most patients present with advanced disease, constitutional symptoms, and generalized lymphadenopathy visible on CT. Large B-cell lymphomas affect females more often than males. These lymphomas tend to grow rapidly and can cause acute symptoms, including SVC syndrome. Lymphoblastic lymphoma is an aggressive high-grade lymphoma that affects young males and can progress to acute lymphoblastic leukemia.

Middle Mediastinal Masses

Most of the masses of the middle mediastinum are benign lesions that are congenital cysts of the foregut. However, lymphomas, cardiac and vascular tumors, myxomas, sarcomas, and neural crest tumors can all be seen in the middle mediastinum and are important to exclude before making the final diagnosis of benign mass.

Bronchogenic Cysts

Bronchogenic cysts comprise more than half of all mediastinal cysts. They are lined with respiratory epithelium and contain bronchial glands and cartilaginous plates. Bronchogenic cysts can become filled with serous fluid, mucus, pus, blood, or "milk of calcium." These cysts are usually asymptomatic, although they can cause compression of the airway and present with cough, dyspnea, and localized wheezing. Bronchogenic cysts can become infected and rupture into the bronchus, pericardium, or pleura. On CXR, they appear as spherical, homogeneous well-marginated masses, which sometimes have air–fluid levels. These cysts are usually surgically resected.

Enterogenous Cysts

These cysts arise from the dorsal foregut and are lined by alimentary epithelium. They may contain gastric mucosa and pancreatic tissue. The most common kind of enterogenous cyst is the **esophageal duplication cyst,** which attaches to the esophageal wall or is located in the esophagus. Secretion of gastric and pancreatic enzymes can cause the cyst to hemorrhage or rupture. These cysts look similar to bronchogenic cysts but can be calcified. Because these cysts can become infected, they should be surgically removed.

Pericardial Cysts

Pericardial cysts are uncommon and usually asymptomatic. They are lined with mesothelial cells that arise from the pericardium. These cysts rarely cause cardiac compression and hemodynamic compromise. They appear as well-marginated spherical or teardrop masses around the heart and can be followed clinically. They are only removed if they are symptomatic.

Posterior Mediastinal Masses

Posterior mediastinal masses are usually neurogenic in origin and include an array of benign and malignant tumors.

Neuroenteric Cysts

Neuroenteric cysts contain both neural and enteric tissue. They tend to form in the posterior mediastinum above the main carina, where the foregut and the notochord are closely apposed during embryogenesis. These cysts are associated with vertebral anomalies such as spina bifida, scoliosis, hemivertebra, and vertebral fusion. They are more common in males and are usually discovered in infancy. These cysts appear similar to bronchogenic and esophageal duplication cysts except for their different location.

Nerve Sheath Tumors

Benign nerve sheath tumors are slow growing and comprise the majority of posterior mediastinal masses. They are usually asymptomatic and discovered incidentally on CXR. Most benign nerve sheath tumors are **neurilemmomas** or **schwannomas,** which are firm, encapsulated masses consisting of groups of Schwann cells. Neurofibromas are the other form of benign nerve sheath tumor and are nonencapsulated, friable masses. Multiple neurofibromas are associated with **von Recklinghausen's syndrome (neurofibromatosis).** On CT, nerve sheath tumors appear as sharply marginated spherical or lobulated masses in the paraspinal region. Approximately 10% of tumors grow through the intervertebral foramina and extend into the spinal canal, resulting in a dumbbell or hourglass shape. These tumors can also cause vertebral erosion. They are treated with surgical resection when possible.

Malignant nerve sheath tumors are a group of spindle cell sarcomas common in the posterior mediastinum. They include malignant neurofibromas, malignant schwannomas, and neurogenic fibrosarcomas. These tumors occur with an incidence of approximately 5% in patients with neurofibromatosis. Patients usually present with pain and nerve deficits. Although the treatment of choice is surgical resection, patients with unresectable tumors are treated with chemotherapy and radiation.

Ganglion-Associated Tumors

Preganglionic tumors are benign tumors that arise from sympathetic and parasympathetic cells. They are biologically inactive.

Autonomic ganglionic tumors arise from neuronal cells, rather than from the nerve sheathes, and include ganglioneuromas, neuroblastomas, and ganglioneuroblastomas.

Ganglioneuromas are benign encapsulated tumors that are composed of one or more mature ganglionic cells. They appear as homogenous, well-marginated, oblong encapsulated masses on CT and are asymptomatic in 50% of cases. Symptoms are usually related to compression of nerves or extension into the spinal canal. MRI can be used to assess for intraspinal extension. These tumors are usually surgically resected.

Neuroblastomas are composed of small round cells arranged in pseudorosettes. They are not encapsulated and can have areas of hemorrhage, cystic degeneration, or necrosis. Most of these tumors occur in children aged <5 yrs. These patients tend to present with metastatic disease and have pain, neurologic deficits, Horner's syndrome, and respiratory distress. The tumors can produce catecholamines and vasoactive intestinal peptides that can cause HTN, flushing, and diarrhea. On CT, patients with neuroblastoma have an elongated paraspinous mass that can impinge on nearby structures and cause skeletal damage. Up to 80% of these tumors display various types of calcification. Patients with limited-stage neuroblastomas are treated with surgical resection, whereas patients with advanced stage are treated with chemotherapy and radiation in addition to surgical resection.

Ganglioneuroblastomas have features of both neuroblastomas and ganglioneuromas. These are the least common type of neurogenic tumor. Symptoms are related to compression and intraspinal extension as well as metastasis. Management is similar to that of neuroblastomas.

MEDIASTINAL LYMPHADENOPATHY

Introduction

The lymphatic system of the lungs consists of lymphatic channels that run along the pleura, within the peribronchovascular connective tissue, and within the interlobular connective tissue. Lymph drains centripetally to the mediastinal and hilar lymph nodes, and it is these central, larger lymphatics that are usually visible radiographically, especially when involved by pathologic processes. Abnormal appearance of these lymph nodes may represent pulmonary disease or disease of the lymphatic system, which itself may be primary or secondary.

Nodal Anatomy

Mediastinal lymph nodes can be anatomically classified, the utility of which is primarily for the staging of lung cancers. As a general rule, lymph nodes communicate with adjacent nodal groups, and lymph flows from lateral to medial and then superiorly within the mediastinum.

Hilar nodes drain to carinal nodes, which then drain to paratracheal nodes. The paratracheal nodes drain into the tracheobronchial nodes and then via the bronchomediastinal ducts into the venous circulation. Lymph nodes in the anterior mediastinum as well as those around the esophagus and aorta communicate with the carinal and paratracheal nodes.

Radiographic Assessment

Enlarged mediastinal lymph nodes can often be detected as opacities or irregularities of the mediastinal contour on posteroanterior and lateral CXR. Similarly, **hilar lymphadenopathy** can be seen as prominence and lobulation of the hila unilaterally or bilaterally. Although plain radiography can help identify gross lymphadenopathy, it is limited in its ability to evaluate more subtle changes. Additionally, discernment and characterization of individual lymph nodes and their anatomic position are inexact without further diagnostic studies. Other etiologies of an abnormal mediastinal contour, such as abnormal mediastinal vessels, can be difficult to distinguish on CXR alone.

The spatial resolution that can be achieved with CT scans has made them useful in assessing the nature of lymphadenopathy in the chest. Mediastinal lymph nodes can be well visualized without IV contrast material, whereas the smaller lymph nodes of the hila often require IV contrast administration to be discerned from vascular structures.

Abnormal lymph nodes are often only distinguished by their increased size. CT scanning is limited in that it only views structures in the transverse plane. Thus, lymph nodes that have their long axis oriented vertically may appear smaller than those lying with their long axis in the plane of the CT cuts. As a result, **CT criteria** for enlarged mediastinal lymph nodes are based on the short axis diameter of the node. **Mediastinal** lymph nodes should be considered enlarged if their **short axis diameter** is **>10 mm.** The only exception is the **subcarinal** group of lymph nodes, which are considered enlarged only if their short axis diameter is **>13 mm.**

Specific Patterns of Mediastinal Lymphadenopathy

Although lymphadenopathy is classically thought of as being associated with certain processes such as lung cancer, lymphoma, infections, and sarcoidosis, many diseases that affect the lungs diffusely can result in abnormal lymph nodes. For instance, lymphadenopathy is found in two-thirds of patients with idiopathic pulmonary fibrosis, 40–70% of patients with collagen vascular diseases, and 50% of patients with hypersensitivity pneumonitis. It can also be seen in other lung diseases, such as bronchiolitis obliterans with organizing pneumonia and lymphocytic interstitial pneumonitis. Patients with cystic fibrosis, asbestosis, and cardiogenic pulmonary edema also frequently demonstrate lymphadenopathy.

Calcification of lymph nodes can be seen on both plain radiographs and CT scans. Dense, homogenous calcifications suggest previous granulomatous infection such as histoplasmosis or TB. So-called eggshell calcifications suggest silicosis or coal workers' pneumoconiosis but can also be seen in TB and sarcoidosis.

In most cases, lymph nodes do not enhance on CT scans after injection of IV contrast material. Postcontrast enhancement can be seen in Castleman's disease or with highly vascular metastases, such as thyroid cancer or melanoma. Rim-enhancing nodes are often seen in mycobacterial and fungal infections.

Lung Cancer Staging

Lymph node involvement is crucial in the staging of **non–small cell lung cancer.** Both the presence or absence of lymphadenopathy and its extent significantly alter the prognosis and treatment options for malignancy. The staging system compiled by the American Joint Committee on Cancer stages cancers according to their tumor-node-metastases (TNM) designations, where the N refers to lymph node involvement.

Clinical staging refers to an estimate of the extent of disease that is reached through noninvasive testing. This testing usually involves **CT scanning** of the chest to evaluate pathologic lymphadenopathy. The finding of enlarged lymph nodes as defined above can reflect metastases or reactive changes. This can be further assessed with **PET scanning.** Additionally, CT scanning is not perfectly sensitive for nodal metastases, as lymph nodes harboring micrometastases can be normal in size. Controversy exists regarding the extent to which surgical techniques should be used to achieve accurate pathologic staging.

N0 signifies the absence of nodal metastases. **N1** nodes include subsegmental, segmental, lobar, interlobar, and hilar regional nodal groups (from peripheral to central anatomic location). These nodes lie distal to the mediastinal pleural reflection on the ipsilateral side of the tumor and thus are contained within the visceral pleura. **N2** nodes include the ipsilateral mediastinal and subcarinal regional nodal groups. The **N3** designation reflects involvement of contralateral thoracic nodes or the ipsilateral scalene or supraclavicular nodes. Axillary or cervical lymphadenopathy is classified as **M1** disease.

The **distinction between N2 and N3 nodal involvement** has tremendous therapeutic relevance. Involvement of N2 nodes in the absence of distant metastases is staged as IIIA disease. Stage IIIA disease can be treated with surgery in addition to chemotherapy and radiation in selected cases. Patients with involvement of N3 nodes have at least IIIB disease and generally are not surgical candidates.

KEY POINTS TO REMEMBER

- The superior border of the mediastinum is formed by the thoracic inlet. Its inferior border is formed by the diaphragm. The lateral borders are formed by the pleural reflections.
- Pneumomediastinum, which always needs to be explained, is defined as the presence of air in the mediastinum outside of the normal confines of the respiratory tract.
- Half of all mediastinal tumors are found in the anterior mediastinum, and anterior mediastinal tumors are most likely to be malignant. The "terrible Ts" include thy-

mic tumors, thyroid masses, teratomas (and other germ cell tumors), and T-cell lymphomas.

- CT criteria for enlarged mediastinal lymph nodes are based on the short axis diameter of the node. Mediastinal lymph nodes should be considered enlarged if their short axis diameter is >10 mm with the exception of the subcarinal group of lymph nodes, which are considered enlarged only if the short axis diameter is >13 mm.

REFERENCES AND SUGGESTED READINGS

Allen MS. Presentation and management of benign mediastinal teratomas. *Chest Surg Clin N Am* 2002,12(4):659–664.

Balkan ME, Oktar GL, Oktar MA. Descending necrotizing mediastinitis: a case report and review of the literature. *Int Surg* 2001;86(1):62–66.

DeCamp MM. Congenital cysts of the mediastinum: bronchopulmonary foregut anomalies. In: Fishman AP, Elias JA, Fishman JA, et al., eds. *Fishman's pulmonary diseases and disorders*. Vol. 2. 3rd ed. New York: McGraw-Hill, 1997:1499–1507.

Graeber GM, Tamim W. Current status of the diagnosis and treatment of thymoma. *Semin Thorac Cardiovasc Surg* 2000;12(4):268–277.

Hainsworth JD. Diagnosis, staging, and clinical characteristics of the patient with mediastinal germ cell carcinoma. *Chest Surg Clin N Am* 2002;12(4):665–672.

Kaiser LR, Putnam JB. The mediastinum: overview, anatomy, and diagnostic approach. In: Fishman AP, Elias JA, Fishman JA, et al., eds. *Fishman's manual of pulmonary diseases and disorders*, 3rd ed. New York: McGraw-Hill, 2002:521–534.

Marchevsky AM. Mediastinal tumors of peripheral nervous system origin. *Semin Diagn Pathol* 1999;16(1):65–78.

Markman M. Diagnosis and management of superior vena cava syndrome. *Cleve Clin J Med* 1999;66(1):59–61.

Musani AI, Sterman DH. Tumors of the mediastinum, pleura, chest wall and diaphragm. In: Glassroth J, King TE, eds. *Baum's textbook of pulmonary diseases*, 7th ed. Philadelphia: Lippincott Williams & Wilkins, 2004:883–912.

Putnam JB. The mediastinum: overview, anatomy, and diagnostic approach. In: Fishman AP, Elias JA, Fishman JA, et al., eds. *Fishman's pulmonary diseases and disorders*. Vol. 2. 3rd ed., New York: McGraw-Hill, 1997:1469–1484.

Ritter JH, Wick MR. Primary carcinomas of the thymus gland. *Semin Diagn Pathol* 1999;16(1):18–31.

Roberts JR, Kaiser LA. Acquired lesions of the mediastinum: benign and malignant. In: Fishman AP, Elias JA, Fishman JA, et al., eds. *Fishman's pulmonary diseases and disorders*. Vol. 2. 3rd ed. New York: McGraw-Hill, 1997:1508–1537.

Rossi SE, McAdams HP, Rosado-de-Christenson ML, et al. Fibrosing mediastinitis. *Radiographics* 2001;21(3):737–757.

Strollo DC, Rosado-de-Christenson ML, Jett JR. Primary mediastinal tumors: part I. Tumors of the middle and posterior mediastinum. *Chest* 1997;112(5):1344–1357.

Strollo DC, Rosado-de-Christenson ML, Jett JR. Primary mediastinal tumors: part II. Tumors of the middle and posterior mediastinum. *Chest* 1997;112(5):1344–1357.

Suster S, Moran CA. Neuroendocrine neoplasms of the mediastinum. *Am J Clin Pathol* 2001;115[Suppl]:S17–S27.

Wright CD. Nonneoplastic disorders of the mediastinum. In: Fishman AP, Elias JA, Fishman JA, et al., eds. *Fishman's pulmonary diseases and disorders*. Vol. 2. 3rd ed. New York: McGraw-Hill, 1997:1485–1498.

Wright CD, Mathisen DJ. Mediastinal tumors: diagnosis and treatment. *World J Surg* 2001;25(2):204–209.

31 Pulmonary Consultative Problems in Specific Patient Populations

Daniel M. Goodenberger

INTRODUCTION

The focus of this chapter is on problems that are peculiar to certain patient populations seen by pulmonary consultants.

SURGERY AND TRAUMA

The pulmonary consultant is asked to see patients on general, thoracic, and cardiac surgical services, most often for investigation of pulmonary infection, investigation and treatment of pulmonary thromboembolic disease, and inability to liberate the patient from mechanical ventilation. The principles for the first two are no different than those covered elsewhere in this book, and coverage of the last topic is beyond the scope of this book. There are, however, several specific problems and syndromes that recur with varying frequency.

Flail Chest and Pulmonary Contusion

Flail chest refers to the **mechanically unstable thorax** that is **due to blunt trauma,** most frequently from motor vehicle collision and severe falls. Instability and paradoxical thoracic movement are enhanced by double fractures of multiple ribs, often cited as three or more in sequence. However, the pulmonary problems of flail chest do not occur in isolation, and physiologic circumstances are often worsened by pulmonary contusion and other intrathoracic injuries. Thus, in addition to the risk of respiratory failure due to ineffective ventilation (hypercarbic), the patient may have an increased alveolar-arterial gradient progressing to hypoxemic respiratory failure. Recognition is based on the history and radiographic evidence of thoracic trauma; paradoxical movement (in with inspiration, out with expiration), which may be subtle and overlooked; increasing respiratory distress; and worsening gas exchange. **Treatment** should be **conservative** in most cases. **Pain control** is important; systemic narcotics may have deleterious respiratory effects and can be minimized with the use of intercostal nerve blocks and epidural morphine. The evidence supporting surgical fixation of the flail segment is scant, as is the evidence for prophylactic positive pressure ventilation by ETT (and there is no demonstrable reduction in mortality). Oxygen is administered for hypoxemia. Overt respiratory failure is treated with mechanical ventilation. In some centers, noninvasive positive pressure ventilation by nasal or full-face mask is used to reduce work of breathing when physical signs point to impending respiratory failure, but evidence to support this approach is largely lacking.

Pulmonary contusion may complicate flail chest or it may occur in isolation. It occurs in a significantly large minority of patients with **severe blunt trauma** to the chest. Chest x-ray (CXR) and CT show alveolar infiltrate, which is generally confluent and does not respect lobar boundaries. Appearance of radiographic abnormalities may be delayed for hours. The gas-exchange abnormalities are those of hypoxemia owing to V/Q mismatch, sometimes reaching the severity of true shunt. **Treatment** is **supportive. Oxygen** is administered, **fluid** is given judiciously to avoid increased alveolar edema, and **narcotics** are administered to reduce splinting. **Good-lung-down positioning** may improve oxygenation. In a minority, positive pressure ventilation is required, which may be noninvasive ventilation in mild cases and endotracheal ventilation in the more severely affected, with positive end-expiratory pressure.

Diaphragm Rupture

The most common cause of diaphragmatic rupture is **blunt trauma,** either from a motor vehicle accident or from a severe fall. Most but not all occur on the left side of the chest; this is usually ascribed to protection by the liver on the right. Usually, the diagnosis is made by trauma surgeons before medical or pulmonary consultation. On occasion, however, the diagnosis is obscure before medical input. The history is of blunt trauma, and the picture is usually dominated by other organ system involvement, but occasionally respiratory distress is a presenting symptom. Physical exam may reveal decreased breath sounds on the affected side, bowel sounds on the affected side of the chest, or abnormal abdominal respiratory movements. On occasion, the operator may discover abdominal viscera in the chest while performing tube thoracostomy. CXR abnormality may be limited to an indistinct or elevated hemidiaphragm, pleural effusion, or abnormally high gastric air bubble or colonic gas. Placement of an NG tube may show the tube to be in the left hemithorax. CT exam is generally definitive.

Approximately one-fourth of traumatic diaphragmatic ruptures occur as a result of **penetrating trauma.** In contrast to blunt trauma, these may present months or years after the inciting event, and the presentation may be dominated by bowel obstruction or ischemia. The diagnostic sequence is the same as for diaphragmatic rupture due to blunt trauma. Therapy for both is **surgical repair.**

PULMONARY DISEASE IN PREGNANCY

Asthma

Asthma is among the most common causes for pulmonary consultation in **pregnancy,** complicating approximately 1 of 20 gestations. Consonant with common wisdom, asthma is better, the same, or worse during pregnancy in approximately equal proportions. It is difficult to predict the course during any individual pregnancy, regardless of preconception severity. Maternal asthma is associated with increased prematurity, growth retardation, and cesarean delivery, among other effects. Diagnosis is straightforward and similar to that in the nongravid. Management is likewise similar. After **baseline pulmonary function tests (PFTs),** the patient should be instructed in the measurement of **peak expiratory flow rate** and asked to measure and record it twice daily for the duration of the pregnancy. **Declines of >20%** should be reported promptly to her physician. The patient should also be instructed in **environmental control,** including avoidance of tobacco smoke, animal dander, and dust, as well as any known specific allergens. Skin testing and immunotherapy should not be undertaken during pregnancy, because of the small risk of anaphylaxis. Treatment is similar to that of nonpregnant patients. (See Chap. 9, Asthma, for more information on dosage and administration of the following drugs.) Inhaled selective beta-2 adrenergic agonists may be used for episodic treatment of mild asthma. Metaproterenol has been demonstrated to be safe, and albuterol and terbutaline are also generally considered safe. There is inadequate evidence at present regarding salmeterol, alone or in combination with fluticasone. There is, however, strong evidence that **inhaled beclomethasone** may be used safely on a daily basis for chronic asthma. **Sodium cromolyn** has been demonstrated to be safe. Although nedocromil has not been demonstrated to be safe, animal studies do not suggest teratogenicity. Leukotriene antagonists cannot be recommended for use during pregnancy owing to lack of human data. **Theophylline** may be used during pregnancy, in sustained-release form, to maintain serum levels of 8–12 μg/mL.

The use of **oral corticosteroids** has caused concern principally because of animal data suggesting a causative relationship to midfacial defects (cleft lip). However, there are no human data to support this despite extensive use, and most pulmonary consultants believe the risk of use is far outweighed by the potential for harm to both mother and fetus from uncontrolled asthma. Given that, oral corticosteroid administration is generally managed in the same way as for nonpregnant patients.

Fetal monitoring should be continuous during labor. **Oxytocin** should be used for labor induction; ergonovine, methylergonovine, and F2-alpha prostaglandin analogs may induce bronchospasm. **Fentanyl** should be used in preference to morphine or meperidine for pain relief, as it does not cause histamine release. **Epidural analgesia** is preferred to general anesthesia. When general anesthesia is required, atropine or glycopyrrolate may be used for bronchodilation, and ketamine or halogenated anesthetics are preferred for the same reason.

Pulmonary Edema Syndromes

In the earlier part of the twentieth century, and in much of the developing world, pulmonary edema during pregnancy is often due to valvular heart disease, frequently rheumatic. **Rheumatic mitral stenosis** is the most common valvular lesion and may present for the first time during pregnancy. Pulmonary edema is most likely to occur late in pregnancy or in the peripartum period. Diagnosis by physical exam and CXR may be difficult during pregnancy, but **echocardiography** is highly accurate and should be performed in any woman presenting with pulmonary edema in pregnancy. Management is initially with **diuresis** and **fluid restriction.** Rapid atrial fibrillation must be controlled, and cardioversion may be required. For the patient whose situation is intractable, balloon valvuloplasty may be necessary. Hemodynamic monitoring during delivery is appropriate.

Other valvular lesions are less common. Diagnosis is by a combination of history, exam, and echocardiography. The finding of previously unsuspected **aortic insufficiency** should raise consideration of Marfan's syndrome, and the aortic root should be carefully evaluated, as the risk of dissection is greatly increased.

Tocolytic pulmonary edema is an uncommon complication, usually after ≥ 24 hrs of IV beta-2 sympathomimetic therapy for treatment of premature labor. Treatment consists of discontinuation and diuretic administration.

Toxemia of pregnancy may be accompanied by pulmonary edema, generally immediately postpartum. In addition to general treatment of toxemia, a loop diuretic should be administered.

Peripartum cardiomyopathy may present with pulmonary edema in the last month of pregnancy. The cause remains uncertain. It is more common in older, multiparous, African-American women. **Echocardiography** reveals severe global left ventricular dysfunction and no other cardiac disorders. Treatment during pregnancy includes loop diuretics and digoxin. **ACE inhibitors** are **contraindicated,** and **hydralazine** may be substituted for afterload reduction. **Beta-adrenergic receptor antagonists** may be used as for other forms of heart failure, although it may be preferable to begin after pregnancy is completed owing to potential fetal effects including growth retardation, postpartum apnea, hypotension, and bradycardia. If anticoagulation is considered necessary because of severity of ventricular dysfunction, **heparin** should be used during the last month of pregnancy to avoid the risk of hemorrhage with longer-acting warfarin. Meticulous **fetal and maternal monitoring** is necessary during labor and delivery.

Pulmonary Embolism

The risk of pulmonary thromboembolism is substantially increased during pregnancy. **Risk factors** include prior venous thromboembolism, particularly during pregnancy, prolonged bed rest, cesarean section, and the known genetic and acquired thrombophilia—deficiencies of antithrombin III, protein C, and protein S; mutations of factor V Leiden and prothrombin 20201A; and antiphospholipid antibodies. Diagnosis of deep venous thrombosis and pulmonary embolism may be made substantially more difficult by the pregnancy. An elevated **D-dimer** level is common in pregnancy and therefore **not useful.** ABG abnormalities are neither sensitive nor specific. **Duplex U/S** exam of the leg veins is helpful if positive, but given that approximately 30% of patients with a positive pulmonary angiogram have negative leg venograms, a negative study is not useful. MRI exam of the lower extremities has been espoused by some, but there are insufficient data to support its use. Venography is generally not recommended in pregnant women. If leg studies are nondiagnostic, the clinician must decide on a test for the diagnosis of pulmonary embolism. Many favor **V/Q lung scanning** (with **no ventilation sequence** if the perfusion scan is absolutely normal). The test is easy, and radiation dose to the fetus is low. However, because only a completely normal scan can be considered negatively diagnostic, because the rate of pulmonary embolism in those with near-normal and low-likelihood ratio scans is 16%, and because the ability of clinicians to arrive at a pretest probability is highly variable, the test remains problematic if not normal. For that reason, some clinicians prefer **spiral CT** of the chest using a **pulmonary embolism protocol.** Fetal radiation dose is less than that with V/Q scan, but maternal breast radiation is relatively high. Further studies are required to settle this issue to the satisfaction of all.

Treatment of thromboembolism in pregnancy is generally with **heparin.** Although warfarin is not teratogenic after the first trimester, the prolonged action raises the risk of hemorrhage with uninduced delivery late in pregnancy. For that reason, treatment with IV unfractionated heparin following the standard protocol is generally given for 5 days, followed by bid SC adjusted-dose heparin. Although fewer published experiences are available for consideration, we prefer the use of standard-dose, **low-molecular-weight heparin therapy.** Heparin is discontinued 24 hrs before planned induction or cesarean section; depending on last dose, activity of labor, and other factors, administration of protamine may be considered for unplanned delivery. After successful labor and delivery, standard duration of anticoagulation is completed with warfarin.

Amniotic Fluid Embolism

The syndrome of amniotic fluid embolism is **rare,** and most obstetricians do not encounter it, nor will most consultants. **Risk factors** include older maternal age, tumultuous labor and delivery, cesarean section, uterine laceration, placental abruption, and meconium staining. The presentation is usually that of abrupt cardiorespiratory failure during or shortly after delivery, with shock, hypoxemic respiratory failure, and often DIC. Pulmonary edema becomes radiographically evident within several hours and may progress to ARDS. **Diagnosis is clinical.** The reported retrieval of fetal squames and amniotic debris from the pulmonary circulation by pulmonary artery catheter is not practical. Mortality is high. Management is through **critical care support** with inotropic agents, intubation and mechanical ventilation with high fraction of inspired oxygen and positive end-expiratory pressure, and careful fluid management.

Aspiration (Mendelson's Syndrome)

The large-volume aspiration of stomach contents resulting in acid injury and chemical pneumonitis was described nearly 50 yrs ago. The **major risk factor** is **emergency endotracheal intubation for induction of general anesthesia,** generally for cesarean section. Diagnosis is through the combination of events, hypoxemia and respiratory distress, and diffuse pulmonary infiltrates. **Treatment is supportive,** with supplemental oxygen and mechanical ventilation with PEEP as required. There is no evidence that systemic steroids are useful, and we do not recommend them. Antibiotics should be reserved for documented bacterial infection, which may arise in a sizable minority.

HEMATOLOGIC DISORDERS

Sickle Cell Hemoglobinopathy

The most frequent pulmonary complication of sickle hemoglobinopathy is the **acute chest syndrome.** As with other acute complications, it occurs most frequently in those with **Hgb SS,** less frequently in Hgb SC, and with varying frequency in Hgb S–beta thalassemia. Rarely, under the same circumstances as for crises (high altitude, vigorous exercise), the syndrome may occur in those with Hgb SA. The course may be severe and is the most common cause of death in adults with sickle disease. The acute chest syndrome is a **clinical presentation** comprising chest pain, cough, dyspnea, tachypnea, fever, and new pulmonary infiltrate on CXR. It occurs most commonly in younger adults, who often have a history of one or more prior episodes. Generalized vasoocclusive symptoms precede or accompany the syndrome in more than half. Pneumonia is the cause in approximately one-fifth; the remainder of cases are most likely due to a combination of vasoocclusion with *in situ* thrombosis and bone marrow (fat) embolization associated with bone infarction. Blood cultures should be obtained, although they are infrequently positive. It is often difficult or impossible to sort out the difference between pneumonia and the other causes, although multilobar infiltrates suggest a noninfectious cause. As a result, patients are usually treated both for (community-acquired) pneumonia and vasoocclusive crisis.

When **pulmonary thromboembolism** is suspected, the diagnostic evaluation is very difficult. V/Q scanning does not differentiate *in situ* thrombosis from embolism, and the radiographic contrast used on helical CT is generally considered hazardous in vasoocclusive disease. If noninvasive evaluation of the lower extremities is negative, experience suggests that withholding anticoagulation is not dangerous. Infection from pneumococcus was probably more common before routine immunization, but the spectrum of organisms seems to be similar to that in other populations who have community-acquired pneumonia, including *Haemophilus influenzae, Mycoplasma pneumoniae,* and *Chlamydia pneumoniae.* Consequently, the patients should be **treated,** at least initially, with a **second-generation cephalosporin and macrolide. Treatment for occlusive crisis** includes judicious hydration, oxygen, bronchodilators, and narcotic pain medication. Those who have multiple prior episodes may have developed pulmonary HTN, which should be taken into account. In those who have progressive deterioration despite these measures, many authorities recommend **exchange transfusion** to a target Hgb S <30%. However, the evidence supporting this procedure rather than **simple transfusion** of carefully **cross-matched leukocyte-poor RBCs** to achieve an **Hct of ≥30%** is minimal, and most patients so treated improve. Those who progress to hypoxemic respiratory failure should be intubated and ventilated using the same strategies as for other patients with ARDS. The use of steroids in this setting is not supported by evidence.

On occasion, the consultant is asked to evaluate a patient with sickle cell disease who has chronic pulmonary disease. Most often, there is significant pulmonary restriction, owing to fibrosis and pulmonary HTN, which may be severe. Treatment is symptomatic and supportive, including oxygen for the hypoxemic. There is insufficient evidence to support recommendation of pulmonary vasodilators to those with severe pulmonary HTN.

Bone Marrow and Stem Cell Transplantation

Pulmonary disease after allogeneic marrow and stem cell transplantation is affected by the conditioning regimen (chemotherapy with or without total body irradiation), immunosuppression after transplantation, and chronic graft-versus-host disease (GVHD). **Problems that occur within the first 100 days** include congestive heart failure; bacterial pneumonia (common hospital-acquired organisms plus aspiration owing in part to severe mucositis); fungal infection, particularly with filamentous fungi such as *Aspergillus* sp. and Mucor but also with endemic fungi and Pneumocystis; parasitic infections, particularly Toxoplasmosis; viral infections, particularly respiratory syncytial virus (RSV), followed later by CMV and adenovirus; and idiopathic interstitial-alveolar disease, which may be caused by a combination of radiotherapy, chemotherapy, GVHD, and diffuse alveolar damage. Diffuse alveolar hemorrhage may also occur during this interval.

Other classification systems divide infection in a way similar to that done for solid organ transplantation, and the occurrence of infections roughly parallels that pattern.

The **diagnostic approach,** although relatively stereotyped, should be pursued aggressively. Obtain a **CXR,** and if the anatomic basis of complaints remains obscure, a **chest CT.** If the picture suggests heart failure, obtain an **echocardiogram** and **con-**

sider hemodynamic monitoring. If infection is considered likely, after routine **blood cultures,** proceed rapidly to diagnostic fiber-optic **bronchoscopy.** If posttransfusion platelet counts allow, **transbronchial biopsy** may add to the results of bronchoalveolar lavage. Samples should be sent for bacterial, fungal, and mycobacterial stains and cultures, as well as for viral cultures and PCR. If no diagnosis is made, the most likely diagnosis is ***idiopathic interstitial pneumonia.*** Although open-lung biopsy has been recommended, the added utility is unclear, and it is not routinely done in many centers.

Treatment of fungal infections, including *Pneumocystis*, is as described in Chap. 15, Fungal Pulmonary Infections. **Toxoplasmosis** is generally treated with pyrimethamine and sulfadiazine, with infectious disease consultation. **CMV,** which is increased in seronegative recipients receiving seropositive donation, is treated with ganciclovir, 2.5 mg/kg IV tid, with renal dose adjustment, and IV immunoglobulin, 500 mg every other day. **RSV** is treated with inhaled ribavirin using a small-particle aerosol generator, 6 g/day over 12–18 hrs for 3–7 days. RSV immune globulin is no longer available, but some experts recommend IV immunoglobulin as for CMV. **Adenovirus** and **parainfluenza virus** infections may be treated with inhaled ribavirin as well, although evidence supporting this practice is lacking.

Idiopathic pneumonia and **diffuse alveolar hemorrhage** are customarily treated with corticosteroids but with little evidence of efficacy or information regarding optimal dose.

Respiratory failure requiring mechanical ventilation from any cause has a uniformly **poor outcome,** with ultimate survival of < 3%.

Late complications of hematopoietic transplantation include idiopathic pneumonia; viral infections, particularly CMV; and obliterative bronchiolitis, which is most likely due to chronic GVHD. The onset is insidious, and PFTs show progressive obstruction, starting with tests of small airway function (forced expiratory function 25–75%). Treatment is ineffective, and the course is usually progressive and ultimately fatal.

The pulmonary complications of autologous transplantation are similar to those of allogeneic transplantation. However, CMV and *Toxoplasma* infection occur less frequently, as does obliterative bronchiolitis, and alveolar hemorrhage is more common.

Solid Organ Transplantation

The pulmonary problems following solid organ transplantation (predominantly renal, heart, lung, and liver) are most often **infectious,** in part because there is no pretransplant conditioning regimen. The timing of posttransplant pulmonary infections is customarily divided into three phases, extrapolated from a classic paper dealing with postrenal transplant patients.

Days 1–30

Bacterial infections with *Staphylococcus, Enterobacteriaceae,* and *Pseudomonas* are most common, with other bacteria including *Legionella* being less common. Invasive fungal infection and pneumocystis are unusual.

Days 31–180

The complications are dominated by **opportunistic infections.** These include endemic (histoplasmosis and coccidioidomycosis most often), cryptococcosis, and invasive filamentous fungi, pneumocystis (rate greatly diminished by near-universal prophylaxis), higher bacteria (*Nocardia*), mycobacteria, and viruses. **CMV** is most common in those recipients who are seronegative but are receiving seropositive organs, but prophylaxis has also made major inroads here. Epstein-Barr virus manifests as posttransplant lymphoproliferative disease, which may have onset 2–4 mos after transplant and is treated with reduction of immunosuppression. The diagnostic evaluation is similar to that described for bone marrow transplantation.

Day 180 Onward

Cryptococcus and **mycobacterial disease** continue to occur. **Human herpesvirus-8 infection** may lead to advanced Kaposi's sarcoma. Those requiring chronically high levels of immunosuppression may be at greater risk for these infections. In those who require lower levels of immunosuppression, community-acquired respiratory viruses and community-acquired bacterial pneumonias become more important. Approximately one-third of lung transplant patients develop **chronic obliterative bronchiolitis** similar to that seen in allogeneic marrow transplant, with similar physiology, as a manifestation of chronic graft rejection.

RHEUMATOLOGIC DISEASES

Scleroderma

The lung is frequently involved in scleroderma. The most common manifestation is **pulmonary fibrosis,** which clinically resembles idiopathic pulmonary fibrosis. Physical exam reveals crackles. CXR and CT show peripheral and basilar distribution of interstitial disease, with small lung volumes. PFTs are restrictive, with reduced lung volumes, low DLCO, and exercise oxygen desaturation followed by resting hypoxemia. Many texts recommend performance of high-resolution CT to detect evidence of ground-glass infiltrates, thought to represent alveolitis with a better prognosis. Similarly, bronchoalveolar lavage is often recommended for prognostic purposes, and some authorities recommend lung biopsy. In practice, however, the diagnosis is not often obscure nor is treatment meaningfully affected by these prognostic efforts. There is little evidence to support the use of any medication in the treatment of scleroderma interstitial lung disease. What is available supports the use of both **IV cyclophosphamide** (2 mg/kg qd) plus **prednisone** at an arbitrary dose of approximately 0.5 mg/kg qd. When this combined regimen is used, *Pneumocystis jiroveci* prophylaxis with TMP-SMX should also be given thrice weekly. Dosage is adjusted according to WBC, and UA is closely monitored.

Although esophageal dysmotility might lead to aspiration, in practice this appears to happen infrequently. Pulmonary HTN, when present, is often due to interstitial lung disease.

Limited Scleroderma (CREST)

In CREST syndrome, interstitial disease is much less common, and the picture is more often dominated by pulmonary HTN. Evaluation includes echocardiography, CXR and chest CT, and PFTs. On occasion, right heart catheterization may be helpful, particularly for trials of vasodilators. Treatment is as for primary pulmonary HTN (see Chap. 2, Pulmonary Hypertension).

Rheumatoid Arthritis

Rheumatoid arthritis has a variety of associated pulmonary problems. The most common is **interstitial lung disease,** which closely resembles that seen in idiopathic pulmonary fibrosis. A second form of interstitial lung disease is bronchiolitis obliterans organizing pneumonia. This resembles the idiopathic form (see Chap. 26, Interstitial Lung Disease). Other parenchymal abnormalities include **rheumatoid nodules,** which are generally multiple and vary widely in size from a few millimeters to several centimeters. They occur most often in men with high-titer disease and soft tissue nodules. When complicated by coal workers' pneumoconiosis, the nodules may cavitate, a situation known as **Caplan's syndrome.** Rheumatoid arthritis may also be complicated by **obliterative bronchiolitis,** an obstructive syndrome resembling that seen in marrow and lung transplant recipients. Although its etiology is controversial, this complication seems to have often followed therapy with penicillamine and to have waned as that drug has fallen from favor. **Pleural effusion** is common in rheumatoid arthritis and is an **exudate,** often with a very low glucose. When **chronic,** the effusions may become chyliform **(pseudochylothorax)** and milky appearing with elevated cholesterol, normal triglycerides, and no chylomicrons.

Treatment with immunosuppressives may lead to opportunistic infection, including mycobacterial, fungal, and pneumocystic disease. In particular, **infliximab** and **etaner-**

cept may lead to **reactivation of latent TB** and **fungal infection.** The drugs given for rheumatoid arthritis may themselves lead to interstitial disease. The most common example is **methotrexate,** which can cause a syndrome with cough, dyspnea, fever, eosinophilia, and interstitial infiltrates.

Finally, no discussion of rheumatoid arthritis involvement of the lung would be complete without noting upper airway obstruction owing to **arytenoid joint arthritis.**

Evaluation for the problems above includes **CXR, PFTs,** and **ABG analysis.** It is generally unnecessary to perform bronchoscopy or biopsy when the diagnosis of rheumatoid arthritis–associated pulmonary fibrosis is most likely. However, when the differential diagnosis includes **bronchiolitis obliterans organizing pneumonia (BOOP), infection,** or **drug reaction,** it is prudent to perform **bronchoscopy, lavage, and biopsy. CBC** and **blood cultures** as well as **bronchoscopic cultures** should be obtained. A single nodule may require a needle biopsy. Multiple nodules in the absence of infectious symptoms may be followed for stability. Pleural effusions must be tapped for evaluation. Stridor requires otolaryngologic evaluation.

Treatment regimens for rheumatoid interstitial lung disease are varied and idiosyncratic. They generally contain **daily prednisone** dosages ranging from 0.25 to 1.5 mg/kg/day and often include **IV cyclophosphamide** in the range of 2 mg/kg/day. Unequivocal evidence of efficacy is lacking. BOOP may be treated with oral prednisone (1 mg/kg/day) for 3–6 mos with very slow taper while watching carefully for relapse. Specific infections are treated based on diagnosis. When a **methotrexate pulmonary reaction** occurs, the drug should be discontinued. Administration of corticosteroids shortens time to resolution from about 4 wks to about 2 wks. Pleural effusions usually require no treatment other than the drainage needed for comfort.

Systemic Lupus Erythematosus

The most frequent pulmonary manifestation of SLE is **pleurisy** and **pleural effusion.** The effusion is an exudate. Pleural fluid ANA and lupus erythematosus prep are not usually helpful. Effusions are not usually large and are often bilateral. Response to corticosteroids is usually prompt.

Parenchymal lung disease is less common. **Acute lupus pneumonitis** typically presents with cough, fever, dyspnea, and bilateral infiltrates. It is often necessary to undertake bronchoscopy to differentiate it from alveolar hemorrhage and infection (particularly in those on immunosuppressive regimens). Because of poor prognosis, treatment is usually with high-dose corticosteroids (1.5 mg/kg/day prednisone or the equivalent).

Infection in those **receiving immunosuppressives** is an important consideration. Those receiving corticosteroids and cytotoxic agents are at risk for pneumocystis as well as fungal and mycobacterial disease. In addition to routine radiographic studies and cultures, bronchoscopy with lavage and biopsy should be undertaken early with therapy directed at the organism isolated.

Diffuse alveolar hemorrhage presents with dyspnea, cough, bilateral pulmonary infiltrates, and worsened gas exchange but may not have overt hemoptysis. Bronchoscopy with alveolar lavage is usually sufficient to make the diagnosis. The prognosis is poor, and treatment correspondingly aggressive—high-dose corticosteroids (IV methylprednisolone, 500–2000 mg/day); IV cyclophosphamide, 2 mg/kg/day; and plasmapheresis.

Vanishing lung syndrome is associated with dyspnea and elevated hemidiaphragms and is generally ascribed to severe bilateral diaphragm weakness owing to lupus. Treatment with corticosteroids sometimes leads to improvement.

The problem with antiphospholipid syndrome and venous thromboembolic disease is dealt with in Chap. 21, Pulmonary Embolism and Deep Venous Thrombosis.

Sjögren's Syndrome

The patient with Sjögren's syndrome may have **lymphocytic tracheobronchitis** and **xerotrachea.** However, the most common pulmonary manifestation of Sjögren's is **interstitial lung disease,** which is manifested clinically with cough and dyspnea and radiographically by reticulonodular diffuse interstitial infiltrates. The infiltrates may be due to nonspecific interstitial pneumonia, or less frequently to **lymphocytic interstitial pneumonia.** While the former is more common, the latter is associated with Sjögren's more than any other connective tissue disease. PFTs are generally restrictive. Bronchoscopy, lavage, and transbronchial biopsy may be necessary if the diagnosis is in doubt, particularly if infection is considered. Lymphocytic interstitial pneumonia may be a precursor to pseudolymphoma or even frank non-Hodgkin's lymphoma. Treatment of interstitial disease is customarily with **prednisone** in the dosage range of 1 mg/kg/day for up to 6 mos, followed by tapering.

Polymyositis

Interstitial lung disease in **polymyositis** and **dermatomyositis** is common and highly associated with the presence of **antibodies to histidyl-tRNA synthetase (anti-Jo1).** The pulmonary symptoms of cough and dyspnea may be insidious in onset. The physical findings may be dominated by the primary disease but may also include pulmonary basilar crackles. The appearance radiographically is similar to that in idiopathic pulmonary fibrosis. Areas of ground-glass infiltrates on CT scan may indicate active alveolitis more amenable to treatment but may also be a manifestation of BOOP, which may be seen on biopsy. PFTs are generally restrictive and may be used to follow the course of the disease. Biopsy is generally unnecessary if infection is not suspected.

A more fulminant form of interstitial disease may be seen, particularly in dermatomyositis, with predominant diffuse alveolar damage. This follows a relentlessly downhill course, and is a form of **Hamman-Rich syndrome.**

The disease may also be complicated by **aspiration** due to pharyngeal muscle involvement and by dyspnea due to pulmonary muscle involvement.

Treatment is generally with **prednisone** in doses of 1 mg/kg qd. **Cyclophosphamide** is often added at a target dose of 2 mg/kg/day. We prefer weekly **methotrexate** as initial agent, with doses in the range of 10–15 mg/wk, adjusting dose by disease response.

KEY POINTS TO REMEMBER

- Recognition of flail chest is based on the history and radiographic evidence of thoracic trauma, paradoxical movement (in with inspiration, out with expiration) that may be subtle and overlooked, increasing respiratory distress, and worsening gas exchange.
- The most common cause of diaphragmatic rupture is blunt trauma, either from a motor vehicle accident or from a severe fall. Most but not all occur on the left side of the chest; this is usually ascribed to protection by the liver on the right.
- Asthma is among the most common causes for pulmonary consultation in pregnancy, complicating 1 in 20 gestations.
- The most frequent pulmonary complication of sickle hemoglobinopathy is acute chest syndrome. As with other acute complications, it occurs most frequently in those with hemoglobin SS, less frequently in SC, and with varying frequency in S–beta thalassemia.

REFERENCES AND SUGGESTED READINGS

Blaiss MS. National Institute of Health. Management of asthma during pregnancy. *Allergy Asthma Proc* 2004;25:375–379.

Cullen P, Modell JH, Kirby RR, et al. Treatment of flail chest. Use of intermittent mandatory ventilation and positive end-expiratory pressure. *Arch Surg* 1975;110(9):1099–1103.

Jain P, Sandur S, Meli Y, et al. Role of flexible bronchoscopy in immunocompromised patients with lung infiltrates. *Chest* 2004;125:712–722.

Lamont RF. The pathophysiology of pulmonary oedema with the use of beta-agonists. *BJOG* 2000;107:439.

Mansour KA. Trauma to the diaphragm. *Chest Surg Clin N Am* 1997;7:373–383.
Mendelson CL. The aspiration of stomach contents into the lungs during obstetric anesthesia. *Am J Obstet Gynecol* 1946;52:191.
National Asthma Education and Prevention Program Expert Panel Executive Summary Report: Guidelines for the Diagnosis and Management of Asthma—Update on Selected Topics 2002. National Institutes of Health, National Heart, Lung, and Blood Institute, Publication No. 02-5075, 2002.
Platt OS. The acute chest syndrome of sickle cell disease. *N Engl J Med* 2000;342:1904.
Rubin RH, Wolfson JS, Cosimi AB, et al. Infection in the renal transplant recipient. *Am J Med* 1981;70:405–411.
Sanson BJ, Lensing AW, Prins MH, et al. Safety of low-molecular-weight heparin in pregnancy: a systematic review. *Thromb Haemost* 1999;81:668–672.
Shackford SR, Smith DE, Zarins CK, et al. The management of flail chest. A comparison of ventilatory and non-ventilatory treatment. *Am J Surg* 1976;132:759–762.
Shackford SR, Virgilio RW, Peters RM. Selective use of ventilator therapy in flail chest injury. *J Thorac Cardiovasc Surg* 1981;81:194–201.
Tanaka H, Yukioka T, Yamaguti Y, et al. Surgical stabilization or internal pneumatic stabilization? A prospective randomized study of management of severe flail chest patients. *J Trauma* 2002;52:525–532.
Vichinsky EP, Neumayr LD, Earles AN, et al. Causes and outcomes of the acute chest syndrome in sickle cell disease. National Acute Chest Syndrome Study Group. *N Engl J Med* 2000;342:1855–1865.
Wang JY, Chang YL, Lee LN, et al. Diffuse pulmonary infiltrates after bone marrow transplantation: the role of open lung biopsy. *Ann Thorac Surg* 2004;78:267–272.
White B, Moore WC, Wigley FM, et al. Cyclophosphamide is associated with pulmonary function and survival benefit in patients with scleroderma and alveolitis. *Ann Intern Med* 2000;132:947–954.

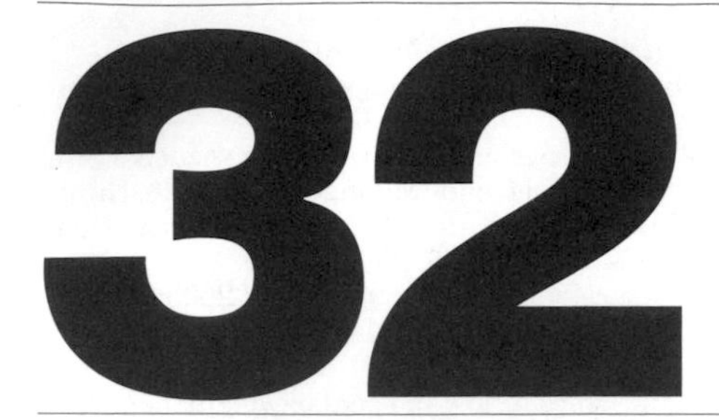

Lung Transplantation

Santhosh J. Mathews and
Elbert P. Trulock III

INTRODUCTION

In 1963, Hardy et al. performed the first lung transplant in a patient with lung cancer. At the time of operation, the tumor could not be fully removed, and a left **single-lung transplant (SLT)** was performed. The patient survived the operation but died 20 days later of renal failure. Between 1963 and 1978, >40 lung transplants were performed in centers around the world, but there were no long-term survivors. Some recipients were probably moribund at the time of transplant, but the causes of death included rejection, infection, and airway complications.

The introduction of **cyclosporine A** (for immunosuppression) around 1980 was a major advance for transplantation. The first successful lung transplants were performed in 1981 as part of combined heart-lung operations for patients with pulmonary vascular disease. In 1983, a Toronto group followed with the SLT for pulmonary fibrosis and performed the en-bloc **bilateral lung transplant (BLT)** with preservation of the native heart in 1986. Subsequently, the en-bloc approach was modified by a Washington University group into the bilateral sequential operation that has been widely adopted. SLT, BLT, living-donor lobar transplants, and heart-lung transplantations are performed for the spectrum of end-stage lung diseases.

This chapter briefly touches on the background of lung transplantation and on common terminology. The primary focus, however, is on postop management of adult lung transplant patients, including a review of immunosuppressive agents and common complications.

THE TRANSPLANTATION SYSTEM

There are three general arms to the organ transplantation system in the United States: the **United Network for Organ Sharing (UNOS), organ procurement organizations (OPOs),** and **transplant centers.** To address the national shortage of organs and problems with donor–recipient matching, the Department of Health and Human Services contracted UNOS to operate the Organ Procurement and Transplantation Network and maintain a national registry for organ matching. OPOs are nongovernmental organizations that harvest organs in their respective service areas and allocate organs based on UNOS policies. As of January 2004, there were 59 OPOs in the United States with variable efficiency in organ procurement. Transplant centers represent the focus and largest membership within UNOS. As of January 2004, there were 257 transplant centers in the United States, and 69 of these were performing lung transplantation. According to UNOS, 925 lung transplants and 27 heart-lung transplants were performed in the United States in 2003.

DONOR SELECTION

Despite numerous measures to facilitate organ procurement and availability, donor organs remain in short supply. Moreover, the donor pool in the United States does not exceed that of other countries that lack legislation supporting transplantation. There were approximately 3900 patients awaiting lung transplantation in January 2004.

TABLE 32-1. STANDARD LUNG TRANSPLANT DONOR CRITERIA

Age <55 yrs
ABO compatibility
Clear chest x-ray
$PaO_2 \geq 300$ mm Hg, ventilated with fraction of inspired oxygen = 1.0, and positive end-expiratory pressure = 5 cm H_2O
$\leq$ 20 pack-yr smoking history
Satisfactory bronchoscopic exam and gross inspection (before harvest)

Adapted from Frost AE. Donor criteria and evaluation. *Clin Chest Med* 1997:18:231–237; and Organ Procurement and Transplantation Network. Policy 3.7: Organ distribution: allocation of thoracic organs. Available at http://www.optn.org/policiesandbylaws/policies/pdfs/policy_9.pdf, revised June 24, 2005.

Given the limitation in the organ pool, donor criteria have become increasingly liberalized. Standard criteria for acceptance are listed in Table 32-1. Donors who do not precisely meet these guidelines may be considered marginal but may nevertheless be suitable depending on the center, surgeon, and recipient. Many of these transplants have proved successful.

All thoracic organ donors are screened with a social and medical history as well as physical exam before harvest. **Medical history** includes the current hospitalization detailing the following: cause of brain death, vital signs, documentation of arrest or hypotensive episodes, use of vasopressors and/or hydration, echocardiogram if available, and ECG. Moreover, **all donors are tested** for HIV, hepatitis B and C, human T-cell leukemia virus type 1, syphilis, and CMV (pretransfusion preferred). Organs that are positive for HIV or human T-cell leukemia virus type 1 are excluded from transplantation, although other infections do not necessarily preclude transplantation. **Malignancy** usually prevents transplantation, as recurrence of the primary tumor in the recipient is of concern. Localized skin cancers, cervical cancer, or neurologic tumors that rarely metastasize are usually acceptable in donor patients.

RECIPIENT SELECTION

The **most frequent conditions** affecting patients referred for lung/heart-lung transplantation are COPD/emphysema (including alpha$_1$-antitrypsin deficiency), idiopathic pulmonary fibrosis (IPF), cystic fibrosis (CF), primary pulmonary HTN (PPH), and Eisenmenger's syndrome. In general, candidates for lung transplantation should be in relatively good health except for their lung disease. When referring a patient for transplantation, the absolute and relative contraindications must be considered (Table 32-2).

All patients generally undergo a **routine evaluation** of their disease. This usually includes complete pulmonary function testing, a measurement of exercise tolerance, and high-resolution imaging of the lungs. Cardiac testing is essential in patients at high risk for coronary disease and may include an ECG, echocardiography, and stress testing. Each transplant center has its own specific evaluation requirements.

To prevent the possibility of hyperacute rejection, donor and recipient are **matched using ABO blood groups.** Recipients are also screened for common alloantibodies. Reactivity against common HLA antigens is a serious barrier to transplantation and is discussed further in the section on rejection.

After evaluation, suitable candidates are placed on the UNOS national waiting list for lung transplantation. In the past, priority for lung organ allocation was determined primarily by waiting time. Under this system, there was a disparity in waiting list mortality among the various underlying lung diseases. Specifically, patients with IPF, CF, and PPH had significantly higher mortality while waiting for transplantation compared to patients with COPD or alpha$_1$-antitrypsin deficiency. Thus, a new alloca-

TABLE 32-2. CONTRAINDICATIONS TO LUNG TRANSPLANTATION

Absolute

Significant dysfunction of major nonpulmonary organs, especially renal dysfunction (which can worsen with immunosuppression). Patients with cardiomyopathy or heart disease refractory to medical therapy or revascularization may be considered for heart-lung transplantation.

HIV infection.

Active malignancy (other than basal or squamous cell carcinoma of the skin). In general, previous cancer should be in continuous remission for 5 yrs before transplantation.

Hepatitis B and C.

Poor rehabilitation potential.

Active extrapulmonary infection.

Relative

Symptomatic osteoporosis (disease must be treated before transplantation).

Ideal body weight <70% or >130%.

Substance abuse (a minimum of 6 mos cessation of alcohol, tobacco, and illicit drugs is needed).

Psychosocial issues and medical noncompliance.

Mechanical ventilation.

Adapted from American Thoracic Society. ATS Guidelines: International guidelines for the selection of lung transplant candidates. *Am J Respir Crit Care Med* 1998;158:335–339; and American Thoracic Society. ATS guidelines: Lung transplantation: report of the ATS workshop on lung transplantation. *Am Rev Respir Dis* 1993;147:772.

tion system was proposed that would consider medical urgency for transplantation. Under this new **allocation policy,** which took effect in May 2005, priority for transplantation is based primarily on **medical urgency** and **expected outcome after transplantation.** These are determined based on several predictors of waiting list mortality and posttransplant mortality, which were identified retrospectively from patients registered on the waiting list in the past few years. Based on these **predictors,** which include diagnosis, pulmonary function test data, oxygen requirement, New York Heart Association functional class, and other objective physiologic and clinical parameters, a lung allocation score is calculated and priority is determined according to this score. The impact of this new system on waiting list outcomes, posttransplant outcomes, and referral practices is uncertain at this time. However, the system is likely to be refined and adjusted over the coming years in an attempt to maximize the benefits of lung transplantation.

Both SLT and bilateral lung transplant (BLT) have been performed for COPD, $alpha_1$-antitrypsin deficiency emphysema, IPF, PPH, and Eisenmenger's syndrome. In contrast, BLT is mandatory for diffuse bronchiectasis associated with CF or other diseases. Heart-lung transplantation is usually reserved for complex congenital heart diseases with pulmonary HTN.

IMMUNOSUPPRESSIVE THERAPY

Immunosuppression strategies vary among transplant centers. Many institutions initially rely on a **triple-drug maintenance regimen** consisting of a **calcineurin inhibitor** [cyclosporine (CSA) or tacrolimus], an **antimetabolite** [azathioprine or mycophenolate mofetil (MMF)], and a **corticosteroid** (methylprednisolone perioperatively followed by prednisone). These agents work on different arms of the immune system to achieve complementary immunosuppression. Postoperatively, some centers use induction therapy with courses of **interleukin (IL-2) receptor antagonists** or **antilymphocyte antibody preparations.** This treatment may reduce the incidence of acute rejection as maintenance immunosuppression takes effect. However, there may be increased risks of infection and posttransplant lymphoproliferative disorders with these agents.

Corticosteroids

Steroids have an antiinflammatory function. They modify B- and T-cell cytokine production, preventing recognition of antigens by T-cells.

- **Dosing:** Variable.
- **Metabolism and excretion:** Hepatic metabolism, including cytochrome P450-3A4 isoform (CYP3A4), and urinary excretion.
- **Interactions:** Barbiturates, phenytoin, rifampin, and St. John's wort decrease corticosteroid effectiveness by inducing CYP3A4. Conversely, inhibitors of CYP3A4, such as azole antifungals and macrolides, may increase steroid levels. Steroids may also increase CSA levels and potentiate aspirin- or NSAID-induced gastritis.
- **Adverse drug reactions:** Complications are common with chronic steroid use and include skin thinning, impaired wound healing, fat redistribution, HTN, hypokalemia, hyperglycemia, adrenal insufficiency, osteoporosis, and mental status changes (ranging from restlessness and poor sleep to agitation and steroid psychosis). Corticosteroids may also increase or decrease the prothrombotic effect of warfarin.

Azathioprine

Azathioprine is a purine analogue that inhibits DNA and RNA synthesis, ultimately blocking proliferation of activated lymphocytes.

- **Dosing:** Initial dosing may be 3–5 mg/kg PO/IV once before transplant, then 1–3 mg/kg PO/IV daily.
- **Bioavailability:** Azathioprine is well absorbed after oral administration. Azathioprine and its metabolite 6-mercaptopurine are 30% bound to plasma proteins.
- **Metabolism and excretion:** Hepatic metabolism and urinary excretion.
- **Interactions:** Allopurinol may reduce metabolism and increase levels of azathioprine. Drugs with bone marrow suppression or toxicity should be avoided, as the effects can be additive. Warfarin levels may increase via unknown mechanisms.
- **Adverse drug reactions:** Bone marrow toxicity can occur (thrombocytopenia, anemia, and leukopenia). GI side effects are seen as well (hepatitis, cholestatic jaundice, and pancreatitis).

Mycophenolate Mofetil

MMF was initially developed as an antibiotic/antineoplastic/antipsoriatic agent. It is a selective, noncompetitive, and reversible inhibitor of inosine monophosphate dehydrogenase, blocking *de novo* purine synthesis. As B and T cells lack the salvage pathway of purine synthesis, they are selectively inhibited.

- **Dosing:** Initial dosing is 1–1.5 g PO/IV qd.
- **Bioavailability:** MMF is given as an ester derivative owing to poor absorption. In this form, it is rapidly absorbed orally. It is 97% albumin bound in plasma.
- **Metabolism and excretion:** MMF is rapidly hydrolyzed to an active metabolite mycophenolic acid (MPA) in the liver. Also, it is later inactivated in the liver by glucuronidation. MPA is eliminated primarily in the urine as MPA glucuronide. In renal failure, accumulated MPA glucuronide may be converted to MPA, causing toxicity.
- **Interactions:** Relatively few drug interactions occur. Antacids may reduce absorption. Cholestyramine and antibiotics that alter gut flora can decrease levels by reducing enterohepatic circulation. Drugs that interfere (e.g., probenecid) or compete for renal tubular secretion may increase MPA glucuronide levels. High doses of salicylates may increase free MPA levels.

- **Adverse drug reactions:** MMF is generally well tolerated with GI side effects being most common (abdominal pain, nausea, vomiting, dyspepsia, diarrhea). These can be overcome by splitting doses or administering the drug with small amounts of food. Bone marrow toxicity is seen as well (anemia, leukopenia, and thrombocytopenia).
- **Monitoring:** Therapeutic monitoring is not routinely performed. Concentrations may be monitored in renal failure or coadministration with CSA.

Cyclosporine

CSA is a fat-soluble fungal polypeptide that inhibits production of IL-2 from CD4+ cells. It binds cyclophyllin in lymphocytes, and the complex then binds calcineurin, inhibiting cytokine gene transcription and lymphocyte proliferation.

- **Dosing:** Initial dosing is 8–10 mg/kg/day split into two doses.
- **Bioavailability:** Oral bioavailability is variable and dependent on the drug formulation (Sandimmune 10–90%, Neoral 30–45%). It is also bile dependent and can be influenced by fat intake, diarrhea, and GI motility. CSA is mostly distributed outside of the blood volume, and the fraction in plasma is 90% lipoprotein bound.
- **Metabolism and excretion:** CSA is extensively metabolized in liver and intestine (CYP3A4). Elimination is primarily by excretion of metabolites in the bile. Only a small fraction is excreted unchanged via GI and genitourinary tracts.
- **Interactions:** Drug interactions are very common as a result of CYP3A4 induction or inhibition. Drugs that decrease CSA levels include rifampin, phenytoin, carbamazepine, phenytoin, St. John's wort, and hydroxymethylglutaryl coenzyme A reductase inhibitors. Increased levels are seen with azole antifungals, macrolides, calcium channel blockers (verapamil and diltiazem; nifedipine has less effect), and grapefruit juice. Many nephrotoxic drugs have synergistic toxicity with CSA. Potassium-sparing diuretics should be avoided owing to the potential for hyperkalemia. Concomitant use of hydroxymethylglutaryl coenzyme A reductase inhibitor therapy increases their risk of myopathy and rhabdomyolysis.
- **Adverse drug reactions:** Renal side effects are common (hyperkalemia, hypomagnesemia, HTN). Metabolic side effects include hyperlipidemia, gout, osteoporosis, hirsutism, and hyperglycemia. Neurologic effects include tremors, peripheral neuropathy, headaches, mental status changes, and, in rare instances, reversible posterior leukoencephalopathy. Gingival hypertrophy (especially in conjunction with nifedipine), a thrombotic thrombocytopenic purpura–like syndrome, and hepatotoxicity can be seen as well.
- **Monitoring:** Therapeutic monitoring is performed due to intra- and interpatient variability of absorption, metabolism, and excretion, as well as the considerable side effect profile. Levels measured include trough, area under the curve, and C2 pseudo-peak levels. Target levels vary with time interval after transplant, organ type, and rejection history.

Tacrolimus

Tacrolimus is a fungal-derived macrolide antibiotic that also inhibits IL-2 production. It binds to immunophyllin, and the drug–protein complex binds calcineurin in a fashion similar to that of CSA.

- **Dosing:** Initial dosing range is 0.1–0.2 mg/kg/day PO.
- **Bioavailability:** Oral bioavailability is poor (20–25%) but not bile acid dependent. It is fat-soluble, and approximately 80% of serum drug is RBC membrane bound.
- **Metabolism and excretion:** Tacrolimus is metabolized in the liver and intestine (CYP3A4). Tacrolimus is excreted unchanged in bile, thus there is no need for adjustment in renal failure or hepatic disease.
- **Interactions:** Similar to those with CSA, but not all mimic CSA. New interactions are also being found.
- **Adverse drug reactions:** Similar to those with CSA.
- **Monitoring:** Trough levels are routinely used (and correlate with area under the curve measurements).

Sirolimus

Sirolimus is a fungal-derived macrolide, also known as rapamycin. Unlike tacrolimus and CSA, which are calcineurin inhibitors, the sirolimus–immunophyllin complex inhibits the mammalian target of rapamycin (mTOR) and blocks cytokine-mediated cell cycling, ultimately inhibiting B- and T-cell function.

- **Dosing:** Initial dosing is 2 mg PO qd. It is diluted with water or juice (except grapefruit juice). A long half-life allows for once-daily dosing.
- **Bioavailability:** Sirolimus is rapidly absorbed after oral administration but has poor bioavailability (approximately 14% with the oral solution but higher with tablets). It is 92% bound to plasma proteins.
- **Metabolism and excretion:** It is metabolized in liver and intestine (CYP3A4). >90% is eliminated via the gut.
- **Interactions:** Similar to those with CSA. There is marked interaction with CSA itself, increasing the levels of CSA by >300%. CSA can be dosed 4 hrs before sirolimus (but this complicates monitoring of blood levels).
- **Adverse drug reactions:** Side effects include HTN. Metabolic effects are similar to those with CSA, but hypercholesterolemia and hypertriglyceridemia are particularly problematic. Bone marrow toxicity may be seen (thrombocytopenia and anemia). Other effects include interstitial pneumonitis and hepatotoxicity. Sirolimus has a black box warning regarding use immediately after lung transplant, as it has been associated with anastomotic breakdown. It can be safely used later (after anastomotic healing), but caution is warranted if other surgeries are required.
- **Monitoring:** Owing to the long half-life, frequent levels are not needed, but monitoring is essential. Target levels also vary depending on whether CSA or tacrolimus is used.

Antithymocyte Globulin

Antithymocyte globulin (ATG) is a polyclonal antilymphocyte globulin used for induction therapy. Atgam is derived from horses, whereas Thymoglobulin is of rabbit origin. There is profound B- and T-cell depletion after administration owing to complement-mediated cytolysis of antibody-coated cells.

- **Dosing:** Atgam: 10–20 mg/kg IV infusion. Thymoglobulin: 1.0–1.5 mg/kg IV infusion. Atgam has a half-life of 6 days, whereas Thymoglobulin has a half-life of 30 days. Thymoglobulin is approximately 10 times more potent than Atgam.
- **Adverse drug reactions:** There are numerous reactions, including flulike symptoms secondary to cytokine release syndrome (IL-1, IL-6, tumor necrosis factor-alpha). These symptoms can be attenuated with premedication (using a combination of prednisone, acetaminophen, diphenhydramine, and IV fluids). There is a potential risk of infection and posttransplant lymphoproliferative disorder (PTLD), but the data in lung transplantation are variable. Leukopenia is the most serious complication of therapy. Thrombocytopenia may complicate therapy, and anaphylaxis is documented, but rare.
- **Monitoring:** Some centers monitor CD3+ levels to gauge adequacy of therapy.

Muromonab-CD3

Muromonab-CD3 (OKT3) is an antilymphocyte agent that may be used as induction therapy (most commonly for drug sparing of other agents). It is rarely used in lung transplantation today. It is a murine monoclonal antibody against CD3 antigen that essentially renders T cells immunologically incompetent and depletes them in minutes to hours. CD3+ cells begin to reappear within 48 hrs of discontinuation of therapy. Therapeutic failure may occur owing to human antimurine antibodies or increased antibody clearance. A cytokine release syndrome has been seen. There is the same risk of infection and PTLD that occurs with other antibody preparations.

Interleukin-2 Receptor Antagonists

IL-2 receptor antagonists are chimeric murine–human monoclonal antibodies. They bind the IL-2 receptor on the surface of activated T lymphocytes and inhibit proliferation and differentiation of T cells. Basiliximab is a true chimeric antibody (25% mouse), whereas daclizumab is a humanized antibody (10% mouse).

- **Dosing:** Basiliximab has a half-life of approximately 14 days, whereas daclizumab has a half-life of approximately 30 days. Basiliximab is given as a 20-mg IV infusion once before transplant and then again on the fourth day posttransplantation; Daclizumab is given 1 mg/kg IV at the time of transplantation and then 1 mg/kg IV at 2-wk intervals as needed.
- **Adverse effects:** Both agents are less immunogenic and have fewer side effects than does ATG or OKT3. Side effects are generally similar to placebo, but there remains a theoretical risk for infection and PTLD. A severe, acute hypersensitivity syndrome (including a pulmonary edema/ARDS-like picture) can occur with basiliximab and is a contraindication to continued use.

Other Therapies

There are a number of other agents that have been used as part of induction therapy, maintenance immunosuppression, or rescue therapy. Alternative immunosuppressive approaches have been developed to treat refractory cases of rejection. For example, extracorporeal photochemotherapy is used as adjunctive therapy in the treatment of rejection, whereas total lymphoid irradiation is a salvage therapy used in refractory rejection. Leukopenia is a major side effect of both therapies.

INFECTION IN THE LUNG TRANSPLANT PATIENT

Infection is a **primary source of morbidity and mortality** in the transplant population. Compared to other organ transplant patients, lung transplant patients are especially prone to infection. The combination of immunosuppression, denervated lung, impaired lymphatic drainage, abnormal mucociliary clearance, and suboptimal cough reflex all contribute to susceptibility to infection. Donor organs may also be a source of infection. Infections may play a role in the subsequent development of rejection.

Perioperatively, it is standard procedure to treat with broad-spectrum antibiotics pending culture results from the donor and recipient. When using **empiric therapy,** the Washington University in St. Louis group prefers **cefepime** and **vancomycin with or without clindamycin** if indicated.

Bacterial Pneumonias

Bacterial infections, especially pneumonias, account for **>50% of infection-related transplant deaths.** Most of these infections occur within the **first 2 wks** after transplantation but also reemerge later in the setting of bronchiolitis obliterans (BO). **Gram-negative rods** are consistently the most common bacterial organisms involved. *Burkholderia* and multidrug-resistant *Pseudomonas* species are a considerable problem in transplant recipients with CF who are colonized with these organisms before transplant. There is no consensus regarding management of these multidrug-resistant infections in the perioperative period, and institutions vary their prophylaxis based on individual culture data and sensitivities. Lung transplant patients are more prone to *Legionella* infection, but the rates of infection are widely variable among institutions.

Listeria and *Nocardia* are also uncommon, and these organisms can potentially be prophylaxed against with TMP-SMX. TB is an uncommon infection in lung transplant patients; however, treatment of infection can be problematic owing to frequent interactions between antimycobacterial agents and immunosuppressive therapies. Patients undergoing transplantation should receive a tuberculin skin test and receive appropriate therapy before surgery.

Cytomegalovirus

CMV is a member of the betaherpes virus group and is the **second most frequent infection** in lung transplant patients. CMV infection in a transplant patient can be acquired via an allograft from a seropositive donor, transfusion of seropositive blood products, or activation of latent disease in a seropositive recipient. Infected patients may be symptomatic or asymptomatic, and the overall risk of developing either infection or disease is 50%. This risk is adjusted based on prophylactic regimens as well as seropositivity of both the donor and the recipient.

Clinical Presentation

Patients may present with a variety of syndromes, including colitis, gastroenteritis, and hepatitis; but **pneumonitis** is the most common manifestation. While CMV pneumonia may be confused with acute rejection, it is unusual in the first 3–4 wks after transplantation, and the average time to onset is 7–8 wks after transplantation. Symptoms include low-grade fever, cough, and shortness of breath. Decreased pulmonary function may be noted on testing, and chest x-rays may demonstrate perihilar infiltrates, interstitial edema, or pleural effusions.

Diagnosis

- **Viral culture:** Shell-vial culture can rapidly determine active infection in 24–48 hrs via fluorescent antibodies to CMV antigen. Culture can be obtained from bronchoalveolar lavage (BAL) fluid, blood, or urine.
- **PCR:** Quantitative PCR is now widely used, but there is no standardized assay. Hence, threshold levels vary from assay to assay, and between centers.
- **Bronchoscopy:** Transbronchial biopsy is the preferred method for diagnosis of CMV pneumonitis. However, CMV pneumonia can be diagnosed based on culture positivity and clinical presentation.

Prevention

No consensus has been reached regarding **CMV prophylaxis.** Vaccination with live attenuated virus has yet to be tested in lung transplant patients. Passive immunoprophylaxis with CMV hyperimmune globulin or polyvalent immunoglobulin has had mixed results but is used at some centers. The most common method of prophylaxis is **antiviral therapy**—i.e., **ganciclovir** or **human CMV Ig.** A preemptive approach can be advantageous as it treats patients identified via a rapid screening test before development of overt disease. The Washington University in St. Louis group uses the following approach:

- A prophylactic strategy is used for donor-positive, recipient-negative recipients. Ganciclovir, 5 mg/kg IV qd, is administered for 10–12 wks.
- A preemptive strategy is used for other transplant patients. A CMV buffy coat is monitored once a week for the first 3 mos. Patients with CMV-positive buffy coats are treated with ganciclovir, 5 mg/kg IV bid, for 2–3 wks.

Treatment

Acyclovir has no role in the treatment of CMV infections, and ganciclovir treatment for 2–3 wks is the therapy of choice. The major side effect is leukopenia. Relapses are frequent after therapy and can be attenuated by maintenance therapy for 3–6 wks after treatment. The possibility of ganciclovir resistance must be considered in recipients who do not respond to therapy. Strategies in these patients include the addition of CMV Ig and/or foscarnet. However, nephrotoxicity is common with foscarnet use, especially when used in conjunction with calcineurin inhibitor therapy.

Fungal Infections

Given the availability of effective therapy, transplant centers have a low threshold for treating fungal infections given their high morbidity and mortality in overt disease states. Most centers generally take a preemptive approach to treating candida and aspergillus infections. No consensus exists regarding prophylaxis. *Candida* infections occur most frequently (43–80%), followed by aspergillus (20–50%). Other fungal infections are much less common.

Candida

Before development of effective therapies, candidal infection was associated with a high mortality. Donor organs are frequently colonized, and infection is common in immunosuppressed patients. *Candida* pneumonitis is rare. Locally invasive and disseminated disease can be treated with fluconazole, caspofungin, or amphotericin B, but despite these therapies, bloodstream infection with candida is still associated with a high mortality. Because **azole antifungals increase cyclosporine levels,** therapeutic monitoring and dose adjustment are necessary. Resistance is also an increasing problem, and drug susceptibilities are variable. *C. krusei* is resistant to fluconazole, and *C. glabrata* and *C. tropicalis* have high minimum inhibitory concentrations, often requiring the use of other agents. *C. lusitaniae* is usually resistant to amphotericin B, and *C. guilliermondii* is often resistant to both amphotericin B and caspofungin. In general, **caspofungin** is now preferred over amphotericin B. When **amphotericin B** is used, **liposomal preparations** are preferentially used, as they reduce the nephrotoxicity associated with the drug.

Aspergillus

Aspergillus is contracted via inhalation of spores, and disease can be devastating in the immunosuppressed patient. *A. fumigatus* is the most commonly isolated species. Patients may be colonized with aspergillus, or develop bronchitis, pneumonia, or disseminated disease. Early posttransplant colonization has been identified as a risk factor for the development of invasive disease. Infection can be detected clinically by **screening sputum** or **BAL fluid for hyphae,** but invasive pneumonia is **confirmed only by biopsy** (transbronchial or surgical). Bronchitis can be treated with **itraconazole** or **inhaled liposomal amphotericin B** (with which there is limited experience). Disseminated disease is usually treated with liposomal amphotericin B, but nephrotoxicity is a major source of morbidity, especially in conjunction with cyclosporine use. **Voriconazole** may be superior to amphotericin B in invasive disease, whereas **caspofungin** may prove to be a less toxic option for refractory disease.

Pneumocystis jiroveci *Pneumonia*

Infection with *Pneumocystis jiroveci* (formerly *P. carinii*) is uncommon as the result of widespread **routine prophylaxis with TMP-SMX.** TMP-SMX may also prevent *Nocardia* and *Listeria* infection. Prophylaxis is accomplished with one double-strength tablet 3 times a week. Suggested treatment for *Pneumocystis* pneumonia is TMP-SMX, 15–20 mg of the TMP component/kg/day PO/IV in 3–4 divided doses qd. Alternative prophylactic therapies include dapsone, atovaquone, and inhaled pentamidine, whereas IV pentamidine can be used for treatment.

Other Infections

Epstein-Barr virus (EBV) infection is implicated in development of posttransplant lymphoproliferative disease, as is discussed elsewhere. VZV manifests as **chickenpox** with primary exposure and as **zoster** with reactivation. Seronegative transplant patients should be **vaccinated against VZV** before transplantation. Immunocompromised patients with acute exposure may receive **varicella-zoster Ig** or **acyclovir** to prophylax against, or at least attenuate, the consequences of infection. Respiratory viruses (respiratory syncytial virus, influenza virus, parainfluenza virus, adenovirus, and rhinovirus) have also been a source of morbidity and mortality, and some of these respiratory viruses have been implicated in development of BO syndrome.

LUNG TRANSPLANT REJECTION

Hyperacute Rejection

Within minutes after transplantation, preformed antibodies to graft antigens (**HLA, ABO,** and **other antigens**) bind the vascular endothelium and initiate the host immunologic response. Pathologically, there is thrombus formation, inflammatory cell infiltrates, and fibrinoid necrosis of the vessels. This complication has been essentially eliminated by ABO matching of donors and recipients and by screening for HLA antibodies in the recipients. Despite this, a few cases continue to be reported.

Acute Rejection

Despite current maintenance immunosuppressive therapy, many lung transplant patients still experience one or more episodes of acute rejection, especially in the first 6 mos after transplantation. **After 6 mos, the risk of acute rejection declines.** Although acute rejection is amenable to medical therapy, it is a strong risk factor for the later development of chronic rejection.

Pathogenesis

Acute rejection is primarily a cell-mediated inflammatory cascade that is triggered by recognition of major histocompatibility complex antigens. Pathologically, acute rejection is characterized by a **perivascular and/or peribronchiolar lymphocytic infiltrate,** with the extent of the inflammation into the surrounding tissue determining the grade of rejection.

Clinical Presentation and Diagnosis

Patients present with **nonspecific complaints** that may be difficult to distinguish from infection. These may include shortness of breath, nonproductive cough, low-grade fever, and decline in exercise oximetry and spirometry (flows decrease by >10%). Exam may be notable for crackles or rhonchi, with x-rays demonstrating nonspecific infiltrates, and blood tests showing leukocytosis. However, many patients may be asymptomatic.

Surveillance transbronchial biopsies are used by some transplant centers, primarily in the first year after transplantation, to monitor for silent acute rejection. After this time, the risk of acute rejection is much lower, and the benefit of surveillance is questionable. The practice of surveillance biopsies remains controversial, as it has neither improved survival nor decreased the incidence of chronic rejection.

When **acute rejection** is suspected, **fiber-optic bronchoscopy with BAL** and **transbronchial biopsy** are generally standard practice. Some centers opt for a noninvasive strategy, treating for acute rejection when infection is unlikely and performing biopsy only in refractory cases. **Single-lung sampling** is generally sufficient in both SLT and BLT (as long as both lungs are from the same donor), as acute rejection is a diffuse process. Multiple samples improve the yield. In the case of BLTs where two separate donor lungs are transplanted, both lungs must be sampled as rejection may be unilateral.

The International Society for Heart and Lung Transplantation (ISHLT) proposed **diagnostic criteria for acute and chronic rejection** in 1990 and revised them in 1996. These criteria are based on **severity** and **location** (Table 32-3). Although airway inflammation is part of the spectrum of acute rejection, it alone is insufficient for diagnosis of acute rejection. Its presence may increase the risk of BO (a feature of chronic rejection), which is discussed later.

Treatment

Most centers **treat acute rejection grades of A2 or greater;** practices vary for grade A1, but it is often not treated when discovered in surveillance biopsies in clinically and physiologically stable transplant patients. Generally, acute rejection is treated with **high-dose IV corticosteroids** (methylprednisolone, 0.5–1 g IV daily for 3 days, then oral prednisone starting at 0.5–1 mg/kg/day and tapered over a few weeks). Symptoms generally resolve in 24–48 hrs. Diagnostic follow-up practices are also variable, with some centers repeating biopsies a few weeks after treatment to assess resolution. Refractory cases may require retreatment with steroids, alteration of maintenance immunosuppression, addition of other agents (e.g., methotrexate), antilymphocyte antibody therapy, or, very rarely, total lymphoid irradiation.

TABLE 32-3. CLASSIFICATION AND GRADING OF LUNG ALLOGRAFT REJECTION

A. Acute vascular rejection (vascular rejection of any grade may occur with or without acute airway rejection)
  - A0: None
  - A1: Minimal
  - A2: Mild
  - A3: Moderate
  - A4: Severe

B. Acute airway rejection
  - B0: None
  - B1: Minimal
  - B2: Mild
  - B3: Moderate
  - B4: Severe

C. Chronic airway rejection
  - Bronchiolitis obliterans
    - a: Active
    - b: Inactive

D. Chronic vascular rejection
  - Accelerated graft vascular sclerosis

Modified from Yousem SA, Berry GJ, Cagle PT, et al. Revision of the 1990 working formulation for the classification of pulmonary allograft rejection: Lung Rejection Study Group. *J Heart Lung Transplant* 1996;15:1–15.

Chronic Rejection

Chronic rejection can take two forms. **Chronic vascular rejection** is manifest by atherosclerosis within the pulmonary vasculature, whereas **chronic airway rejection,** the more common of the two types, is characterized by BO.

Pathogenesis

Bronchiolitis obliterans (BO) is a cicatricial process affecting the small airways. Initially, there is a lymphocytic infiltrate in the submucosa. With migration of the infiltrate into the epithelium, epithelial destruction and loss of bronchiolar mucosa follow. Fibroblasts and myofibroblasts, stimulated by this reaction, lay down intraluminal granulation tissue. Some airways may remain patent, whereas others are obliterated. BO is likely the result of a multifactorial insult to transplanted tissue. Table 32-4 lists the risk factors most commonly linked to chronic airway rejection.

Clinical Presentation and Diagnosis

The onset of chronic rejection is insidious, with progressive loss of lung function. Patients may present with progressive dyspnea, cough, wheezing, and low-grade fever. These symptoms may resemble asthmatic bronchitis, usually without improvement after bronchodilators or inhaled corticosteroids.

Histologic confirmation is difficult, and transbronchial biopsies may not offer adequate tissue for diagnosis. In 1993, the ISHLT proposed a clinical description of BO, termed **bronchiolitis obliterans syndrome (BOS),** that relies on **pulmonary function testing** to make the diagnosis of BO. In 2002, an update of the diagnostic criteria was proposed (Table 32-5). As BOS involves the small airways, the midexpiratory flow rates (FEF 25–75) may decline before the forced expiratory volume over 1 sec or forced expiratory volume over 1 sec/forced vital capacity ratio.

TABLE 32-4. MECHANISMS OF CHRONIC AIRWAY REJECTION

Immune mechanisms

Acute rejection: Acute rejection has been noted to be a risk for developing subsequent BO. The risk of BO has been correlated with higher grades of histologic rejection, persistent rejection, or recurrent rejection after treatment. Patients with more than three episodes of acute rejection were also noted to be at increased risk of developing subsequent BO. There is some suggestion that in certain cases, severe acute rejection may lead directly to airway fibrosis.

HLA mismatching: Lung transplants are not HLA-matched with recipients. One series has suggested that the presence of anti-HLA antibodies precedes development of BO. In general, the significance of HLA mismatch remains controversial.

Medication noncompliance: Patients with blood cyclosporine levels <200 ng/mL in one series were noted to be at increased risk for BO.

Nonimmune mechanisms

CMV infection: CMV pneumonitis is a risk factor for developing BO syndrome. Prophylaxis may attenuate this risk.

Hemodynamic factors: Donor "cold" ischemic time at the time of transplantation (between procurement and surgery) increases the risk of BO. Reperfusion injury, after vascular anastomosis, may cause oxidative damage to the allograft tissue. Disruption of the bronchial circulation in the transplanted lung may be a contributing factor.

Non-CMV viral infections: As mentioned previously, respiratory viruses may be implicated in the pathogenesis of BO.

BO, bronchiolitis obliterans.

Treatment

Prevention of chronic rejection is the goal of treatment. As noted, acute rejection episodes clearly play a role in the pathogenesis of BOS. Moreover, infection is implicated as well. Therefore, use of induction therapies, potent immunosuppression, and infection prophylaxis with preemptive antimicrobial therapy may decrease the likelihood of chronic rejection.

As progressive airflow limitation is a hallmark of the disease, **outpatient spirometry** has been used to help with early detection of BOS. Acute declines in spirometry may also be used to monitor for episodes of infection or acute rejection.

Despite these strategies to minimize the risk, the prevalence of **BOS approaches 50% by 3–5 yrs** after lung transplantation. BOS is usually treated with augmented

TABLE 32-5. CLASSIFICATION OF BRONCHIOLITIS OBLITERANS SYNDROME (2002)

BOS 0: FEV_1 >90% of baseline and FEF_{25-75} >75% of baseline

BOS 0p: FEV_1 81–90% of baseline and/or $FEF_{25-75} \leq$ 75% of baseline

BOS 1: FEV_1 66–80% of baseline

BOS 2: FEV_1 51–65% of baseline

BOS 3: $FEV_1 \leq$ 50% of baseline

BOS, bronchiolitis obliterans syndrome; FEF_{25-75}, midexpiratory flow rate; FEV_1, forced expiratory volume over 1 sec.
Modified from Estenne M, Hertz MI. Bronchiolitis obliterans after human lung transplantation. *Am J Respir Crit Care Med* 2002;166:440–444.

immunosuppression, but there is no consensus about therapy. Although immunosuppressive therapy may stabilize lung function in some cases, the overall results of treatment have been disappointing. The management of BOS is confounded by the presence of mild bronchiectasis and chronic infection, usually with *Pseudomonas*. Appropriate antibiotic treatment for infectious exacerbations is essential in these patients.

POSTTRANSPLANT LYMPHOPROLIFERATIVE DISORDER

PTLD is a well-recognized complication of solid organ transplantation. Most PTLD falls in the spectrum of **non-Hodgkin's lymphoma** and is predominantly of **B-cell lineage.** PTLD is often, although not always, associated with EBV infection. B lymphocytes are transformed by EBV infection and undergo uncontrolled clonal expansion in the setting of drug-induced T-lymphocyte suppression.

The incidence of PTLD after lung transplant has been in the range of 6% at Washington University, with the presentation and pattern of organ involvement related to the time of onset after lung transplantation. **Disease in the thorax,** and involvement of the **allograft itself,** has been typical of cases **within the first year** after lung transplant. **Extrathoracic sites,** especially the GI tract, have predominated in cases **after the first posttransplant year.**

In the first year, PTLD is often identified as a **pulmonary nodule, pulmonary infiltrate,** or **lymphadenopathy** on routine chest radiograph. Later cases in the GI tract have presented as **nonhealing ulcers, bowel perforations, GI bleeding,** and **masses.** Deescalation of immunosuppression is the first step in management. Other approaches include surgical excision, rituximab, and conventional chemotherapy.

OTHER COMPLICATIONS

Lung transplant patients are at **higher risk for developing malignancy** than are individuals in the general population. Squamous cell carcinoma of the skin is more common, as are cancers of the cervix, anogenital region, and the hepatobiliary system. Routine cancer screening and prevention are therefore essential.

Lung transplant patients seem to be at **higher risk for venous thromboembolism** and hypercoagulability, but the mechanism is unclear. **GI complications** also prove to be a source of morbidity posttransplantation. Patients often have chronic gastritis, peptic ulcer disease, and gastroparesis. Secondary malnutrition can lead to a number of other systemic problems.

Recurrence of primary disease can occur in the engrafted lung. The list of diseases that have recurred includes sarcoidosis, bronchoalveolar carcinoma, lymphangiomyomatosis, Langerhans' cell histiocytosis, pulmonary alveolar proteinosis, diffuse panbronchiolitis, and giant cell pneumonitis.

OUTCOMES

Survival after transplant is a complicated issue. Initial differences in **1-mo survival** usually reflect perioperative mortality associated with the **complexity** and **severity** of the surgery for each disease type. For example, in the UNOS Annual Report Data, patients transplanted for COPD had a 90% 3-mo survival as compared to 84% for PPH and 82% for IPF respectively. These outcomes must be considered in light of the fact that patients with conditions like PPH and IPF would have higher mortality without transplantation when compared to a patient with COPD.

A number of risk factors have been identified as **risk factors for a high 1-yr mortality.** Those carrying highest risk are patients with PPH [odds ratio (OR), 2.74], ventilator dependence (OR, 2.42), sarcoidosis (OR, 2.15), retransplantation (OR, 2.03), IPF (OR, 1.91), and dependence on IV inotropes (OR, 1.91). Other risk factors include other non-COPD diagnoses, seropositive CMV donor (into a CMV-negative recipient), and donor history of recipient diabetes mellitus. In the ISHLT data, there was no evidence to suggest that recent infection in the recipient, cause of donor death, procedure type, or HLA mismatch was a significant factor in 1-yr mortality. Advanced age may be a factor.

Retransplantation is infrequent and accounts for <4% of lung transplants in the ISHLT registry. The most common reasons for performing this procedure are premature failure of the graft, severe airway complications, and chronic rejection. Often, patients who need a second graft are no longer suitable candidates for transplant. Moreover, patients who are transplanted a second time tend to have poorer outcomes as compared to the primary lung transplant population.

KEY POINTS TO REMEMBER

- The most frequent conditions affecting patients referred for lung/heart-lung transplantation are COPD/emphysema (including alpha-1-antitrypsin deficiency), IPF, CF, PPH, and Eisenmenger's syndrome.
- The new allocation system for transplantation makes transplantation for subacute conditions, such as AIP, possible.
- The introduction of immunosuppression (cyclosporin A) was a major advance for lung transplantation. Immunosuppressive therapy regimens are complicated and require close monitoring to avoid side effects.
- Complications after lung transplantation are common. BOS (chronic airway rejection) occurs in approximately 50% of all transplant patients and is responsible for significant morbidity and mortality.

REFERENCES AND SUGGESTED READINGS

Alexander BD, Tapson VF. Infectious complications of lung transplantation. *Transpl Infect Dis* 2001;3:128–137.

American Thoracic Society. ATS guidelines: lung transplantation: report of the ATS workshop on lung transplantation. *Am Rev Respir Dis* 1993;147:772.

American Thoracic Society. ATS guidelines: international guidelines for the selection of lung transplant candidates. *Am J Respir Crit Care Med* 1998;158:335–339.

Bando K, Paradis IL, Similo S, et al. Obliterative bronchiolitis after lung and heart-lung transplantation. An analysis of risk factors and management. *J Thor Cardiovasc Surg* 1995;110:4–13.

Estenne M, Hertz MI. Bronchiolitis obliterans after human lung transplantation. *Am J Respir Crit Care Med* 2002;166:440–444.

Estenne M, Maurer JR, Boehler A, et al. Bronchiolitis obliterans syndrome 2001: an update of the diagnostic criteria. *J Heart Lung Transplant* 2002,21:297–310.

Ettinger NA, Bailey TC, Trulock EP, et al. Cytomegalovirus infection and pneumonitis. Impact after isolated lung transplantation. Washington University Lung Transplant Group. *Am Rev Respir Dis* 1993;147:1017–1023.

Frost AE. Donor criteria and evaluation. *Clin Chest Med* 1997:18:231–237.

Hausen B, Morris RE. Review of immunosuppression for lung transplantation: novel drugs, new uses for conventional immunosuppressants, and alternative strategies. *Clin Chest Med* 1997;18:353–356.

Haverich A, Görler A. Modern immunosuppression strategies in lung transplantation. *Curr Opin Organ Transplant* 1999;4:249–253.

Husain AN, Siddiqui MT, Holmes EW, et al. Analysis of risk factors for the development of bronchiolitis obliterans syndrome. *Am J Respir Crit Care Med* 1999;159:829–833.

International Society for Heart and Lung Transplantation Website. Available at: http://www.ishlt.org. Accessed October 17, 2005.

Jaramillo A, Smith MA, Phelan D, et al. Development of ELISA-detected anti-HLA antibodies precedes the development of bronchiolitis obliterans syndrome and correlates with progressive decline in pulmonary function after lung transplantation. *Transplantation* 1999;67:1155–1161.

Kelly K, Hertz MI. Obliterative bronchiolitis. *Clin Chest Med* 1997;18:319–338.

King-Biggs MB. Acute pulmonary allograft rejection: mechanisms, diagnosis, and management. *Clin Chest Med* 1997;18:301–310.

Malouf MA, Chhajed PN, Hopkins P, et al. Anti-viral prophylaxis reduces the incidence of lymphoproliferative disease in lung transplant recipients. *J Heart Lung Transplant* 2002;21:547–554.
Maurer JR,Tewari S. Nonpulmonary medical complications in the intermediate and long-term survivor. *Clin Chest Med* 1997;18:367–382.
Organ Procurement and Transplantation Network. Policy 3.7: Organ distribution: allocation of thoracic organs. Available at: http://www.optn.org/policiesandbylaws/policies/pdfs/policy_9.pdf. Accessed October 17, 2005.
Patterson GA. Indications: unilateral, bilateral, heart-lung, and lobar transplant procedures. *Clin Chest Med* 1997;18:225–230.
Reilly JJ. Chronic lung transplant rejection: bronchiolitis obliterans. Available at: http://www.uptodate.com. Accessed October 17, 2005.
Reilly JJ. Evaluation and treatment of acute lung transplant rejection. Available at: http://www.uptodate.com. Accessed October 17, 2005.
Schulman LL, Weinberg AD, McGregor CC, et al. Influence of donor and recipient HLA locus mismatching on development of obliterative bronchiolitis after lung transplantation. *Am J Respir Crit Care Med* 2001;163:437–442.
Straathof KC, Savoldo B, Heslop HE, et al. Immunotherapy for post-transplant lymphoproliferative disease. *Br J Haematol* 2002;118:728–740.
Trulock EP. Cytomegalovirus infection in lung transplant recipients. Available at: http://www.uptodate.com. Accessed October 17, 2005.
Trulock EP. Indications; selection of recipients; and choice of procedure for lung transplantation. Available at: http://www.uptodate.com. Accessed October 17, 2005.
Trulock EP. Infectious complications other than cytomegalovirus following lung transplantation. Available at: http://www.uptodate.com. Accessed October 17, 2005.
Trulock EP. Overview and outcomes of lung transplantation. Available at: http://www.uptodate.com. Accessed October 17, 2005.
Trulock EP. Procedure and postoperative management in lung transplantation. Available at: http://www.uptodate.com. Accessed October 17, 2005.
Trulock EP, Edwards LB, Taylor DO, et al. The registry of the International Society for Heart and Lung Transplantation: twentieth official adult lung and heart-lung transplant report—2003. *J Heart Lung Transplant* 2003;22:625.
United Network for Organ Sharing Website. Available at: http://www.unos.org. Accessed October 17, 2005.
Williams TJ, Snell GI. Early and long-term functional outcomes in unilateral, bilateral, and living-related transplant recipients. *Clin Chest Med* 1997;18:245–257.
Yousem SA, Berry GJ, Cagle PT, et al. Revision of the 1990 working formulation for the classification of pulmonary allograft rejection: Lung Rejection Study Group. *J Heart Lung Transplant* 1996;15:1–15.

Index

Note: Page numbers followed by *t* indicate tables; those followed by *f* indicate figures.